Pain in Childbearing and its Control

Key Issues for Mid and Women

Second Edition

Rosemary Mander

Emeritus Professor of Midwifery
School of Health in Social Science
University of Edinburgh

With a contribution by

Dr Jennifer M. Tocher

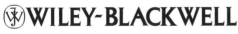
A John Wiley & Sons, Ltd., Publication

This edition first published 2011
First edition published 1998
© 1998, 2011 Rosemary Mander

Blackwell Publishing was acquired by John Wiley & Sons in February 2007. Blackwell's publishing programme has been merged with Wiley's global Scientific, Technical, and Medical business to form Wiley-Blackwell.

Registered Office
John Wiley & Sons Ltd, The Atrium, Southern Gate, Chichester, West Sussex, PO19 8SQ, United Kingdom

Editorial Offices
9600 Garsington Road, Oxford, OX4 2DQ, United Kingdom
2121 State Avenue, Ames, Iowa 50014-8300, USA

For details of our global editorial offices, for customer services and for information about how to apply for permission to reuse the copyright material in this book please see our website at www.wiley.com/wiley-blackwell.

Wiley publishes this book in a variety of electronic formats. ePDF: 9781444392050; ePUB: 9781444392067

Library of Congress Cataloging-in-Publication Data

Mander, Rosemary.
Pain in childbearing and its control / Rosemary Mander, with a contribution by Jennifer M. Tocher. – 2nd ed.
    p.   ; cm.
  Includes bibliographical references and index.
  ISBN 978-1-4051-9568-3 (pbk. : alk. paper) 1. Anesthesia in obstetrics. 2. Pain–Treatment.
3. Analgesia. 4. Labor (Obstetrics). I. Tocher, Jennifer M. II. Title.
[DNLM: 1. Analgesia, Obstetrical. 2. Anesthesia, Obstetrical. 3. Labor, Obstetric. 4. Pain–therapy.
WO 450]
  RG732.M29 2011
  617.9'682–dc22

2010031136

A catalogue record for this book is available from the British Library.

Set in 10/12.5pt Times by SPi Publisher Services, Pondicherry, India
Printed and bound in Malaysia by Vivar Printing Sdn Bhd

1 2011

Contents

Acknowledgements

I would like to say 'thank you' to Jo Murphy-Lawless, Sally Ferguson, Cheri Van Hoover, Margitta Beil-Hildebrand and LauraJane Yeates. Also to Iain D. Abbot, who produced the drawings and to whom I am so grateful for so much that words are beginning to fail me.

Introduction to the second edition

The dynamic nature of care in childbearing never ceases to be a source of amazement.

This dynamism manifests itself in a multiplicity of ways. Care providers, such as midwives, appear to both extend and intensify their skills and their areas of interest to address different aspects of the life of the childbearing woman. Because of my own developing range of interests and because of care providers' increasing interest in and understanding of the emotional aspects of childbearing, I aim, in this second edition, to further extend my approach to pain. In the first edition, the focus was predominantly on physical pain, with some attention to other forms of 'suffering'. This orientation reflected the then developing focus on what was becoming known as 'perinatal pain' (Niven & Gijsbers 1996).

Midwives' and others' ideas have moved on from the groundbreaking work of this admirable team of researchers. Thus, in this edition I will seek to develop my approach to what I called suffering. I will be giving more and more appropriate attention to emotional and other non-physical forms of pain. In this way, this book will meet the needs of a wide range of midwives, as well as other practitioners and students.

Pain as real

Through the medium of this book, I seek to present the reality of pain in childbearing. I will be discussing the extent to which pain is perceived by some disciplines as invariably negative. It may be interpreted as little more than just another medical problem which is caused by injury, surgery or disease; thus, it is viewed as demanding to be treated and resolved by whatever technical or pharmacological means are available. This impression is dominated by the masculine, medical and confrontational analogies of fighting and battle, seeking to convince us that pain needs to be defeated, by all the interventions in the medical armamentarium. Hence, the library catalogue presents me with titles such as: *Defeating Pain*, *The Challenge of Pain*, *The Conquest of Pain* and *Victory over Pain*. Such warlike views of pain are too simplistic to be acceptable, even less useful.

On the other hand, there are those who regard pain in childbearing as referring only to labour pain. I will be arguing that labour pain is uniquely and qualitatively different from any other form of pain known to humanity. Because labour pain is associated with healthy processes which are more than likely to lead to a satisfactory outcome, it has been

Pain in Childbearing and its Control, Second Edition. By Rosemary Mander. Published 2011 by Blackwell Publishing Ltd. © 1998, 2011 Rosemary Mander.

described in terms of being a 'positive pain' or 'pain with a purpose' (Kitzinger 1996). This view of pain can be helpful.

As well as the possibly appropriate general focus on the pain of labour, I will argue that there are other forms of pain associated with childbearing. Some of these forms of pain may be associated with pregnancy-related pathological conditions. Some of them will be associated with the physiological changes of childbearing and, probably because of this association, tend to be neglected. I will be arguing, though, that there are still other forms of pain which the childbearing woman may encounter. These forms of pain may not be generally regarded as pain as usually understood. So the meaning of the term 'pain' may need to be deconstructed in order to understand how these phenomena justify such a label. These feelings may include the woman's reaction to her childbearing experience or other events. Equally, these feelings may be associated with human interactions, perhaps with those who provide care or those with whom she is in a loving relationship. In this book I will argue that such pain may be as real as the universally-recognised pain of physiological labour. But unlike healthy labour pain, these feelings will carry serious and long lasting consequences for the woman and those near to her.

Thus, I aim through this book to adopt a balanced approach to the topic of pain in childbearing. This approach will show pain as a real experience. I will be including both the positive as well as the negative aspects of pain, irrespective of how it has originated and who is experiencing it.

Women's experiences

It may be that women's experiences vary between the two extreme representations of pain mentioned above; but the limited research into the woman's experience of childbearing pain and the methods used to control it is an example of a reluctance to view pain as a part of the complete childbearing experience. Our previous narrow focus on, for example, the techniques used to relieve or remove the woman's pain has inhibited a complete or 'holistic' understanding of the woman's experience of childbearing. Such inhibition has been facilitated by the 'inexpressibility' of physical pain and the way in which pain splits the sufferer from those close by (Scarry 1985). Scarry goes on to remind us that this split is partly due to the 'unshareability' of pain, which is aggravated by the limitations imposed by language, especially English; as Virginia Woolf observed in this context, 'language at once runs dry' (1925). These phenomena have contributed to doubts as to the existence of childbearing pain, discussed in Chapters 5 and 6, which are compounded by professional reluctance to believe the accuracy of the sufferer's narrative. For these reasons, and perhaps in self-defence against reality shock, the woman sufferer may be overlooked, further weakening her already excruciatingly vulnerable position.

Thus, the political nature of pain emerges. Scarry's focus on the balance of power in the relationship between the sufferer and the attendant may be less than relevant in the context of childbearing. Or is it? To what extent are the 'caring professions' in a position to assist the childbearing woman to reduce or control her experience of pain? I intend that this book should illuminate a wide range of aspects of this situation in order to help you, the reader, to answer this question.

Orientation

This approach that I have outlined is partly a response to the reviews of the first edition of this book. While they were almost invariably positive, one of the reviewers criticised my approach for being too hard on medical practitioners. If it applies, I make no apology for any such approach; I am not entirely convinced, though, that such criticism is justified. This reviewer complained that I was too vigorous in my condemnation of our medical colleagues, while being too lenient with my fellow midwives. Such a comparison merits closer attention.

The crucial difference is found in the nature of the professionals' contribution. The midwife's unique selling point (USP) is his or her non-interventional support of the woman experiencing healthy childbearing. For this reason, the midwife may be censured for sins of omission, involving his or her cautious use of, for example, pharmacological pain remedies. Our medical colleagues, whose USPs depend on their actively intervening in what may be physiological processes, may be guilty of committing sins of commission. This is an altogether different scenario because there is a risk of actually creating pathology in an otherwise healthy situation. This grave possibility raises the spectre of iatrogenesis. Perhaps unfortunately, this is a concept which will re-emerge regularly, but hopefully not too frequently, throughout this book.

Thus, the balanced approach, for which I strive in this book, will take full cognisance of all aspects of the human and technical environment in which childbearing happens. That said, the question remains of what is meant by the term 'childbearing'. Although, giving birth is obviously crucial to childbearing, this term clearly encompasses more than labour and birth. This is the reason why I choose to use it. Throughout this book, childbearing is used to include any aspect of reproduction, beginning with the woman or couple thinking about conceiving a baby through to her or their establishment of parenting.

The midwife's experience

This book seeks to focus on the experience of pain faced by the childbearing woman. This focus is entirely appropriate. Given my remit, though, of extending the boundaries of my approach to pain, another aspect deserves to be at least considered. This aspect is the pain or suffering endured by the midwife providing care for the childbearing woman. In Chapter 2 I discuss the implications of the system of 'Care' for the woman and draw attention the institutionalised regime, common to many countries, which has been graphically termed 'iatrogenic rape' (Lesnik-Oberstein 1982). While the woman's experience has attracted attention, if not remedies, the experience of the midwife working with her tends to be disregarded. It is not impossible that the compliance demanded of the woman (Kirkham 1989; Svensson et al. 2007) may also be required of the midwife attending her. Thus, midwives with appropriate aspirations and expectations may find their achievements seriously curtailed by the system within which they practise, engendering feelings of suffering and pain at their failure to actualise these expectations. The midwife who stands up for the ideals which he or she knows to be achievable may find him or herself the butt of 'horizontal violence' from colleagues who, similarly oppressed, are no longer able to raise their heads above the parapet. While measures are being begun to address these systematic challenges, the problem of the midwife's pain may not be easily resolved (Mander et al. 2010).

The chapters

Although the analogy of the journey is over-used to the point of being hackneyed, I use it for this book's theoretical framework because it emerged crucially from a research project focusing on women's perceptions of their experience of giving birth (Halldorsdottir & Karlsdottir 1996). Thus, in this book Part I, 'Before the Journey's Commencement', establishes the context for childbearing and the pain experience; this includes historical, cultural, theoretical and research related issues. Part II concentrates on 'Beginning the Journey', which comprises childbirth education, including the extent to which it prepares the woman for her complete childbearing experience, and pain in pregnancy. Part III, 'The Journey', focuses on labour. Despite the increasingly tenuous link between labour and pain as interventional pain control becomes more effective, I include in Part III the issues and the interventions which may be applied to many types of pain. These topics fit together because the experience of labour and the desire to address pain are probably equally universal. In Part IV, I consider the period after the birth for the woman and child as 'The Journey's End'. The conclusion is included in Part IV and draws together the themes which emerge.

Because of the 'bad press' which the term 'drug' tends to attract, throughout this book I endeavour to use the word 'medication' when discussing pharmaceutical products.

Part I

Before the Journey's Commencement

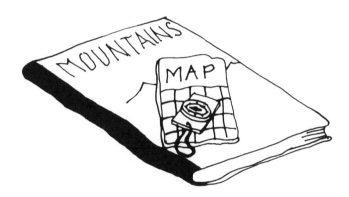

Chapter 1

Pasts and peoples

General background

When thinking or writing about any form of pain, I have a tendency to generalise my ideas. I don't think that I am unique in this respect. This is an inevitable way of attempting to manage an otherwise unmanageable concept. As the reader, though, you should keep in mind the artifice of such a strategy. Pain is above all an individual phenomenon. Only the person experiencing it is able to really know what that pain is like. Other people may think that they know what the pain is like. They may have experienced pain in the same part of the body, or possibly due to a similar cause, in the past. Alternatively, they have witnessed or even provided care for a number of people and think they know what a person who is experiencing this form of pain looks like. All of these people, whether they are experienced or whether they are witnesses, are mistaken. They are making assumptions which are either weakly founded or totally unfounded. Obviously, such unfounded assumptions carry serious implications for the person actually experiencing the pain.

For the present, though, I feel obliged to encourage the reader to keep at the forefront of his or her mind this 'health warning':

> Do not allow yourself to be lulled into assuming that you know what another person's pain is – that way lies danger.

This health warning applies not only to modern day experiences and practices. I venture to suggest that such a cautious approach should be applied equally to former peoples in their own times and settings.

In this chapter I plan to trace, first, the ways in which attitudes to pain have developed in certain societies over time. This section does not claim to be comprehensive because there are some societies whose literature is not accessible to me for linguistic reasons. In order to trace these developments, it is necessary to consider the major pain theories, together with significant exceptions. These historical views are then applied to childbearing pain. The second part of this chapter turns the focus to the association between culture and pain-related experiences and practices. This cultural orientation leads, inevitably, to consideration of the meanings which may be attributable to experiences of pain.

Pain in Childbearing and its Control, Second Edition. By Rosemary Mander. Published 2011 by Blackwell Publishing Ltd. © 1998, 2011 Rosemary Mander.

Historical attitudes to and interpretation of pain

Ideas about pain and its control inevitably develop as society changes. As a result, even relatively recent ideas quickly become outdated. On the other hand, deeply held, perhaps ancient, ideas about pain in general and specific forms of pain may surface to manifest themselves in certain circumstances. I suggest that an experience as intense as childbirth is one of those circumstances.

Esther Cohen's analysis (1995) of early historical attitudes to pain demonstrates not only the crucial cultural component of pain, but also the temporal developments within those cultures. In his unique paper, which has stood the test of time, Donald Caton (1985) outlines how some of the attitudinal changes did or did not actually happen. His paper provides a useful framework for this section. Caton traces the gradual change from regarding pain as a mystical or divine intervention, possibly an emulation of a suffering deity, to a natural, secular phenomenon. Simultaneously pain was transformed from being considered generally, if convolutedly, beneficial. It has since come to be regarded as a universally destructive phenomenon.

In prehistoric tribal societies magical influences were held to be responsible for non-traumatic painful experiences (McKenzie & Parris 1997). Beliefs in these magical influences allowed women healers and the shaman or medicine man to assume powerful positions in attributing the cause and necessary punitive actions to remedy the pain. Such mystical convictions were gradually superseded by a trust in or fear of deities. In a similar way, in some cultures pain has been attributed to the absence of balance, or to the frustration of desires (Main & Spanswick 2001).

According to Caton (1985), early Greeks and Jews perceived pain as having a dual role. The first role of pain was to convey divine punishment to those who transgressed. McKenzie and Parris point to 'the curse of Eve' (see below) as an example of such divine intervention (1997: 2). Thus Greeks, such as Homer, attributed pain to arrows released by the gods. Such forms of external attribution were not uncommon and were similarly applied to a range of disease processes. The second role of pain in this setting was considerably more positive. Together with punishment, pain carried with it the opportunity for the person to show remorse for whatever 'sin' was said to have caused the pain. In this way, the penitent was able to achieve healing through cleansing, which brought redemption from the original transgression.

Similar ideas persisted from the fifth century CE through to the Enlightenment; under Judaeo-Christian influence, pain continued to be interpreted as divine retribution for wrong-doing. Through this powerful link spiritual leaders emerged as comforters and healers. Thus began the long-standing connection between the church and public health. Fundamental to these ideas was the church's dependence on the dogma of original sin, which materialised in woman's inherently evil nature (Yee 2003). Inevitably self-inflicted pain was eventually substituted for spontaneous pain in a form of 'pre-emptive strike' to prevent disease by appeasing or propitiating the deity. Thus, an element of magical thinking developed. During the Spanish Inquisition this concept was extended to inflict pain on others to achieve their purification (Glucklich 2001). Therefore, pain's dual role as both punishment and redemption emerges. These combined magical and mystical ideas became expanded by logic and observation, such as of substances to ease pain. These observations led to suspicions that human-controlled phenomena were involved and not just superhuman agencies. Such observations included public health measures, like isolation, which occasionally limited the spread of bubonic plague.

From about 1600 the age of faith made way for the age of reason. A link became established between the study of nature and the understanding of divine laws. Thus, the scientific approach to knowledge emerged. Divine laws became relatively less significant, to the extent that the contribution of the deity was eventually questioned by the influential thinkers of the enlightenment. Up to this time changing attitudes had resulted in only minimal changes in treatment, because the methods available were so limited.

These two fundamentally important functions of pain underwent a series of transitions, not necessarily synchronously, with the Renaissance, the Age of Reason and the Age of Revolution. But, by the nineteenth century social changes were leading to philosophers, such as Jeremy Bentham (1748–1832), to consider pain as a totally natural phenomenon, devoid of either divine causation or redemptive capacity. With the increasing power of medical practitioners in the nineteenth century, aspirations to becoming a scientific discipline completed the transition to pain being regarded as predominantly secular. Without actually mentioning the terms, Caton implies the association between the changing perceptions of pain and the relative changes in the power base of the occupational groups regarded as professions. He eventually reaches the obvious conclusion that, through the self help and complementary health movements, both the causation and the remediation of pain have been comprehensively secularised through the assumption of responsibility for any pain by the affected individual. Thus, moral or religious interpretations of pain appear to have become largely obsolete in sophisticated settings.

Pain theory

In contemplating the theory on which our understanding of pain is founded, we need to remember that pain theories are precisely that. Their role is to facilitate our understanding of the relationship between two or more variables. Theories, like the comprehension which they engender, are in no way fixed or immutable. Thus, our understanding of pain needs to be regarded as dynamic. In the same way that 'ropes' and 'bells' (see specificity theory below) currently seem archaic, in the future it is not impossible that 'gates' (see currently accepted pain theory below) may similarly be viewed as anachronistic.

Our understanding of pain has clearly increased as human knowledge of anatomy and physiology has developed. I have shown, in the previous section, that there have been other influences; these include religious, philosophical, political and social aspects. In prehistoric settings, attitudes to pain would barely have justified the term 'theory'.

Bonica and Loeser (2001) outline the role of the ancient Greeks (fourth–fifth century BCE), such as Aristotle, in seeking the underlying sources and mechanisms of pain. The contribution of the brain and central nervous system was variably recognised, competing with the heart for priority. In ancient Rome (third century BCE), Galen was able to recognise nerve fibres as having a role in the transmission of pain sensations. By the Middle Ages, the part played by the central nervous system was being modified by perceptions of humoral functions.

Specificity theory

Although the term was not widely used until after the work of Schiff in the mid-nineteenth century, René Descartes was the original 'key philosopher' (Wall 1999: 20) who introduced the concept of dualism, which led eventually to specificity theory. Descartes (1596–1650) sought an anatomical and physiological explanation of the sensation of pain which had been recognised by Aristotle. Descartes employed the newly developed scientific method to find this explanation. By dissection and introspection, he came to regard the human body as no longer the 'temple of the soul' as espoused by the all-dominant church. Descartes proposed regarding the human body as a machine, controlled by physical principles (Melzack 1993). His dissections identified nerve fibres, on the basis of which he concluded that a specific system transmits impulses from cutaneous pain receptors to a cerebral pain centre. This mechanism was considered analogous with 'pulling on one end of a rope makes a bell ring which hangs at the other end to strike at the same instant' (Wall & Jones 1991). This approach to pain is summarised by the well-known drawing of the 'Boy with Foot in Fire'. Cartesian dualistic ideas continued to influence knowledge and therapy until well into the late twentieth century (Wall 1999). While Descartes is often blamed for modern mechanistic approaches to health, Mark Zimmerman considers that he does not deserve such a bad press (2005).

In the light of Charles Bell's (1774–1842) recognition of the separate flow of sensory information through channels in the spinal cord, in 1842 Johannes P Müller developed the doctrine of specific nerve energies. These energies were thought to comprise coded or symbolic messages which could be transmitted only by sensory nerves to the brain. A major flaw in this earth-shattering realisation was the belief that one single sense of touch encompasses all forms of pain.

Maximilian Von Frey developed Müller's work and combined it with physiological observation and newly introduced staining techniques to identify four types of cutaneous receptor organs or 'modalities'. This theory persisted in affirming direct links to an appropriate cerebral centre and, on the basis of surgery, such pain 'pathways' were identified in the anterolateral or dorsal quadrant of the spinal cord.

The strength of these forms of specificity theory lies in their physiological specialisation. The multiplicity of weaknesses of specificity theory, though, includes the psychological assumption of straight-through transmission and the absence of any allowance for personal or temporal variation in pain perception. This approach to pain has been blamed for the medicalisation of pain and, hence, impeding understanding and more effective remedies (Bendelow & Williams 1998).

Pattern theory

The weaknesses of specificity theory were clearly apparent to clinicians, so a search was begun to illuminate the complexity of transmission. The results comprise 'pattern theory'.

Following pathological observations, Alfred Goldscheider (in 1894) hypothesised that, together, central summation in the dorsal horn and stimulus intensity are the critical determinants of pain. John Bonica (1990a) referred to this as 'Intensive (Summation) Theory', but the emphasis was clearly on the stimulation spatially or temporally of non-specific receptors. The earliest, or peripheral, pattern theory focused on intense peripheral stimulation being interpreted centrally as pain; physiological specialisation was effectively ignored. The lack of any theory addressing phantom limb/body pain was recognised by William Livingston, who in 1943 refined pattern theory to produce the central summation theory; a pattern of incremental and reverberatory circuits were thought to explain the otherwise inexplicable phantom pain experienced by amputees.

A still more complex hypothesis was advanced by Willem Noordenbos in 1959 in the form of the sensory interaction theory, according to which a rapidly conducting fibre system inhibits synaptic transmission in a more slowly conducting pain-carrying system. This theory further proposed a multi-synaptic afferent system within the spinal cord. Thus, the physiological stage was set for the gate control theory (see 'Currently accepted pain theory' below).

Affect theory

Integrated into other pain theories is one which for centuries stood alone as the only explanation of pain. This is the 'affect theory' of pain, which defines pain as an emotion, rather than as a sensation (Melzack & Wall 1991). Affect theory is closely linked with what Bonica (1990a) termed the 'Fourth' theory of pain, which differentiates the neuro-physiological perception of pain from the cognitive aspects of the response to pain, as determined by a range of factors including culture and previous experience.

Psychological/behavioural theory

This chronic form of pain reflects disconcerting trends in general psychology, being sum-marised in terms of 'pain as behaviour'. It relates to the forms of pain sometimes known as 'psychogenic' and incorporates a response to cues which are part of the individual's environment. These forms of behaviour may be associated with triggers which led to the original pain experience (Fordyce et al. 1988).

Fear-avoidance model of pain

This model of pain, formulated by Johan Vlaeyen and colleagues in 1995, may not be unrelated to the psychological/behavioural theory (above). It essentially comprises fear of aggravating pain giving rise to the avoidance of certain beneficial activities (Moffett et al. 2004). Randomised controlled trials using this approach to pain show that it is amenable to non-pharmacological intervention, but that any benefits demonstrated tend to be temporary.

Currently accepted pain theory

The pain theory which is most widely and generally accepted was developed during the early 1960s by Ronald Melzack and Patrick Wall (1965). More recently another pain model has been introduced which is particularly relevant to midwifery, which will more appropriately be considered in detail in the light of the discussion on cultural aspects of pain (below).

Gate control theory

It is clear that, in the history of pain theory, the role of the central nervous system was insignificant, to the extent of the cerebral contribution being negligible. This imbalance was redressed by Melzack and Wall in the early 1960s, using new technology which permitted the electronic recording of individual nerve cells' activity. This work combined Melzack's study of the psychology of the somatic senses with Wall's interest in the physiology of the pain pathways to address certain paradoxes in our understanding of pain (Wall & Jones 1991: 129):

> the variable relationship between injury and pain
> that innocuous stimuli may elicit pain
> the location of pain discrete from the site of damage
> pain in the absence of injury or after healing
> changes in the nature of pain over time
> intractable pain with/without obvious cause.

Melzack and Wall built on the already well-recognised phenomenon by which gentle stimulation inhibited pain sensation to draw up the gate control theory of pain (Melzack & Wall, 1965); it explains persuasively the psychological aspects of pain, the physiology of pain transmission and the modulating influences. The gate control theory emphasises the body's in-built pain control mechanisms and provides a feasible explanation for the non-intervention or low-tech approaches to pain control, including psychological methods, back-rubbing and transcutaneous electrical nerve stimulation (TENS; Chapter 8).

This theory may be briefly summarised thus:

(1) The passage of nerve impulses from afferent fibres to spinal cord transmission cells and thence to local reflex circuits and the brain is modulated by a spinal gating mechanism in the dorsal horn. As with all central nervous system (CNS) synapses this transmission is controlled by mechanisms which either facilitate or inhibit the passage of the impulse.

(2) The spinal gating mechanism is influenced by the relative amount of activity in large diameter (low threshold myelinated afferent) fibres and small diameter (high threshold myelinated A-delta and unmyelinated C) fibres: activity in large fibres tends to inhibit transmission (close the gate) while small-fibre activity tends to facilitate transmission (open the gate).

(3) The spinal cord gating mechanism, which is now thought to operate in a number of sites including lamina 2 of the substantia gelatinosa of the dorsal horn, is influenced by nerve impulses descending from the brain.

(4) A specialised system of large diameter, rapidly conducting fibres (the Central Control Trigger) activates selective cognitive processes that then influence, by way of descending fibres, the modulating properties of the spinal gating mechanism.

(5) When the firing rate or output of the spinal cord transmission cells exceeds a critical level, it activates the Action System - those neural areas that underlie the complex, sequential patterns of behaviour and experience characteristics of pain. The critical level

is determined on an individual basis by the person's brain, and is dependent on a range of factors, such as previous experience (Melzack & Wall 1991; Melzack 1993).

The impact of the publication of the gate control theory was 'astonishing' in terms of both its vigour and viciousness; although Melzack maintains that its greatest effect lay in its emphasis on the dynamic role of the CNS, especially the brain (Melzack 1993). In the context of childbearing, this theory assists our understanding of how the emotions which childbearing women experience, such as confidence or fear, as well as cognitions, such as knowledge or meaning, affect the woman's pain experience.

Further hypotheses

The gate control theory has impacted profoundly on the subsequent development of both knowledge and its application. The two major effects are that, first, simplistic pain theories are no longer acceptable and, second, an holistic orientation to all aspects of pain is recognised as essential. There has also been some progress with addressing the persisting paradoxes of pain.

Phantom pain

Phantom pain is usually considered to be associated with the loss of a limb. Because such pain may occur after the loss of other body parts, such as following mastectomy, it may be known as phantom limb/body pain (PL/BP). The theory of a 'neuromatrix' has been developed (Melzack & Katz 2006) which serves to explain the continuing nature of these sensations. This 'psychological template' includes cerebral structures and continues to function after the loss of the body part.

This continuing neuromatrix results in sensations of a phantom in most people who lose a part. These sensations are not necessarily unpleasant, but up to 85% of amputees experience pain and may find it distressing, limiting and disabling (Brodie et al. 2007). The neuromatrix theory takes account of previous pain experiences and interventions which have or have not been effective. This orientation makes this theory particularly appropriate to women in labour (Trout 2004). The research in this area tends to be weak in terms of methods and responses. It is clear that distressing phantom pain conditions urgently need more, and more, authoritative, research attention.

Prolonged pain

In association with the gate control, observations of small, unmyelinated afferent or C nerve fibres were observed to behave in an unusual way (Wall & Jones 1991). Following an initial episode of acute and severe pain, those C fibres arising in deep visceral or joint tissues were found to show increasing activity, recognised as slowly increasing pain. These authors further suggest some cerebral control of this impulse-triggered prolonged pain. They give as an example the pain of a twisted ankle, which is initially sharp but is followed by a vague ache. It is also suggested that this mechanism may be relevant to surgery.

Alongside the gate control and impulse-triggered prolonged pain mechanisms, Wall and Jones (1991) propose that damaged nerve fibres may engender prolonged pain due to local escape of chemicals normally transported only within the axon. This prolonged pain, termed 'transport-controlled prolonged pain', has been attributed to nerve growth factor. Again, C fibres appear to contribute crucially, perhaps by diagnosing a local problem, for which reason they have been labelled 'chemical pathologists'.

A midwifery model

Nicky Leap's midwifery understanding of labour pain and its control is widely regarded as a development of pain theory (1996). The status of this development, though, is uncertain because of Leap's focus on the *care* of the woman in labour. Despite this uncertainty and because of this model's decisive influence on the ideas which are discussed in this book, I outline the model at the end of this chapter.

Summary

It is apparent from this discussion that our understanding of pain has developed beyond all recognition since Aristotle and that it is continuing to do so. In the same way as we now understand that pain is not a simplistic concept, we know that our understanding of it must also be multifaceted, multidisciplinary and dynamic. It may be that, in historical terms, an understanding of the nature of pain has not been necessary in order to treat it. This situation is changing and our increasing understanding is facilitating more suitable methods of helping people, and particularly childbearing women, to cope with pain.

Cultural aspects

It may be that childbearing and the associated pain are one of the few common experiences shared by the various component groups which comprise the current global society. Although the experience is common, attitudes to it and their expression vary hugely and not invariably predictably. This chaotic situation is further complicated by the varying backgrounds, experiences and attitudes of those providing care during childbearing. In this section, I examine the cultural inputs into and perceptions of this conundrum of pain. I first consider the nature of culture and the factors which have been shown to influence it. I move then to the cultural factors that affect the sufferer's pain expression and carers' pain perception. Next are the cultural factors impinging on childbearing in general and the associated pain in particular. The themes emerging from this material are drawn together by considering the meaning of pain.

In considering culture in the present context, it is necessary to draw heavily on North American literature. Such heavy reliance should carry with it a further health warning on the grounds of our transatlantic cousin's preoccupation with the 'other'. This leads to a neglect of the impact of what may be termed the 'dominant' culture.

The meaning of culture

'Culture' is a term which carries many meanings; for this reason it is necessary to contemplate the sense in which I use it. Like so many abstract concepts, culture may exist at a variety of more or less abstruse levels. All too often, assumptions may be made about a person's culture from his or her physical appearance. This view is worryingly over-simplistic and carries the likelihood of racial stereotyping and racism.

In contrast Charalambos Tsekeris (2008), who studied culture in a Greek context, emphasises culture's socially-inherited nature and the extent to which it features shared ideals. The complexity of culture is clearer in the unwritten and unstated assumptions and values which determine the behaviour of the members of the relevant group. These assumptions are powerfully influential in controlling behaviour, and may be the only visible manifestation of group membership. While culture describes complex abstractions, terms like 'ethnic/ity' are marginally clearer. These terms refer precisely to a person's racial origin; however, such straightforward terms become less comfortable when the word 'group' is added, as this introduces political nuances.

There are certain factors that have been shown to influence culture.

Geography

There is a tendency to consider culture merely in terms of geographical origin. This is one of the traps which ensnared Zborowski in his still ground-breaking work on the cultural components of pain responses (1952). In a New York setting, he collected data on pain expression by patients of four ethnic backgrounds. The groups were selected following discussion with clinical staff, because staff found difficulty coping with the differing reactions to pain. The groups comprised Italians, Jews, Irish and a group long settled in the USA but of northern European extraction, entitled 'Old Americans'. The data were collected qualitatively by open-ended interviews with patients, observations of them while in pain and interviews with staff caring for them.

Mark Zborowski's work is frequently and appropriately criticised for his superficial and one-dimensional approach, together with the creation of 'cardboard characters instead of describing real people' (Kleinman et al. 1992: 2). Despite such criticisms, Zborowski's work did break new ground in the study of pain.

Thus, Zborowski made partial use of geographical origin as a proxy for culture; however, others have been more discriminating in their interpretation of geographically based culture (Lasch 2000). Such reassurances, though, leave the reader with concerns that occasionally culture may be used as a method of stereotyping 'immigrants coming from non-traditional regions such as Southeast Asia and Latin America' (Lasch 2000: 16). This process is surely counterproductive if individualised care is the aim.

Religion

These two examples (Zborowski 1952; Lasch 2000) show the extent to which culture is associated with geographical origin. This association is supported by an observation made prior to an authoritative attempt to measure the link between pain and culture, which identified 29 cultural groups whose pain responses had been researched (Lipton & Marbach 1984). Religion and skin colour as well as geography featured as determining characteristics in five groups. Geographical origin and religious persuasion may be thought to be synonymous, but these authors state that such groups are few. The major religions influence culture by, for example, advocating pain acceptance, adopting either prospective or retrospective approaches; examples are the Muslim 'kismet' (destiny), Hindu 'karma' (reincarnated burden) or the Christian atonement.

The significant relationship between religious persuasion and geographical origin has emerged in North American pain studies (Sternbach & Tursky 1965). The weakness of such research is found in religious persuasion and geographical origin being so similar in their determination of culture that they are interchangeable. This point was brought home forcefully to me when a woman of North African extraction was criticising the NHS staff's limited understanding. Her comments were unsurprising until she asserted 'You Christians'. I was taken aback as I certainly do not regard my religious orientation as a prominent characteristic. For her, though, Western European was clearly synonymous with Christian, supporting my argument that culture is inextricably and equally linked, at least in observers' minds, with religion and geographical origin.

Education

With hindsight, I realise that the North African woman was simply applying a cultural stereotype to me, which I considered inappropriate. Thus, the usual stereotyping found in maternity care was reversed. Jo Green and her colleagues (1990) support this contention that stereotyping is invariably unidirectional. The stereotyping on which they focused was the woman's education relative to her involvement in childbearing decision-making. While their data supported the positive aspects of the stereotypical 'educated' woman, this supremely trustworthy study refuted the usual negative stereotypes of the less-educated woman.

Socio-economic class

This authoritative study persuaded Green and colleagues that education is inextricably linked to a person's cultural orientation. These researchers further considered whether social class is associated with education and culture, discussing stereotypes of 'uneducated working class women' (1990: 127). They dismiss social class (determined in the classic style by the male partner's occupation) as not 'a very good indicator of women's attitudes' (1990: 128).

While Green et al. have clearly debunked the myth of the stereotypical 'working class woman', James McIntosh's research (1989) found that she was alive and, if not well, at least residing in Glasgow. McIntosh argued that women in lower socio-economic groups have their own shared perspectives of and attitudes to childbearing which are culture-bound. In his sample of 80 women, half belonged to social class IIIb and the remainder to social classes IV and V. He claimed to have identified the stereotypical working class woman who is 'less opposed to medical intervention and control and less likely to espouse the cause of natural childbirth'.

The culture of social class was explored prior to a study of women's reproductive lives by Emily Martin (1989). She believes the crucial difference to be the reliance of middle class families on paid outside help and support; whereas 'working class' families are more likely to be able, or need, to pool their own resources.

The comments by Green, the argument by McIntosh and observations by Martin combine to demonstrate that socio-economic class brings with it a range of features which contribute to a unique culture.

Gender

It is not unknown for female health care staff to scoff at men's limited tolerance of pain. Although possibly politically incorrect, gender differences in pain perception are becoming recognised. The authoritative work of Gillian Bendelow and Simon Williams recognised that the 'conditioned stoicism' of men renders them less well able to cope with pain (1998: 207). Clearly, the experience and the expression of pain may be worlds apart. These researchers, however, argue that it is women's perception of pain as natural, as opposed to men considering it abnormal, which allows women to both tolerate and, only when necessary, articulate pain.

At a more physiological level, the work of Zsuzsanna Wiesenfeld-Hallin in Sweden (2005) sought to investigate the general finding of a greater sensitivity to pain among women. She found differences in the neurological 'wiring' which may serve to explain such differences. The rationale which she suggests relates to men's susceptibility to wounds through their time-honoured roles as hunters and warriors. For this reason, she maintains that men are more vulnerable to somatic pain compared with women, whose reproductive pain is more visceral.

Other influencing factors

In the same way as Wiesenfeld-Hallin leads us to contemplate the socio-cultural influences on pain perception, Cecil Helman (2007) focuses on whether the expectations of society lead to cultural acceptance or non-acceptance of pain. His examples include, first, the groups who live in war zones and who accept battle-wounds and their pain as, not merely inevitable, but actually admirable. Moving into a rather different social climate, Helman then suggests that cultures which are able to control pain effectively tend to find pain unacceptable. Thus, certain groups in countries such as the USA 'welcome analgesic drugs'.

Culture and pain

The links between pain responses and culture are well-recognised, as reflected in the widely used though somewhat limited definition of pain, which allows for cultural variations in pain perception:

> An unpleasant sensory and emotional experience associated with actual or potential tissue damage, or described in terms of such damage. (International Association for the Study of Pain 2009)

The cultural variations of pain perception have been demonstrated through a series of research projects undertaken by various disciplines adopting different perspectives. I now review some research findings relating to the client's expression and the carer's perception.

The person in pain

Focusing on the difficulty of making cultural comparisons of pain expression, Helman (2007) sought to distinguish public from private pain. Public pain involves some form of articulation, whereas private pain foregoes such expression. Exemplifying the latter, he cites the 'stiff upper lip' so admired by 'Anglo-Saxon' peoples and the anecdotal absence of pain behaviour among warriors. Alternatively, this distinction may reflect either the lack of sensitivity of the observer or a physiological shock reaction, rather than non-verbal/verbal behaviour in the sufferer. Even so, Helman concedes that 'an absence of pain behaviour does not necessarily mean the absence of private pain'.

The first 'observations' of the cultural implications of pain were made by 'missionaries, travelers and other laymen (and even some medically trained persons)' (Wolff & Langley 1977: 313). These observations were based on assumptions that so-called 'primitive' peoples are less sensitive to pain than their 'civilised' counterparts (Morris 1991: 39). Reflecting the thinking then prevalent, genetic inheritance was held responsible. The missionaries and their fellow travellers probably had in mind gruesome initiation ceremonies and other rituals (Soikava et al. 2005). In these ceremonies, apparently painful behaviours typically produce no recognisable pain response in the 'celebrant'. As distinct from more humdrum everyday pains, these mystical ceremonies demonstrate the significance of culture; thus, the meaning of the situation, event and other unique factors are crucial in the perception, interpretation and expression of pain (Glucklich 2001).

Despite the tendency to draw conclusions about the cultural factors associated with a person's perception and expression of pain, some anthropologists remain healthily sceptical about the validity of research findings (Wolff & Langley 1977). Exemplifying Zborowski's study (1952), these critics bemoan the continuing lack of experimental data supporting a cultural component of pain. They regret the lack of sound anthropological research on pain responses, blaming this on existing experimental studies being anthropologically naïve, and completed anthropological studies lacking the experimental rigour to permit valid conclusions.

As critiqued in 'Geography' (above), an unprecedented study focusing on pain and culture sought the differing perceptions, interpretations and expressions of pain by patients and by staff (Zborowski 1952). Zborowski sought to illuminate the acceptability or otherwise of pain behaviour as viewed by staff and patients of differing cultural backgrounds. The immediate spur to this study was the seemingly infinite potential for conflict associated with differing attitudes to pain. Zborowski focused on four 'ethno-cultural' groups of patients. The sample comprised: Jews (n=31), Italians (n=24), Irish (n=11) and Old Americans (n=26). Additionally, there were 11 patients of unstated ethnic origin. A qualitative research design involved interviews with the patients, staff and 16 healthy respondents, which were recorded on 'wire' and transcribed. There is no indication of how the observational data were organised.

The Italian and Jewish patients had been perceived as demonstrating similar emotional responses to pain, and this was interpreted as meaning that they had a 'lower threshold of pain' than other groups. Zborowski found that the situation was more complex than that. Although the responses to pain appeared similar, the underlying attitudes were diametrically opposed. The meaning and implications of the pain were the prime concern of the

Jewish people, whereas it was the immediate experience that concerned the Italians. Thus, analgesia solved the Italians' problems, but the Jewish people perceived analgesia, not just as no solution, but as actually causing more problems by masking any potentially threatening symptoms. The Italian and Jewish patients were perceived by the American/ ised staff as vocalising pain excessively to attract attention. The staff responded to what they considered to be an over-emotional reaction by minimising their assessment of these patients' pain; thus, articulation was interpreted as histrionics and was counterproductive in gaining sympathy and treatment. Pain expression in these groups further differed according to whether the pain occurred at home or in hospital. The differences were determined by the tendency of the Italians to adopt a more macho and the Jewish people a more manipulative orientation. Thus, although these two groups exhibited similar pain behaviour, it derived from different attitudes to pain, served differing functions and sought to achieve different ends. The Old American patients, however, were perceived by staff as being compliant and demonstrating the stiff upper lip approach to pain. Members of this group thought it pointless to fuss about their pain and believed it necessary to behave like a 'good American'. This group considered emotional displays counterproductive.

These attitudes suggest a future orientation in the Jewish patient, compared with a present-time orientation in the Italian. Each group of patients expressed confidence in the staff, investigations and hospitalisation; while this was greatest in the Old American, the Jewish patient tended to be more sceptical and pessimistic.

Not surprisingly, Zborowski (1952) identified individual differences between members of each of the four groups and sought the reasons for within-group variation. Some individual differences were attributed to the patient's degree of 'Americanisation', which correlated with the duration of time since the patient, or their forebears, had immigrated. It is generally recognised that the behaviour of migrants changes when they reach their destination. The attitudes and behaviour associated with pain are more deeply held and ingrained than others and, hence, change more slowly. Zborowski observed that the pain behaviour of the Jewish and the Italian patient may be similar to the Old American if the patient is third generation but, although behaviours may adapt, underlying attitudes persist. Also, recognising the individuality of adherence to 'the old ways', distinction may be made between ideological and behavioural ethnicity (Brodwin & Kleinman 1987). The latter is the everyday version, whereas the former emerges for 'religious holidays and political rallies'. The extent to which these forms of ethnicity are amplified by migration remains open to conjecture.

The gradual change in the behaviour of ethnic groups and the even slower change in underlying attitudes led Zborowski to explore how cultural attitudes to pain are transmitted. He concluded that early influences within the family are crucial. He suggests that 'appropriate' childhood behaviours are rewarded and, hence, reinforced. In contrast, other more 'inappropriate' behaviours are disregarded, or even punished, to obliterate them from the child's repertoire. In the context of encouraging appropriate behaviour, pain behaviour is likely to have been learned within the family of birth as a coping mechanism. 'Secondary gains' act as reinforcers, from which the sufferer benefits; examples include controlling situations, justifying dependency, punishing others and avoiding sex.

Zborowski is certainly guilty of further racial stereotyping when describing certain groups of women as overprotective and rewarding of more dependent behaviour (Kleinman et al. 1992). Zborowski's creation of 'cardboard characters', serving to dehumanise the subjects and their experience of pain, is also criticised. Despite these limitations, Arthur Kleinman and his colleagues recognise this study's contribution to founding the study of culture and pain expression, in itself no mean feat.

More recently, aspects of Zborowski's much-criticised study have been endorsed by researchers in England (McAllister & Farquhar 1992), who also found that people of different cultures adopted differing attitudes to their health problems. Asian women (n=23) were compared with 'white indigenous' women (n=14) regarding their perceptions of health/illness causation. The relevant differences, attributed to culture, were that Asian women were less concerned about the causes of illness, and this was associated with greater confidence in medical and other health advisors. The Asian women attributed their health problems to psychological factors, such as stress, and to the UK climate. The white indigenous women, however, were more likely to blame lifestyle, including smoking and employment. These attributions reflect a weakness in this study recognised by the researchers; this is the way that the white indigenous women's views related to health promotion material to which they were exposed, and which could not be read by many of the Asian women. Despite this, the cultural differences in attitudes to health, identified by Zborowski (1952), appear to be endorsed.

A contrary rationale for cultural differences in pain behaviour depends less on the individual and what they have learned from family than on their experience (Craig & Wyckoff 1987). These writers argue that the person in pain decides consciously whether to articulate their distress and seek help. This decision is based on their estimation, using previous experience, of what best advances their own interests. This interpretation of pain behaviour is reminiscent of the learning-free, forward-looking expectancy theory (Lewin 1935) in which the individual scrutinises all aspects of the situation, including cultural, to calculate how to achieve their most desired outcome. Thus, a decision emerges about whether the pain is made public or kept private. Regardless of the decision, the sufferer conforms to culturally determined rules governing emotional displays, rather than allowing any reflex pain behaviour. Having suggested an alternative to the solely cultural interpretation of variations in pain behaviour, these researchers focus on the dangers of cultural stereotyping in pain assessment. While Zborowski identified major differences in attitudes to health and pain behaviour between cultural groups, he also noted differences within those groups. These inter- and intra-group variations are of a similar magnitude, but the reader is warned that stereotyping reduces their significance and renders care and treatment less relevant to the individual. A phenomenon which may aggravate stereotyping is the preparedness of a minority group to withhold information from the dominant group for fear of being labelled as 'weak', 'mad' or just 'different'. These researchers maintained that this applies in therapeutic as well as research settings.

The carer and his or her perception of the client's pain

As mentioned already (see 'The Meaning of culture'), concern about the potential for conflict between staff and patients served as the spur to the original, though flawed, study of pain expression (Zborowski 1952). That the attitudes of staff continue to arouse anxiety is demonstrated by continuing research in this area. This anxiety began with research by Lois Davitz and her colleagues (1976), which examined the association between nurses' cultural backgrounds and their beliefs about patients' pain. This study found that Korean and Japanese nurses assessed the physical pain and the psychological distress as equally high. The American nurses were similarly consistently low in their estimation of both forms of suffering. The Puerto Rican nurses, however, linked low levels of physical pain with high levels of psychological distress. In spite of these discrepancies, all the nurses agreed on their estimation of children's psychological distress as being less than adults. Similarly, they agreed that female patients experienced more pain than males, which may be associated with the totally female sample of nurses.

This research (Davitz et al. 1976) focused on the culture as determined by nurses' geographical origins. As mentioned already, culture has been shown to include a number of facets, which were neglected by these researchers. Particularly disturbing is their non-recognition of an occupational culture. Reassuringly, such recognition is now demonstrated by North American writers warning of the dangers of ethno-centrism or beliefs of the superiority of one's own ethnic group (Davidhizar & Giger 2004). The spectre of stereotyping clients to predict pain behaviour emerges. Thus, we are alerted to the likelihood that 'personal biases can influence reactions' (2004: 53).

An example of such culturally unacceptable behaviour was identified in a childbearing situation (Bowler 1993). Referring to the phenomenon as 'making a fuss about nothing', Isobel Bowler found that midwives, who were invariably Northern European in origin, thought that Asian women made 'too much noise' and constantly grumbled about minor symptoms. The continuing existence of such stereotyping is confirmed by Michelle van Ryn and StevenFu (2003).

Although the cultural background of caring staff in terms of their geographical and ethnic origin has been studied, the staff culture *per se* has not attracted as much research attention as it deserves (Green 1993). This contrasts with the culture of the work group, in general, which has been studied assiduously in more manual occupations (Argyle & Colman 1995). One notable exception to this lack of research is found in the ethnographic study of a labour ward (Hunt & Symonds 1996). These researchers reflect on how the culture of hospitals has moved on from the deprivation of the Victorian era, and has been superseded by an open, public and idealised, yet sanitised, atmosphere.

Another, serendipitous, observation of the impact of culture arose out of an evaluation of a Danish Alternative Birth Centre (ABC). Because of the small size of the ABC and its popularity, a number of women had to be refused admission and gave birth in the 'obstetrical ward' (Skibsted & Lange 1992: 185). The ABC-refused women matched the women who gave birth in the ABC in their socio-demographic characteristics, but their behaviour in labour and interventions matched the 'obstetrical ward' group. The authors appropriately conclude that the staff and environment influenced the ABC-refused women to conform to the obstetrical practice. Thus, the culture of the obstetrical ward staff and the environment in which they practised was demonstrated to have overcome the aspirations and education of the ABC-refused women.

The carer's care

The role of the person providing care has been shown to be pivotal in addressing the problem of the client's pain. Whether carers accept and function optimally in this role, though, is quite a different matter. Writing about nurses in a postoperative setting, Alfhild

Dihle and her colleagues (2006) recognise that their 'unique opportunity' to treat pain effectively may be missed. The attitudes mentioned already contribute to the effectiveness of pain control, but these are aggravated by factors such as inadequate knowledge, incomplete assessment and adherence to a medical model of care (Walker et al. 1995).

The nurses interviewed and observed by Dihle and her colleagues were clearly knowledgeable about the principles of caring for a patient in pain; they were able to explain the appropriate procedures and how scrupulously they followed them. During the observation phase, however, these researchers identified a 'discrepancy' (2006: 475) between the nurses' perceptions of how pain was managed and the reality of the nurses' performance in practice. On the basis of this discrepancy, Dihle and colleagues argue that it constitutes a barrier to effective pain control. Thus, as well as the two factors mentioned above, 'the usual traditions or habits' are more likely than adequacy of knowledge or completeness of assessment to determine the effectiveness of pain management. It is clear that research into pain assessment and the education of carers are of limited value when compared to the culture of the clinical environment.

Culture and childbearing

Having considered the cultural significance of pain to the person experiencing it and to the staff, and before focusing on the cultural implications of pain in childbearing, we examine the cultural importance of childbearing itself. I suggest that the cultural aspects of childbirth have become significant for two reasons. The first relates to the intrinsic importance of birth to all human societies, which may be summarised as the anthropological argument. The second reason relates to a phenomenon currently emerging in the UK, if not in other societies; this is the political connotations of health in general, and childbearing in particular, among ethnic minority groups. These issues are becoming widely recognised and may be linked with accusations of racism.

Anthropology

Preceding her ethnographic study of birth in four cultures, Brigitte Jordan (1978) discussed culture's contribution to the experience of childbirth. She, first, differentiated the almost inextricable pathophysiological and social components of childbirth. The differing practices and customs surrounding childbirth support her argument that it is the critical nature of childbirth, represented by perceived risks of trauma or death, which lends this event its significance. Thus, unchallengeable packages of childbirth practices become culturally established. The cultural mores which evolve control a diversity of childbirth practices, such as who may be present (Jordan 1978) or what the woman eats or drinks (Cheung 1996).

Jordan also focused on how knowledge of others' childbirth practices may change or even improve practices prevalent in the West. She argued that experimentation with changing practices, such as medication or birth position, may expose the researcher/ practitioner to accusations of unethical practice and perhaps to litigation. She suggested that understanding other cultures' practices may facilitate the 'unavoidable change of contemporary ways of doing birth' (1978: 4).

Emphasising the significance of childbirth, Jordan regretted the absence of suitable data. She blamed this deficiency on the low status and female-oriented nature of birth. Perhaps as more female researchers become involved in this area, easier access and more data will emerge. Currently available data are of poor quality, she maintained, due to researchers' tendency to assume a medical orientation.

Politics of culture

Analysing maternity care provision for 'black' women, Anne Phoenix (1990) reminded us that the majority of UK maternity carers are white. Hence, discriminatory attitudes develop and become institutionalised (Ahmad 1993). Such discrimination has been shown to focus on those perceived to be less suitable to bear children, such as the unmarried, the very young and those with children already. Phoenix argues that black women have been stereotyped, particularly as belonging to the latter category, resulting, she argues, in discrimination in the form of institutionalised policies. One example (Phoenix 1990) is the automatic categorisation of black women as 'at risk' on the grounds that certain groups have higher perinatal mortality rates (Ahmad 1993). Such categorisation inevitably affects the woman's care as Asian women's categorisation is thought to be due to their reluctance to accept care which they consider culturally inappropriate (Parsons et al. 1993). Further examples of institutionalised discriminatory policies include the non-recognition of the need for interpreters, resulting in the husband or son translating the woman's intimate health history. Another example is staff's difficulty with non-British names, resulting in confusion and danger (Parsons et al. 1993).

The political nature of culture manifests itself most disconcertingly clearly in the maternal death statistics (Lewis & Macfarlane 2007). Despite being suitably cautious about their data, these authors conclude that for black African women, and marginally less in black Caribbean and Middle Eastern women, the maternal mortality rate is significantly higher than that for white women. Thus, for the former groups of women her culture, in the form of her social situation, is more likely to impact on her survival than her long term health.

Pain, culture and childbearing

Having related culture to both pain and childbearing, I now integrate these strands by focusing on cultural aspects of pain in childbearing, about which there is little research (Vangen et al. 1996). This neglect is largely due to Western clinicians, whose childbearing practices are regarded as a 'gold standard' by other 'less advanced' societies (Jordan 1978: 35). Thus, childbearing has become medically dominated and the woman has become a patient. Jordan further identified that the medical attitude to disease, as another problem to be resolved by intervention, has been applied to pain. The relevance of such an approach is uncertain and was seriously questioned by Jordan.

To support her argument, Jordan compared childbearing women in the USA, Holland, Sweden and Yucatan. Because the American woman must convince her carers that she needs medication to control her pain, she must display her need, leading to high levels of 'noise and hysteria in American obstetric wards'. Mayan women in Yucatan, though, accept that pain is part of the childbirth experience. The woman prepares herself for pain, which is regarded as usual, healthy and finite. Jordan found similar attitudes in Holland; Dutch women, she stated, accept childbirth pain and believe that nature will take its course. Hence, analgesia is 'neither expected or required' (Tasharrofi 1993). Van Teijlingen (1994) linked British women's attitudes to pain in labour to their adherence to a medical model of health, reminiscent of the American woman's (Jordan 1978). To explore this comparison, Senden and colleagues (1988) compared the expectations and experiences of labour pain in women in Iowa (USA) and Nijmegen (Holland). In a sample of 256 women, a large majority of Dutch women (79.2%) did not use analgesia; this applied to only 37.6% of American women. The proportion in each group showing satisfaction with their pain control and the fulfilment of their expectations showed no significant difference. These authors, like Jordan (1978), attributed their findings to the confidence of Dutch women in the successful functioning of their bodies.

In contrast to the observations by Jordan, Bonica (1990a, 1994) reported his unpublished observational data of 'eight thousand women in the USA and almost three thousand in other countries'. On the basis of these somewhat questionable data he refuted the contention that the expression of pain varies between women in different cultures. The method of collecting these data is not described, so the rigour of Bonica's approach is uncertain, as is the significance of his findings.

In the same way as other researchers have demonstrated the dynamic nature of culture in terms of the response to pain, Sheila Hunt and Anthea Symonds (1995) recount the changing cultural attitudes to childbirth pain in the UK. In the course of their study of the culture of a labour ward these researchers identified how, in the mid 1930s, the status of birth as 'natural' was rejected; simultaneously the pain of birth became less acceptable to women. Thus, attitudes that still prevail in Holland and Yucatan virtually disappeared in the UK. Such attitudes to pain and its control reflect a more longstanding movement towards the acceptance of the medical view of childbearing (Edwards 2005).

The attitude of women in India appears to have much in common with those in Holland and Yucatan (Jeffery 1989), in that the absence of pain control is not problematic but irrelevant. Jeffery's ethnographic study found that 'intense' pain is regarded as beneficial, through the all-too-obvious connection with speedier birth. The articulation of pain is also culturally controlled, through excessive vocalisation being linked with 'shamelessness'; thus, women are encouraged to 'accept the pains, calling on God's name'.

Examining pain behaviour, Schott and Henley (1996) discuss the extent to which racial stereotypes may cease to apply, due to the intensity of childbearing pain or local influences. They comment on the UK tendency to value quiet, elevated to institutional policy (Chapter 12) but which reduces the possibility of a woman using sound as a coping mechanism.

More recent research endorses Jeffery's observation. In a study of 137 labouring women, significant differences appeared in analgesia use between Pakistani-born (Punjabi) and Norwegian-born women (Vangen et al. 1996). Of the 67 Pakistani women, 30% received no analgesia, compared with only 9% of the 70 Norwegian women. There is no suggestion that the Pakistani women's labours were any less painful. The researchers emphasised the communication difficulty between the Norwegian midwives and the Pakistani women, a large majority (82%) of whom spoke little or no Norwegian.

Socio-economic backgrounds also differed markedly. The Pakistani women tended to receive analgesia, if any, which required minimal communication or instruction, such as intramuscular pethidine rather than nitrous oxide and oxygen or epidural analgesia. These findings are supported by a recent study in Germany (David et al. 2006) which suggests that Western stereotypes of Asian women may not be accurate; however these researchers do not show whether language or culture, or a combination, are responsible for the differing analgesia use.

Despite the shortage of research-based material on this topic, that which exists shows the considerable variation in and implications of the expression of childbirth pain between and within cultural groups over time.

Meanings

Throughout this chapter, the importance of the meaning of pain has become clear. I make no apology for this because of the impossibility of dissociating any pain from what that experience means (Morris 1991: 34). In this chapter the meaning of pain has emerged in the grisly initiation rituals, the celebrant's interpretation of which constrained his perception and expression of pain. Zborowski (1952) suggested that certain ethnic groups were more concerned with the meaning and implications of the pain than its treatment; however, for others the immediate experience was the major concern. Ascribing a meaning to pain constitutes both a legitimation (Bendelow & Williams 1998) and a coping mechanism, which may apply no less to childbearing pain than to the other acute and more long term forms.

In 2000, I sought to unravel the complexity of labour pain and drew conclusions about the fundamental significance of the meaning which the woman attaches to her pain. This significance included the inevitable negativity with which labour pain is all-too-frequently associated. As Drew Leder observed, pain's meaning may be the very incarnation of 'the unhappy, the bad, the wrong' (1986: 259). This short term negativity may be linked with the longstanding and medically-fostered association between pain, pathological processes and death, which have been linked with punishment, atonement and redemption (Caton 1985; Morris 1991: 36).

Understanding the meaning of labour pain may bring the realisation of physical and emotional achievement, which Lynn Callister and her colleagues termed 'self-actualisating' (2003: 147). Perhaps disconcertingly, though, as well as providing meaning, pain carries the potential to obliterate the meaning of phenomena which help us to make sense of our lives (Leder 1986).

Since 2000, a phenomenological study in New Zealand has demonstrated the dynamic nature of the meaning of labour pain and the role of the midwife in facilitating the woman's understanding of the meaning (Vague 2003). This research clearly shows how the woman's interpretation of the meaning of pain and the midwife's response to her interpretation develops as the woman moves forward in her labour.

These dynamic developments include not only changes in the woman's perception of the meaning of her pain, but also changes in her self-perception. The woman's ability to comprehend the pain of birth and her adjustment, is transformatory in that it brings with it confidence in her ability to mother the new arrival (Mander 2010).

Leap's midwifery model

Because of pain's complexity, it is unsurprising that most models (see 'Pain theory' above) have over-simplified the pain experience. This observation applies most particularly to childbearing pain. Nicky Leap drew on midwifery expertise to introduce a refreshingly different model of pain. Her qualitative study involved interviews with midwives experienced in attending home births (Leap 1996), on the basis of which Leap proposed the existence of two pain paradigms. Differing fundamentally from previous models, these two approaches were entitled 'pain relief' and 'working with pain' (Leap 1997, 1998, 2000; Leap & Anderson 2004).

While seeking strenuously not to equate pain relief with the medical model, Leap's efforts are less than convincing. Pain relief involves early well-meaning offers to the woman of a menu of pain control methods; possibly during childbirth education or else in early labour. Although not intended to, these offers persuade the woman of her likely need for these interventions (Evans 2006). Thus, a self-fulfilling prophecy materialises. One factor, causatively associated with pain relief, is a staff culture of difficulty in coping with a woman who is clearly articulating her pain:

> Some midwives give pethidine because they don't like the fuss and noise and the agitation and the fact that the woman won't settle down. I think that sometimes the midwife isn't coping with the pain either. They think that the woman isn't and actually they're not.
>
> Midwife in Leap 1996: 48, her emphasis

Difficulty in coping is aggravated by a low tolerance for noise in labour areas. The result, which some of us have encountered, is the midwife being reprimanded by her colleagues for noises emanating from the birthing room.

Thus, the 'pain relief menu' originates as well-meaning, to the point of humanitarianism, but it insidiously carries subliminal messages. This approach becomes increasingly directive; to the extent of persuasion being exerted to encourage the woman's acceptance of hi-tech pain control. Such persuasion is exerted by staff who had been sympathetic to the woman's aims and ideals. Thus, the woman is in a 'double whammy': let down by her assumed supporters and vulnerable to any persuasion being applied.

The midwives distinguished pain relief from working with pain (Leap 1996: 50). This concept emerged from the midwives' acceptance that some pain is fundamental to physiological labour. Accepting this reality meant that the midwives were able to acknowledge the woman's pain and its articulation without assuming pathology or needing to remedy it. The 'abnormal' pain of a complicated labour was clearly differentiated from 'normal' pain.

Working with pain was tied into the midwives' philosophy of confidence in the woman being able to birth physiologically. They deplored any diminution of the woman's confidence in her body and close companions and sought to re-establish that confidence:

> If you can build up confidence in women that they can definitely get on and do this, then I think they will. (Midwife Leap 1996: 65)

Unsurprisingly, Leap's work has contributed significantly to the UK campaign to reinstate the culture of normality of childbirth (Downe 2004).

Thus, through this ground-breaking research, the importance of culture in pain and its control is, yet again, emphasised.

Chapter 2

Experiences and observations

In this chapter I address the experience of pain and its observation by two groups whose input is crucial to both our knowledge and our practice: researchers and carers. It is necessary, first, to clarify the nature of this ubiquitous phenomenon.

Defining pain

In order, in this section, to examine pain in broad terms, it is helpful to consider some of the recent attempts to define 'pain'; this definition is important before moving on to consider one much-neglected aspect of pain – emotional pain. The first example of a definition is found in a traditional medical textbook:

> Pain is that sensory experience evoked by stimuli that threaten to destroy tissue, defined …
> as that which hurts (Mountcastle 1980: 391).

This definition's problems relate mainly to the apparently inevitable link between pain and tissue damage. Such a link is too tenuous and too variable to be useful, while the obvious 'organic' emphasis in this definition limits the possibility of other forms of pain.

Merskey prepared a more complete definition in an effort to encompass both 'organic' and 'psychogenic' pain, which was subsequently adopted by the fledgling International Association for the Study of Pain (IASP) (Bonica 1990a: 18):

> An unpleasant experience which we primarily associate with tissue damage, or described in terms of tissue damage, or both.

This definition went on to state:

> Pain is always subjective. Each individual learns the application of the word through experiences related to injury in early life.

The introductory words have recently been modified, in the interests of inclusiveness, to read:

> An unpleasant sensory and emotional experience associated with actual or potential tissue damage, or described in terms of such damage. (IASP 2009)

Pain in Childbearing and its Control, Second Edition. By Rosemary Mander. Published 2011 by Blackwell Publishing Ltd.   © 1998, 2011 Rosemary Mander.

Although some women might regard 'unpleasant' as an understatement of their experience of childbearing pain, this definition is sufficiently vague to encompass a range of pain perceptions. While the IASP definition is generally and somewhat complacently accepted, brave souls have criticised its reliance on verbal ability (Cunningham 1999) and have received short shrift (Derbyshire 1999). The IASP definition's persistent focus on pathological and organic pain is another source of criticism, and the need for debate is recognised (Jensen & Gebhart 2008).

The difficulty of devising an adequate and complete definition of pain has been attributed to its dubious homogeneity (Bendelow & Williams 1995). This may be attributable to linguistic deficiencies, which has been contrasted with the multiplicity of terms for other important concepts. An apocryphal example is the variety of Inuit words for the phenomenon which Anglophones know as 'snow' (Szasz 1957: 10). Thus, the absence of applicable words means that 'pain' must be qualified by suitable adjectives to make its meaning more comprehensible.

In a nursing context, Margo McCaffery coined a definition of pain which is useful both temporally and qualitatively:

> Whatever the experiencing person says it is, existing whenever he or she says it does.
>
> (1979: 18)

While this definition does expand the experiences which are included in the concept of pain, the implied focus on *physical* pain persists. This tunnel vision is addressed by Ronald Melzack and Patrick Wall, who emphasised our limited understanding of pain, leading them to offer:

> a category of experiences, signifying a multitude of different, unique experiences having different causes, and characterised by different qualities varying along a number of sensory, affective and evaluative dimensions (1991: 46).

Despite the somewhat unreconstructed IASP definition, Melzack and Wall's move towards a biopsychosocial understanding of pain is gaining ground (Quintner et al. 2008).

Emotional aspects of pain

By scrutinising its history in Chapter 1 it became clear that pain has traditionally been envisaged as an emotion associated with previous sin. René Descartes' ideas at the beginning of the enlightenment introduced the distinction between bodily and other forms of pain, including guilt, tribulation and similar mental pain (Glucklich 2001). The acceptance of Descartes' scientific ideas about a mind-body split was gradual. This is evidenced by its absence from philosopher John Locke's writing (1632–1704), which did not distinguish between pain which 'is physical and that which is mental'. A century later, though, Jeremy Bentham (1748–1832) had accepted the Cartesian distinction between physical suffering and mental anguish (Caton 1985).

The development of appropriate tools means that the concept of mental pain is now able to be differentiated from the less complex depressive states (Orbach et al. 2003).

Thus, throughout this book, I seek to consider pain in terms of Melzack and Wall's more inclusive definition (1991). In this section, however, I concentrate on those forms of pain that are thought to feature a significant emotional component and to a lesser extent, if any, physical aspects. The term 'suffering' is becoming appropriately used to describe such feelings:

> Suffering involves experiencing yourself on the other side of life as it should be.
>
> Frank 2001: 355

Although Iain Wilkinson's admirable analysis of suffering from a sociological view-point assumed the comparability of pain and suffering (2005), it fell to Arthur Frank to clarify similarities. The defining feature of suffering is found in its total negativity which, in turn, renders the experience beyond the capability of human expression, making it unspeakably isolating. Wilkinson probed the complex relationship between pain and suffering, arguing that there are situations where bodily pain is not felt as suffering (2005: 21); for some women, childbearing may be one such example. Likewise, suffering some form of unrecoverable loss may not feature bodily pain. Thus, the link between suffering and bodily pain is tenuous. Clearly, suffering carries a spiritual dimension, as explained by Eric Cassell: a 'state of severe distress associated with events that threaten the intactness of the person' (1998).

While non-physical pain or suffering may be ascribed to pathological or psychiatric processes (Merskey 2005), I deplore this latter assumption. Partly because it has been attributed to ignorance, I give no credence or further attention to the possibility of that pain which has been referred to as 'psychogenic' (Melzack & Wall 1991: 32).

The mind/body split

Before focusing on emotional pain or suffering, we should consider the concept of mind/body dualism. Our understanding of pain has long been held back by this concept, for which Descartes has, perhaps unfairly, been held responsible (Cervero 2005) and which has subsequently been embraced by our medical colleagues (Bendelow & Williams 1995). Concluding his philosophical investigation into pain and pleasure, Thomas Szasz (1957) pleads for a re-examination of Cartesian dualism. While Melzack and Wall's gate control theory (1965) might have answered Szasz's plea by ending the Cartesian mind/body split, this is not the case, as evidenced by later major texts omitting material relating to affective aspects of pain (e.g. Bonica 1990). The persistent legacy is the scientific or, more precisely, medical understanding of pain as purely physical. This understanding, preferred as it is to all others, impedes acceptance or utilisation of a holistic interpretation of pain (Bendelow & Williams 1995: 161–2). This mind/body split has been associated with the tendency noted already to ascribe the emotional component of pain to psychiatric conditions rather than regarding the pain experience as one complete entity. While making no apology for attributing the persistence of this concept to certain disciplines, we recall that the nature of pain itself aggravates the dichotomy by alienating our minds from our bodies, thus perpetuating Cartesian dualism (Bendelow & Williams 1995).

Suffering

In order to consider pain which is predominantly emotional and which merits the term 'suffering' (Frank 2001), I examine first its healthy and pathological forms. I next move on to suffering which is more directly associated with bodily pain and, finally, I discuss how suffering may manifest itself during childbearing.

Healthy suffering

Suffering tends to be constructed in terms of social suffering visited on entire populations (Benatar 1997); mass rape, genocide and famine come all too easily to mind. As well as these appallingly familiar examples, it is necessary to contemplate others' suffering, including not only people with health problems, but also physically healthy individuals, who tend to be neglected (Benatar 1997: 134). Pain may not endure the same voiceless-ness (Morris 1996), but suffering, as a form of emotional pain, certainly brings an 'unsharability' common to other forms of pain (Wilkinson 2005: 16).

Healthy suffering is regarded by some as an oxymoron; for example, Margaretha Strandmark argues that suffering is a form of ill health due to the potentially pathological powerlessness it inevitably brings (2004). On the basis of her phenomenological research, Strandmark argues that the absence of three levels of hope (spiritual, aspirational and physical) leads to destructive feelings and, hence, to guilt and shame.

Under certain circumstances, though, suffering may be a challenging but healthy response to the difficult or distressing situations which we meet throughout our lives.

Thus, Nathan Cherny has defined suffering as

> an aversive experience, characterized by the perception of personal distress which is gener-ated by adverse factors that undermine quality of life (2005: 7).

Suffering may feature bodily pain but, on the one hand, this is a far from necessary component, while on the other, the sufferers may find themselves being taken way 'beyond the physical' (Morse 2001: 47). Jan Morse, who regards suffering as an 'emotional pain response', (2001: 47), laments the tendency of medical researchers to focus on bodily pain. Thus, suffering and emotional pain comprise a response to the person's environment and to the other actors sharing it. A complex interplay of emotions becomes established with the other actors, together with recollections of past bitter experiences. These may include bereavement or loss of personal faculties, affection or self-esteem. Emotional pain may manifest itself in physical form or may present as altered body language or as symptoms, such as enuresis or other regressive behaviour. This healthy, if unwelcome, experience of suffering is an unavoidable fact of life. Such pain increases as the sufferer ages, largely because it is an association with loss (Cherny 2005). These losses may be through death or other forms of separation, by loss of income/employment, relationships or meaning to life.

Some authorities, such as Gillian Bendelow and Simon Williams (1995), refer to grief as a form of emotional pain. The fundamental link between attachment and loss engendering painful grieving is widely accepted (Bowlby 1969; Mander 2006) and grief has appropriately been termed 'the cost of caring'. Grieving is essentially healthy and beneficial, and enables adjustment to the losses confronting us as we move through life (Marris 1986). Grief facilitates progress, possibly not directly, from the initial feelings of distraught hopelessness, eventually achieving some degree of resolution or integration which permits our usual functioning for a large part of our lives. Although grief may be viewed as apathetic passivity, it is better regarded as a time during which the person actively strives to complete the emotional tasks to be faced; the phrase 'grief work' encapsulates this active striving.

The stages of grief through which the person needs to work have been recounted in various ways, but Elisabeth Kübler-Ross's, albeit limited, typology is well-known and useful (1970). Individual variation combined with a 'one step forwards two steps back' progression inevitably determines grieving. The initial denial response of grief constitutes a defence mechanism which protects from the full impact of realisation. This helps to insulate from the unthinkable reality, allowing a 'breathing space' in which to marshal our emotional resources. As denial ceases to be effective, awareness of the reality of loss dawns; simultaneously powerful emotional reactions and their physical manifestations materialise, featuring sorrow, guilt, dissatisfaction, compulsive searching and anger. Realisation dawns in waves as the grieving person plays for time by 'bargaining' with her- or himself to delay accepting reality. The despair of full realisation of the loss eventually supervenes, bringing apathy, poor concentration and bodily changes. Although we may never 'get over' the loss, after eventual acceptance we normally integrate it into our experience of life. This process is complex, involving slow progress and setbacks, in the form of oscillations and hesitations. The ultimate degree of 'resolution' or 'integration' is recognisable in the bereaved person's ability to think realistically and with equanimity about the weaknesses, as well as the strengths, of the lost relationship.

The healthy suffering of grieving matters, mainly because it contributes to the balance or homeostasis in the life of the bereaved person. The emotional pain of grief is crucial in helping us to begin recovering from the effects of loss.

Pathological suffering

As with many arbitrary distinctions, the boundary between healthy and pathological suffering may be unclear. Grief, mentioned above, exemplifies how the physical manifestations of healthy suffering in the form of sorrow may be difficult to distinguish from true depression (Ogrodniczuk et al. 2003). A commonly experienced mental illness, depression, constitutes a good example of pathological suffering. While the suffering involved in depression takes a variety of forms, in addition to the characteristic lowering of mood, the experience is often explained by the sufferer in terms of pain, for which Humphry Osmond and his colleagues used the term 'mood pain' (1984: 5). Depression as a form of pain, if needing substantiation, appears in the personal experience of Canadian author Marni Jackson:

> I now think of depression as pain. It's a kind of living death, a non-feeling that is its own sort of agony. The problem was, I always knew exactly how dead I was, how my mind had shut down. There was still this consciousness of what I was losing. Everybody who is depressed is aware of what they've lost. That's the real hell of it. (2003)

This disconcertingly personal statement shows clearly how, though in no way physical, the person suffering the pain perceives it as very real. Such accounts are supported by research which focuses on the pathological anguish of depression associated with work-related stress experienced by certain workers (Shurtz et al. 1986). Similarly, anguish has also been identified in other psychiatric conditions (Rosenbaum et al. 1994). The inclusion of mental illness as a form of pain is certainly justified by the symptoms that a depressed person is likely to encounter. Even if Harold Merskey's limited definition of pain is used, the symptoms fall well within the scope of an 'unpleasant experience' (Bonica 1990a: 18, above). I discuss pathological suffering in childbearing below.

Body-related suffering

While considering the suffering that a person may face in the absence of physical pain, we should recall that mental suffering not uncommonly co-exists with physical and other pain. The concept of 'total pain' (see below) was introduced by Cicely Saunders to emphasise the complexity of the physical, emotional, social and spiritual components of the suffering inherent in advanced cancer (Clark 1999). On the basis of this concept, she argued that effective pain control is impossible until each aspect has been adequately addressed. The role of the multidisciplinary team, comprising carers and family in this situation, is to plan care, taking account of the range of factors that impinge on the person's pain experience.

An emotional vicious circle is likely to develop and escalate when the person experiencing physical pain becomes anxious or depressed due to inadequate pain control. Such mental suffering lowers the patient's pain threshold, thus exacerbating the original problem. The 'conspiracy of silence' in which staff and family may collude, supposedly in the patient's interests, further aggravates any anxiety relating to their condition or other matters. The pain is exacerbated by spiritual concerns, which fill the mind of the person who recognises the proximity of death. Memories of previous losses, unfinished business, unsatisfactory relationships, feelings of guilt and the meaninglessness of life emerge, further reducing the person's coping ability. Thus, total pain may be summarised in the words of one for whom Saunders provided care: 'All of me is wrong' (Clark 1999: 733).

Emotional pain in childbearing

While childbirth is widely regarded as a happy event, we must bear in mind that some degree of emotional pain or suffering not uncommonly features. This suffering may be as mild as the momentary regret which a mother encounters on learning that her baby is not of the gender for which she was hoping (Mander 2006); or it may be something more. The process of adaptation to motherhood has been explained in terms of suffering, which interferes with the woman's other relationships and needs time for these to be renegotiated (Barclay et al. 1997). These researchers warned, however, of the difficulty of differentiating maternal suffering or distress from the more serious emotional pain that is depression (Barclay & Lloyd 1996).

Healthy suffering in childbearing

A mother experiences a healthy reaction of suffering if there is some form of loss associated with her childbearing. This might comprise miscarriage, stillbirth or the neonatal death of her baby (Mander 2006). Less likely to come to mind, but still engendering grief, are the losses associated with the birth of a baby with a disability, relinquishment of a baby for adoption or a diagnosis of infertility. Such suffering has been extended to include that which the mother invariably experiences as an inevitable consequence of loving, or even anticipating loving, her child (Marck 1994). These 'mothering pains' are said to begin after the physical pains of childbirth are completed, but last indefinitely.

Usually disregarded, the pain of recognising an unwanted or unplanned pregnancy is often assumed to be short-lived. Similarly disregarded, perhaps because of its political sensitivity, is the suffering which a woman encounters in association with termination of pregnancy (TOP). Despite this disregard, a detailed account of the experiences of women having TOP shows the less-individualised care provided for such women (Moulder 1998). Adopting 'respectful caution' (1998: 92) rather than genuine engagement, staff assume that the woman is firm in her decision and will make her needs known. This 'hands off' approach is apparent in the staff's acceptance of the woman's decision, their assumption that TOP is a minor intervention and their certainty of the woman's responsibility for her own well-being.

Environmental suffering

While ordinarily assumed to be supportive, the environment in which the woman lives and is required to give birth may actually be responsible for causing or aggravating her painful suffering. This happens at different levels.

Sexual discrimination In its widest sense the environment in which the woman functions is far from being a level playing field. The concept of inequality, which disadvantages women, may serve to aggravate other hardships. In the global context, the increasing numbers of female-headed households (FHHs) has been linked to low incomes in both developing and developed countries (SIDA 2001). This trend has been termed the 'feminisation of poverty' which, in turn, renders women and their babies more vulnerable to poor perinatal outcomes. This scenario, on the other hand, has been criticised as little more than a self-fulfilling prophecy, serving to divert financial resources away from those who need them most (Chant 2003).

The system of 'care' At a systematic level in health services, such as the UK NHS, birthing, originally a sociobiophysical process, has been reduced to an industrial one (Kitzinger 2006: 56). Thus, the birthing woman may be traumatised to the extent of what has been termed 'iatrogenic rape' (Lesnik-Oberstein 1982). The long-term nature of the distress caused by such trauma is addressed in a UK context by Jean Robinson (2007) and by Kathleen Kendall-Tackett in a North American setting (2004). That such trauma is by no means exceptional emerges in the work of a nurse-therapist who describes it as 'culturally commonplace' (Sorenson 2003: 259). While Sheila Kitzinger argues that the entire culture of childbearing has been rendered less humane, research attention has been focussed most precisely on the negative impact of vaginal examination (Hilden et al. 2003; Bergstrom et al. 1992; Stewart 2005).

Intimate Partner Violence (IPV)   On a personal level, suffering during healthy childbearing may, initially, appear unrelated to the violence visited on the woman by her current or previous partner. The tendency of pregnancy to serve as a catalyst to such abuse has for too long been denied by health care personnel, as found by research into the attitudes of senior staff:

> disbelief and reluctance to accept domestic violence as an issue for health professionals.
>
> Bewley 2002: S3

Jay Silverman and colleagues' research found that the both maternal and neonatal effects of IPV were wide-ranging (2006). In the UK Confidential Enquiries into maternal deaths, though, the potential for appalling outcomes following 'domestic abuse' have been demonstrated (Lewis 2007).

Pathological suffering and childbearing

While depression is rarely said to feature bodily pain, the distressing nature of it is well-recognised (Littlewood & McHugh 1997). There is no reason to believe that depression causes any less suffering when associated with childbearing, than at other times in the life cycle. Depression before the birth during pregnancy is now, somewhat belatedly, beginning to attract the research and clinical attention which it has long deserved (Freeman 2007).

The term 'postnatal depression' (PND) remains more familiar, though. The term itself is a source of considerable debate among mental health practitioners, being distinct according to some from postnatal distress (Miller et al. 2006). Its value to those working with childbearing women, though, is that 'PND' differentiates the relatively inconsequential mood lability, or 'blues', from hugely significant changes.

Like the appropriateness of the name, the condition's incidence is uncertain. This is because of the problem of making a diagnosis, which is compounded by sufferers' difficulty seeking help due to guilt or fear of stigma. Although an incidence of around 10–15% is quoted (SIGN 2002), this may be an underestimate, as Penelope Leach suggests that 'up to 60% of new mothers experience some form of PND' (Welford 1996).

A range of causes has been suggested, including genetic, psychodynamic, socio-cultural, obstetric and hormonal factors. Knowledge of the causes is of limited value, though, when the benefits of focusing interventions on vulnerable women are so uncertain (Dennis & Hodnett 2007). Despite the questionable benefits of prophylactic interventions, the socio-familial causes and effects of PND attract appropriate attention, including that of feminists. The male-determined societal expectations of motherhood are thought to engender in women unrealistically romantic views of childbearing. When women fail to achieve such romanticised expectations, a male-dominated medical system diagnoses the woman's disappointment as psychiatric pathology. Thus, the pain of PND serves to exemplify the oppression of women (Littlewood & McHugh 1997). It may be that more realistic views of motherhood are needed, rather than the pronatalist attitudes currently prevailing. Midwives are ideally situated to facilitate such realism.

Total pain

Never having experienced labour, it is through being with women in childbirth that I have formed the impression that the transition phase of labour may equate with 'total pain' (Mander 2002). UK textbooks have only recently started to mention that time in labour known as the 'transition phase' (Downe 2009), although North American texts have traditionally done so (Bobak & Jensen 1993). Sheila Kitzinger defines transition as:

> the very end of the first stage of labour ... It is often the most difficult part of labour, but may last for only a few contractions. (1987: 223)

It is my observation that the woman begins to despair of her ability to complete her labour as she wishes; this happens at the time when her contractions are especially intense, in preparation for the birth. As a result, the woman feels there is little she can do to help herself. This psychological low point in combination with seemingly interminable and unproductive pain correlates with the mental and physical pain labelled 'total pain' by Cicely Saunders (see above, Ong & Forbes 2005; Clark 1999).

The characteristics of 'the transition' include:

> You may suddenly lose your ability to keep things in perspective.
> You may no longer be able to keep on top of your contractions.
> You may shake uncontrollably.
> You may find yourself very confused mentally; you may want to go home, feel irritated with those around you, and find it difficult to cooperate (Tucker 1996: 154).

The transition, however, has been described more objectively:

> Expresses sense of extreme pain
> Expresses sense of powerlessness
> Shows decreased ability to listen or concentrate on anything but giving birth.
>
> Vogler 1993: 471

At this time the midwife is challenged to maintain rapport, while supporting the woman through this supremely demanding phase.

Summary

In this section I have demonstrated that emotional pain should be considered alongside other, perhaps more easily recognisable, forms of pain. I have indicated situations in which a person is likely to experience emotional pain, which may be known as 'suffering', including those associated with childbearing. Although non-physical forms of pain tend to be dismissed, possibly on the grounds that to remedy them is particularly challenging, their significance should not be underestimated.

This is supported by a longstanding comparison:

> Mental pain is less dramatic than physical pain, but it is more common and also more hard to bear. The frequent attempt to conceal mental pain increases the burden: it is easier to say 'My tooth is aching' than to say 'My heart is broken' (Lewis 1940: 144).

Assessing pain

The lack of recognition of emotional pain leads us, quite appropriately, into considering the assessment of pain. In the sections on culture and pain theory in Chapter 1, I demonstrated the crucial yet challenging role of pain assessment. I now explore the issues associated with the measurement and assessment of pain. I begin by examining the main problem, meaning the widely recognised *under*estimation of pain by care providers in general (Kappesser et al. 2006; Idvall & Brudin 2005), and evidence that a similar situation exists in maternity (Sheiner et al. 2000). I next look at the rationale for assessment and instruments to assess pain, emphasising acute pain. Finally, I contemplate the relevance of these instruments to maternity care.

Traditional observation

The difficulty which is encountered in a nursing context in assessing and remedying the patient's pain is due to the innate fear of pain which lurks inside us all (McCaffery 1983). Such fear engenders denial of the patient's pain and is compounded by two other factors, which apply particularly to on-demand or *pro re nata* (prn) medicine administration. First is medical under-prescription of analgesia, in terms of both the dosage and the frequency of administration. The second and compounding factor, attributable to poor knowledge, is the nurse's tendency to further reduce the patient's analgesia by administering the medication in smaller doses and even less frequently than prescribed (McCaffery 1983).

Margo McCaffery's longstanding observation has been endorsed by research in England (Willson 2000) which showed that the complex interrelationship of patient and carer characteristics cannot be ignored. The nurse's tendency to underestimate the patient's pain was reiterated by a Scottish study, finding that over 70% of nurses 'accepted' that they did this (Lloyd & McLauchlan 1994). The nurse's reluctance to administer analgesia post-operatively emerged in the majority of nurses, who agreed 'that it should be used for as short a time as possible'. As previously identified by McCaffery and endorsed by Heather Willson (2000), almost one-quarter of these nurse respondents were concerned that the medication carried addiction risks.

McCaffery's hypothesis of nurses' denial of patients' pain as self-protection may apply to midwives (Niven 1992). Kate Niven pursued this argument to contemplate the damage that the midwife's unsympathetic attitude causes to the mother–midwife relationship. For this reason, or for fear of addiction, systemic pain medication in labour has been demonstrated as providing inadequate analgesia.

To ascertain the perceptions among women, midwives, obstetricians and anaesthetists of analgesic effectiveness, Linda Rajan (1993) re-analysed others' data (Chamberlain et al. 1993). Rajan found that generally the staff assumed pain control to be satisfactory to the woman, whereas the women experienced it as inadequate. This applied, typically, when pethidine was used. However, the reverse held when nitrous oxide and oxygen (N_2O & O_2) in the form of a premixed gas was used and the women found it more effective than perceived by staff. Unlike the nurse administering inadequate medication due to denial, Rajan suggests that the midwife's different knowledge base explains these findings. She maintains that the midwife compares the woman's observed pain with the extremely painful abnormal labours which she has attended, and provides analgesia proportionate to the *appearance* of pain. The woman, on the other hand, compares her pain with other pain she has experienced, which pales into insignificance by comparison, and expects pain medication proportionate to that. These mismatched expectations remain unarticulated and self-perpetuating, being exacerbated by socio-cultural and linguistic differences. The discrepancy between women's and staff's perceptions is aggravated by the greater congruency between the perceptions of individual staff members; this compounds the woman's frustration at finding that her pain perception is accepted by no one among her carers. Rajan's observations were endorsed by an Australian study (Baker et al. 2001), which identified midwives' tendency to underestimate the woman's pain as it becomes more severe (Idvall & Brudin 2005). The factors which lead to inaccurate estimation of pain have been found to be exacerbated by experiential and cultural differences between the carer and person in pain (Sheiner et al. 2000).

Others have identified the midwife's concern about using pain medication, such as in Sweden where Ulla Waldenström found that the midwife's concern related not to addiction risks, but to the drug's effect on the labour and the baby (1988). The Swedish midwives compensated for their reluctance to administer medication by their certainty of the benefits of their presence.

A serious omission from the literature is the midwife's assessment of either the woman's pain or the effects of any drugs/techniques. Except for Angela Baker and colleagues (2001) who employed the short form McGill Pain Questionnaire, no pain assessment instruments are mentioned, leading to the conclusion that none have been used. While basic pain assessment tools feature in postoperative care, they appear to have no place in labour. Even Adela Hamilton only mentions the midwife's responsibility for 'monitoring the effects of these [drugs]' (2009: 506) with no mention of any formal assessment. In view of these omissions, it is necessary to examine the reasons for using such tools and what form they take, before considering their place in maternity care.

The rationale for assessment of pain

Pain assessment matters in both clinical and research settings. In this section I consider first the clinical aspects, before addressing research. Assessment is primarily associated with interventions to address pain. This involves facilitating the coping mechanisms of the person in pain, with or without the use of extraneous interventions such as medication. The meaning of the pain to the individual is likely to affect, first, her ability to cope with it and, second, the support and other interventions which may help. After the intervention(s) a re-assessment evaluates their effectiveness and provides the basis for planning future therapy.

Adopting a multidisciplinary orientation, John Loeser (2005) emphasises the multiplicity of disciplines involved in caring for a person with pain, particularly if it is long term; examples include physiotherapists, social workers and occupational therapists as well as nursing and medical personnel. This approach carries the need for shared interdisciplinary understanding of the patient's pain experience, which is facilitated by using recognised assessment instruments. Although pain assessment instruments may be criticised for spurious objectivity, subjective assessments tend to be particularly unreliable. Thus, pain assessment can only improve the carer's evaluation of this most personal, private and subjective of all human experiences.

In order to write about the various aspects of pain, I have separated the assessment of pain from the interventions that are used to either prevent or remedy it. Such a separation is totally artificial and clearly has no place in practice. Similarly, pain assessment may be undertaken routinely, without affecting patient care, to the detriment of that care. Collecting information which is not utilised to enhance care obviously raises serious ethical problems. This 'health warning' applies equally to pain assessment instruments of uncertain reliability or validity (Strong et al. 2002).

Instruments for assessing pain

The science of pain measurement has been termed 'dolormetrics' (Rollman 1983) and it incorporates a wide range of approaches, varying in technical complexity. The close relationship between research and practice in this area is illustrated in two ways. First, the assessment instruments in clinical use may also be used to measure pain in laboratory-based and other research. The second example of these close links materialises in the use of some tools, originally experimental pain research instruments, which have become, rightly or wrongly, part of clinical practice. We should, however, question the clinical value of pseudo-scientific research jargon such as 'pain threshold', meaning the point at which pain is just perceived, and 'pain tolerance', meaning the point at which pain is no longer able to be borne. Such supposedly 'objective' measures are of questionable value clinically, even in one individual when biological stability or constancy are uncertain.

For these reasons the measuring instruments have changed to rely increasingly heavily on self-assessment by the person in pain. Despite this change, it is sometimes necessary for the carer to make the first move to open up the topic of pain. Observation may lead the carer to suspect pain, even though the person has not verbalised her pain, or may even have denied it. In describing the many pain assessment instruments, it is necessary to remember that these techniques are in no way exclusive. For this reason, after considering the principal measures, I examine those instruments that comprise a combination. This multiplicity of techniques reminds us that patients may encounter more than one pain at a time, requiring each pain to be assessed separately.

Physiological indicators

While physiological sequelae of pain, such as tachycardia and perspiration, may be useful indicators of its intensity, they lack specificity. Many physiological, psychological and pathological phenomena, like pain, alter the heart rate, rendering such observations futile.

Attempts to incorporate such indicators into a pain measurement scale have resulted in the usual underestimation of pain (Lowe 2002).

Self report verbal descriptors

Traditional forms of pain observation have tended to rely on verbal interaction. These have developed into systematic formats which are applied interactively or in writing. Verbal descriptors are usually used in combination with other approaches. These may combine verbal and numerical scales, the best known being the McGill Pain Questionnaires (MPQs) (see 'A combination of methods'; Melzack 1975). While self report is the 'gold standard' (Strong et al. 2002: 126), because of its subjectivity, this strength is also a weakness. A long-recognised problem in using words to denote, particularly, the intensity of pain is their variability of meaning between individuals; thus, what constitutes severe pain to me, may only be moderate to you. This makes verbal rating scales less robust, although they may be preferable in some situations (Loos et al. 2008). In therapeutic settings, though, the problem of precision is less significant than in research, but our multicultural society requires clinicians and researchers to take account of the user's language skills. I discuss the difficulties associated with neonatal pain in Chapter 11.

Numerical scales

To clarify the relationship between the various degrees of pain, descriptive words often have numerical values added. This may result in a 'painometer' (Gaston-Johansson 1999) or a pain thermometer (Ware et al. 2006). The importance of the 'anchor words', to indicate the extremes of the pain experience, cannot be over-emphasised; examples are 'no pain' as the minimum and 'pain as bad as it could possibly be' as the maximum. Despite this, people in pain may still experience difficulty in ascribing numbers to an experience as human as pain. For research purposes, establishing the relationship between the intervals is crucial to permit statistical calculations.

Visual Analogue Scales

Whereas numerical scales are subdivided to indicate differing levels of pain, often with words attached to each level, a *Visual Analogue Scale* (VAS)(Blumstein & Moore 2003) provides only anchor words at each extreme. If words are used to indicate imprecise levels without numbers, the scale is known as a 'Graphic Rating Scale' (ten Klooster et al. 2006). The absence of numerical indicators increases the sensitivity of these scales, but the lack of fixed points may offer patients more freedom of choice than they can handle, resulting in difficulties. As with many assessments, the electronic form of the VAS is proving helpful to clinicians (van Duinena et al. 2008).

Other single assessment tools

For people who may encounter difficulty with numbers and/or words, *Faces Rating Scales* (FRS) have been shown to overcome these obstacles (Fadaizadeh et al. 2009). The FRS comprises seven facial expressions of pain, which range from 'happy' (score 0) to 'agonised' (score 6). With a view to speedily assessing pain in children with limited verbal skills, *Colour Analogue Scales* (CAS) have been shown to discriminate between different degrees of pain (McConahay et al. 2005).

Gender-free *Body Outlines* (anterior and posterior) permit the user to indicate the location of the pain. These instruments do not require anatomical literacy or common language. They carry the disadvantage, however, of being two-dimensional and being unable to indicate the pain's superficiality/internality. To overcome this weakness, the user may be requested to add an 'E' (external), 'I' (internal) or 'EI' (both) to pinpoint the pain more precisely.

A combination of methods

The MPQs (Melzack 1975) combine body outlines and verbal descriptors with numerical values attached. These instruments evolved out of the recognition of the multidimensional nature of the pain experience and that instruments which focused solely on the intensity of pain were too restrictive (Melzack 1983). The MPQs seek to determine intensity, quality and duration of the person's pain and facilitate diagnosis, assist therapeutic decisions and evaluate interventions' effectiveness (Melzack & Katz 1994).

In the original MPQ, information about the nature of the pain was sought through offering the patient 78 words describing the pain. These words originated from those frequently used by patients and carers to describe pain. They are subdivided into 20 groups, which were based on statistically-derived levels of agreement between respondents. From these words the patient chooses those that best describe her pain. The words cover sensory aspects of pain, such as 'tugging', affective aspects, such as 'fearful', evaluative aspects, such as 'unbearable', and miscellaneous aspects, such as 'wretched'.

Using an MPQ provides quantitative information in the form of scores indicating the sensory, affective and evaluative dimensions of pain. These are the Present Pain Intensity (PPI), the Pain Rating Index (PRI) and the Number of Words Chosen (NWC). These scores are used to evaluate the effectiveness of pain interventions (Melzack 1975).

Its virtually ubiquitous use supports the claim that the MPQ is 'valid, reliable, consistent and, above all, useful' (Melzack & Katz 1994). Inevitably, though, this instrument is not without its critics. Some criticisms relate to its origins, having been developed initially to facilitate understanding and communication between researchers (Melzack 1975). Despite this, MPQs are used increasingly frequently in clinical settings.

Common understanding, however, is jeopardised by the differing forms of the MPQ; only the body outlines and the presence of 78 words are common and consistent features, suggesting limited comparability (Wilkie et al. 1990). A serious criticism of the MPQ relates to its heavy reliance on vocabulary; this renders it irrelevant to certain groups and has spurred the veritable growth industry in non-verbal tools mentioned already. The instructions for using the MPQ questionnaire are contained in the original journal paper (Melzack 1975); but they are neither well-detailed, comprising a critique of patients' comprehension rather than precise instructions, nor easy to follow, as is crucial if being applied clinically.

The skewed distribution of MPQ scores, rather than the normal distribution claimed by Melzack has been criticised (Wilkie et al. 1990). As the bias is to the left it is possible that this instrument, as with traditional methods, may underestimate pain. Because of the time taken to use the original, the short form McGill Pain Questionnaire (SF-MPQ) was developed (Dworkin et al. 2009; Melzack 1987). However, the limited applicability of this instrument to the increasingly important neuropathic pain has seriously curtailed its usefulness. This limitation is further aggravated by its lack of sensitivity to small but significant changes over time and after therapeutic interventions. This criticism has resulted in yet another generation of the MPQ (Dworkin et al. 2009). Despite the increasing recognition of non-physical pain, reflected in the IASP definition (2009), the limited relevance of MPQs to such pain is another source of criticism (King 2000).

Pain assessment tools in labour

I focus here on the assessment of labour pain, because other childbearing pain is probably comparable with other experiences of pain, whereas labour pain is unique. As I mentioned above in the section on 'Traditional observation', while midwives monitor the woman's pain and her response to interventions, they do not use formal assessments; although this observation is contradicted by Baker and colleagues, who assert that the SF-MPQ is used 'routinely' for assessing labour pain (2001: 171). It is necessary now to consider what progress has been made in labour pain assessment and whether any such progress benefits either the labouring woman or those who care for her. Because more attention has been given to research in this area, I examine this first.

Problems in applying an MPQ in labour were first demonstrated by a large study (n = 141) to evaluate 'prepared childbirth' (Melzack et al. 1981). It was applied once when labour was established, but this was problematical, causing variations in the data, as the precise stage of labour was unknown. Obviously, questionnaire completion is only possible between contractions, preventing the usual fundamentally important focus on *current* pain.

Despite these difficulties, an MPQ has been used in other labour pain research. A smaller study involved completion once labour was established and again within 2 days (Niven & Gijsbers 1984). Women with experience of non-childbearing pain showed lower scores, indicating perceptions of less pain, than non-experienced women. Refuting criticisms that the MPQ is 'cumbersome', the researchers contend that it is recommended, being both acceptable and valid.

A more challenging Australian protocol produced less sanguine findings (Baker et al. 2001). These researchers admit that their plan to apply the SF-MPQ quarter-hourly throughout labour was 'demanding' (2001: 176). Unsurprisingly, as labour progressed women became unwilling or unable to continue participating; only one woman completed the SF-MPQ in the second stage. Despite this, the researchers claim credit for the frequency of observations.

A marginally less intrusive form of data collection was applied in Germany to assess women's pain and 'fitness' during labour and their perceptions of participation (Gross et al. 2005). A coloured VAS using sliding scales was offered to the woman every 45 minutes to represent her current feelings of pain and of fitness. A majority of women declined one or more measurements. Even though only 28 (56%) participants completed the evaluation, their views about participation are particularly important because women's views about involvement tend to be disregarded. Twenty-one women evaluated their participation wholly positively, with seven expressing mixed views. Negative comments reported that the assessments were 'bothersome' or 'irritating' (2005: 126). Surprisingly, six women welcomed the, sometimes insufficient, distraction of being assessed. These researchers conclude that longitudinal prospective measurements are feasible in labour, linking them to the feedback provided for the women. Mechthild Gross and colleagues' work suggests that data collection in labour may serve to evaluate and improve pain and other interventions.

Researching pain

Origins

The ground-breaking event in the history of controlling childbearing pain was the first administration of ether to a woman in labour by James Young Simpson in 1847 (Mander 1998a). The research basis of Simpson's subsequent introduction of chloroform, like so many in obstetrics, was scanty to say the least, being undertaken in Simpson's dining room. So chloroform's lethal side effects (Knight & Bacon 2002; Mander 1998a) went on to maim and kill generations of childbearing women. Thus under-researched, the medical control of childbearing pain became established. In this section I consider whether the research basis of this aspect of maternity care has developed in 160 years.

Victorian preoccupations with pharmacological substances inevitably produced a back-lash, in Grantly Dick-Read's (1933) ideas on natural childbirth. Research featured in neither Dick-Read's nor his opponent's teaching. The former emanated from his jingoistic, eugenic and religious convictions (Kitzinger 1989), while his opponents claimed women's support (Lewis 1990; Gutmann 2001).

Physiological research

Realisation in the middle ages that the brain rather than the heart is central to pain perception preceded Descartes' (1596–1650) use of the then new scientific method to study and mechanise the human body. His theory led to belief that specific superficial nerve endings led, via the dorsal horn of the spinal cord and the anterolateral spinothalamic tract, to cerebral pain centres. The 'intensive' or 'pattern' theories emerged to contradict this specificity theory, being advanced by various physiologists and psychologists. Based largely on animal experiments, the gate control theory seemed to resolve this contradiction (Melzack & Wall 1965; Chapter 1, 'Currently accepted pain theory').

Psychological research

The gate control theory suggested that various factors affect the individual's perception of pain intensity (Melzack 1993), some of which are not physiological, but psychological. In childbearing, social support is one such moderating factor (Mander 2001).

In the twentieth century Dick-Read, on the basis of his experience, argued that fear engenders or at least aggravates labour pain. The relationship between anxiety and pain is now being given the research attention which is much-needed (Escott et al. 2004).

The surprise finding that women's satisfaction does not necessarily correlate with the most effective pain control emerged from a longstanding study investigating epidural analgesia (Morgan et al. 1982). This distinction between effective pain control and a satisfactory birth experience dawned as a revelation and illuminated issues of control, which became increasingly significant.

Pain intervention research

Since the National Birthday Trust (NBT) in the UK published the results of its national study in 1993, researchers have, unfortunately, not been inclined to replicate this work (NBT; Chamberlain et al.). This was a descriptive prospective study involving mothers and partners as well as midwives and medical staff. Aiming to demonstrate methods used and circumstances of their use, comparisons were sought between consumers' and staff's views. Side effects of methods were investigated, using a 6-week follow-up (Wraight 1992).

Despite serious sampling and methodological difficulties (Mander 1998c), the researchers drew conclusions relating to the organisation of maternity services and reflect satisfaction among mothers with pain control (Chamberlain et al. 1993). Additionally, the closure of small maternity units was recommended 'unless geographically necessary' (1993: 117), as was the encouragement of women to accept epidural analgesia for operative deliveries and also the availability of 'non-medical volunteers' to stay with women in labour. The research basis of such recommendations remains unclear.

Since this ill-fated attempt to chronicle a UK-wide picture, greater and more appropriate reliance has been given to meta-analyses and systematic reviews, such as those in the Cochrane Database.

Unfortunately and probably unsurprisingly, Donald Caton and his North American colleagues did not learn from the UK experience. The result was a much-hyped project to examine 'The Nature and Management of Labor Pain', using a series of specially commissioned systematic reviews (Caton et al. 2002). As well as a number of variably informative findings, the steering group commented in the 'Implications for Research':

> By and large, the comparison groups in available studies of the effects of pain relief methods reflect needs and interests of physicians and other caregivers rather than those of laboring women ... few comparisons are available to help inform women about the choices and options that they face. It would be very helpful for women to understand the advantages and disadvantages of epidural or opioid analgesia relative to such options as nitrous oxide, labor support, and other nonpharmacologic methods. (2002: S130).

Apart from the slightly patronising tone of this conclusion, it is necessary to observe that it was hardly necessary to undertake a series of systematic reviews to reach this conclusion. As long ago as 1994 a plea was made that research is needed to:

> give women the information they need to be able to make fully informed decisions about pain control in general and epidurals in particular. (Mander 1994: 14).

Pain research issues

Thus, on both sides of the Atlantic, the need for research to answer women's questions has been identified. Women users of the maternity services may be regarded by some as a 'hard to reach' group. The importance, however, of involving women in setting the research agenda to ensure that women's needs are addressed and that the research is truly woman-oriented cannot be overstated.

It may be argued, while recognising that much of the research mentioned in this chapter has been quantitative, that the research agenda, in order to accommodate women's needs more effectively, should include a more qualitative orientation. Such a change in research approach would clearly require a major sea-change among both researchers and funding bodies.

Conclusion

This chapter has shown the veracity of the first part of the observation by Baker and her colleagues, who argued that it is: 'inherently difficult for care providers to accurately assess and effectively manage pain' (Baker et al. 2001: 172)

The extent to which the latter part of this statement holds true remains to be seen.

Chapter 3

Medication: constraints and consequences

Although the midwife utilises many interventions in her care, which have been shown to be variably beneficial, it is his or her use of medicines that traditionally has been most stringently controlled. Further, midwives in a range of educational and other settings find the consequences of ignorance of or disobedience to these controls being impressed on them. In this chapter we consider the constraints, especially the legislative framework, within which the midwife practises and is able to prescribe and administer medicines to the woman for whom he or she cares. We look, first, at the reasons for the legislation and, second, at what it comprises. Third, we examine the operation of the legislation and, then, how the legislation relates to an area which is of increasing interest, that is, complementary interventions. An important constraint on the midwife's administration of medicines is their fetal and neonatal effects, which is examined next. Finally, there is some discussion of the consequences of non-adherence to the legislative constraints.

The rationale for legislation

Because the search for the magic bullet has long been abandoned, it is common sense to consider both the benefits and hazards of any form of medication. They are sensibly perceived as a double-edged sword, imparting both advantages and dangers. Legislation is intended to allow the benefits to accrue, while limiting the effects of any dangers. Unfortunately the reactive, rather than proactive, nature of legislation is all too frequently a matter of shutting the stable door after some tragic event. An example is the Medicines Act (1968) which reached the statute book as a reaction to the thalidomide *debacle*, and which used hindsight to protect consumers; such protection was by introducing statutory controls to enhance the safety of new medications.

Another reason for the legislation controlling medicines is protection in a wider sense. This reason is particularly relevant in the present context because of the risk of addiction to many of the drugs which midwives administer. Thus, legislation aims to reduce the risk of addiction in both consumers and staff. While a clearly laudable aim, it may be necessary to question why these substances are the subject of legislation, when many agents

Pain in Childbearing and its Control, Second Edition. By Rosemary Mander. Published 2011 by Blackwell Publishing Ltd. © 1998, 2011 Rosemary Mander.

that are similarly dangerous are not. Thus, some drugs such as alcohol and tobacco, which are dangerous and probably addictive, are subject to comparatively lax legislation.

Yet another rationale may apply in the context of the role of the midwife, which some regard as having increased autonomy. It may be that the price for such autonomy is the increasingly stringent control of certain aspects of practice.

The regulations

The framework which guides and controls the midwife's actions in relation to drugs comprises both legislation and publications by the statutory body, which carry the weight and force of legislation.

- They derive originally from the Medicines Act (1968) which was primary legislation facilitating a regulatory framework for a series of subsequent statutory instruments.
- The Misuse of Drugs Act (1971), together with amendments in 2001, aimed to outlaw the illegal supply or possession of controlled, or Schedule 2, drugs.
- The Prescription Only Medicines (Human Use) Order (1997) established the criteria for legal prescriptions. More relevant in the present context, it permits midwives to possess and administer certain medications in the course of their professional practice. These are diamorphine, morphine, pethidine and pentazocine. The concept of a Patient Group Direction (PGD) was also regularised.
- The NMC's 'Standards for medicines management' (2008a) covers the classification of drugs, and the supply, surrender, recording and destruction of drugs.
- The Midwives Rules and Standards (NMC 2004) and the NMC Code of Professional Conduct (NMC 2008b).

These regulations mean that a midwife on registration is permitted to supply, and administer, as appropriate on his or her own initiative, substances specified in the medicines legislation under 'Midwives Exemptions' using Midwives Supply Orders (MSO) (NMC 2005) as long as it is part of the midwife's professional practice. This legislation permits the midwife to supply/administer without needing a Patient Specific Direction (PSD) or medical prescription. Where any medicine is not included in the exemption list then, a prescription, a PSD or Patient Group Direction (PGD) is necessary (NMC 2005). In order to comply with this legislation, the midwife must address four issues; these are authority, ability, context of activity and competency.

The transparency of these regulations has unfortunately been wasted on certain agencies. This has led to midwives being unable to obtain a supply of medications, to them not having suitable prescribing courses available and to established protocols not taking account of midwifery practice (NES 2006). While recommendations have been made to resolve the tunnel vision of these agencies and organisations, these difficulties do not appear to take priority.

Practices that may be regarded as the extended role of the midwife, such as topping up epidural analgesia, are controlled by the Midwives Rules (Macintyre & Schug 2007; NMC 2004: 19).

The Midwife's role in certain specific situations

There are a number of situations in which the midwife's role regarding medicines deserves special attention.

Legislation and Regulations relating to complementary medicines

Although some people may think that homeopathic and other complementary remedies are of so little effect that they must be harmless, this has by no means been established. That the reverse may be the case evidences the need for better education (Tiran 2005).

Midwives and other health care personnel need to accept the popularity of complementary and alternative (CAM) approaches to health care, if only to avoid alienating women who are already using such remedies (Tiran & Mack 2000). In such a more open environment the risks of any adverse drug interactions caused by undisclosed self-treatment, would be greatly reduced. Equally risky would be treatment by a practitioner who is inadequately prepared to apply the treatment being offered. For this reason, the formalisation of education and qualification of a range of complementary therapists is proceeding apace. Academic criteria aim to ensure a suitably firm base in the biological and other sciences as well as focussing on the specific therapy. The practice of complementary interventions by allopathic practitioners would be as deplorable as the possibility of a complementary practitioner offering allopathic services. Thus, the need for regulation of these mushrooming disciplines has resulted in the oversight of groups such as aromatherapists by the Health Care National Training Organisation (HCNTO) (2006).

The regulation of CAMs therapists, though, is appropriately regarded as a mixed blessing (Stone & Lee-Treweek 2005). On the one hand, such perceived endorsement may facilitate the professionalisation of the therapists involved; but on the other hand it may threaten the 'slippery slope' (2005: 54) of establishment interference. Such a threat brings the possibility of dissatisfied practitioners breaking away to form splinter groups, resulting in seriously weakened professional groups. As some groups of midwives, such as the independent midwives, have found to their cost, many occupational groups now find themselves being more tightly regulated. This unnecessarily firm regulation represents a knee jerk reaction to certain well-publicised scandals in allopathic medicine. CAMs practitioners also find themselves in this potentially precarious position (Stone & Lee-Treweek 2005: 53–4).

Because of their potential risks, complementary remedies are subject to regulation in the same way as allopathic medicines. The regulations controlling the midwife's use of complementary remedies are also included in Guidance following Rule 7 in the Midwives Rules which states:

> Homeopathic and herbal medicines are subject to the licensing provisions of the Medicines Act 1968. A number of these however, have product licences but have not been evaluated for their efficacy, safety or quality and you should look to the best available evidence to inform women.

> A woman has the right to use homeopathic and herbal medicines. However, if you believe that using the medicines might be counterproductive you should discuss this with the woman.
>
> NMC 2004: 20

The NMC's view of CAMs may be reflected in the paragraph which follows immediately:

> If you are aware that a woman is self administering illegal substances you should discuss the health implications for her and her baby with her. You should also assist her by liaison with others in the multi-professional team to gain further support or access to detoxification programmes. (NMC 2004: 20).

Additionally, the NMC document entitled 'Standards for medicines management' (2008a) spells out the regulations under the Medicines Act (1968) covering these remedies. The quality, safety and efficacy of all medicines are controlled at entry to and removal from the market by the Medicines Act (1968). Because many complementary medicines were already on the market when the Act came into operation in 1971 they are covered by special arrangements which were applied to drugs already existing. These drugs were granted Product Licences of Right which exempted them from additional scrutiny.

Fetal and neonatal effects

There are a number of situations in which the potentially harmful effects of a medication on the fetus or neonate may influence the woman's or her health care providers' treatment decisions. The example which probably comes most easily to mind is the use of systemic opioid analgesics during labour and their effects on the respiratory centre and other neonatal behaviour.

The woman with HIV/AIDS is another example. In this case the childbearing woman may be advised to take antiretroviral therapy in order to reduce the viral load and, hence, the risk of transplacental transmission; thus, the risk of the baby being affected would be lowered. The woman and her attendants would need to take into account, first, the risk of causing HIV resistance to antiretrovirals, this would limit their effectiveness should they be needed in the future; second, that it is possible that highly active anti-retroviral therapy may lead to mitochondrial damage; and third, that there is a theoretical risk of carcinogenesis from antiretroviral drugs (Isaacs et al. 2003).

A further example which may need consideration, though it is infrequently discussed, is the treatment of mother with cancer and the effects which the chemotherapeutic medication may have on the cells of the developing fetus (Mander 2010). Consideration of the fetal effects would affect the woman's decision about both undergoing and the timing of chemotherapy.

The woman at risk of or who is being treated for postnatal depression tends to be either discouraged from breastfeeding or encouraged to stop; this is because of the transmission of drugs via the breast milk. The SIGN Guidelines adopt a quite pragmatic approach to this decision:

> the risk of breast feeding in this situation may be over-estimated and the advantages under-estimated. The process of excretion of psychotropic medication is complex, with variation in milk/maternal plasma ratios for different drugs and between foremilk and hindmilk. ... The evidence base is limited due to the small number of breast feeding women who have

been exposed to any specific drug and the lack of any systematic approach to monitoring and registering information about the use of psychotropic medication in breast feeding women. (SIGN 2002)

The general conclusion is that drugs to treat postnatal depression, such as Selective Serotonin Re-Uptake Inhibitors (SSRIs), may be administered while the woman breast-feeds, but the baby should be problem-free and her condition monitored carefully.

Clearly, the woman should be able to discuss the effects of these medications with the midwife, on the basis of which she may make her decision about treatment.

Consequences of non-adherence

In this section, I consider the consequences when a practitioner inadvertently contravenes the regulations or legislation. This is no place to look at the punishments meted out to criminals like Allitt and Shipman (Harvey 2002). In the past medication errors or adverse drug events (ADE) have been regarded variously seriously. Some of us may recall an occasion such as when a nervous and inexperienced midwife helping a senior obstetrician at an assisted birth inadvertently gave him sterile water instead of local anaesthetic to administer. The intervention for which he was using the medication was widely recognised by midwives to be ineffective, but even he was surprised at exactly how ineffective his ministrations were on this occasion! Busy, high stress areas such as ICU, A&E, NNU and labour ward are known to be particularly vulnerable to medication errors. Tragically the outcomes of such errors can be disastrous, as reported by the Confidential Enquiries into Maternal Death:

> [After an assisted birth a woman with an epidural infusion experienced] a grand mal convulsion followed by ventricular fibrillation from which she could not be resuscitated. She had received 150ml of a 500ml bag of 0.1% bupivacaine in saline intravenously in error.
> Cooper & McClure 2007: 109

As these authors later correctly identify, this tragedy was not the sole responsibility of the midwife who connected the wrong bag of fluid to the woman's IV line. It was not purely a drug administration error, but there was a definite element of a systems error involving a range of other factors, including the storage of these fluids.

This specific observation is supported by a Department of Health (DoH) publication which states that such adverse events are invariably associated with a 'multiple breakdown in the system' (2007). The research to which DoH refers provides details of the causes of such incidents, finding that the error is linked to orientation or training issues in 60% of cases. A proportion of these cases are likely to have involved students (Wolf et al. 2009). Unsurprisingly, in view of prescribers' stereotypically illegible handwriting, 40% of incidents feature some form of communication problem. As in the above case, storage or access is at least partly responsible for 35% of incidents. The problems which students encounter in identifying the correct tubing for connecting medications and other therapeutic substances is highlighted. The increasing complexity of health care is likely to aggravate such problems and qualified staff are clearly not immune from such errors.

The other factors identified by DoH (2007) include issues of competency, supervision, labelling or distraction and affect 80% of cases. These data obviously support the DoH contention that a multiplicity of aspects contribute to any single adverse drug event, rather than just one single person's negligence.

This observation has clearly not reached the media or the wider public; in terms of the consequences for the 'perpetrators' of medication errors, it is usual to read in the popular media of individual members of staff being disciplined after any highly publicised adverse drug event. Whether this form of scapegoating is the best way to deal with such incidents has long been the subject of controversy (Arndt 1994).

It is likely that the patient who suffers some form of iatrogenesis from the drug error is not the only victim; Charles Denham argues that there is a 'second victim' (2007: 107) in the form of the staff member who is made to suffer inappropriately severe punishment. In order to promote a healthier working environment, Denham argues that the staff member at the 'sharp end' has a right to expect any action taken to be just, respectful, compassionate, supportive and transparent. In this way, all staff are able to learn from what would otherwise be a totally negative event. On the basis of the development of this healthier working environment, harm to the 'third victim' of the adverse drug incident, the health care system itself, should be avoided. Any health care professional who has been involved in, or affected by such an incident, would surely endorse such an eminently rational approach.

Conclusion

This chapter has demonstrated that medications are something of a double-edged sword. Their nature means that they are a mixed blessing and not only for the person for whom they are prescribed and to whom they are administered. Their potential for harm has been shown to extend to the person who actually undertakes that prescribing and administration; although, hopefully, that potential is less and less likely to be realised.

Chapter 4

Physiology of pain in labour

Dr Jennifer M. Tocher

Nothing begins and nothing ends, that is not paid for with moan. For we are born in other's pain and perish in our own.

Daisy Francis Thomson 1859–1907

The experience of pain is one that all human beings share to a greater or lesser degree over the course of their lifetime. It is a concept that all can articulate and express with a common understanding, however it is also a sensation that is highly individualised and subjective. The experience of pain in childbirth is something that only 50% of the population might have an expectation of ever experiencing and yet many people would be able to give an account of the severity and actual expected experience of this pain without ever having done so.

The purpose of this chapter is to look at the physiology of pain and its manifestations in labour. This will be achieved by explaining the physiology of pain and then looking at this in relation to labour pain. We will then look at the gate control theory of pain (Melzack & Wall 1965), and the part that it plays in the pain of childbirth.

Pain

In its most simplistic form, the pain circuit in the body can be described as follows: pain stimulates pain receptors, and this stimulus is transferred via specialised nerves to the spinal cord and from there up to the brain. The process of nociception describes the normal processing of pain and the responses to noxious stimuli that are damaging or potentially damaging to normal tissue. There are four basic processes involved in nociception (McCaffery and Pasero 1999). These are:

- transduction;
- transmission;
- perception; and
- modulation.

Pain in Childbearing and its Control, Second Edition. By Rosemary Mander. Published 2011 by Blackwell Publishing Ltd. © 1998, 2011 Rosemary Mander.

Transduction of pain

Transduction begins when the free nerve endings (nociceptors) of C fibres and A-delta fibres of primary afferent neurons respond to noxious or harmful stimuli (Tortora et al. 2006). These fibres literally carry the message to the brain that there is a harmful stimulus present which may induce pain or suffering to the body. Nociceptors are exposed to noxious stimuli when tissue damage and inflammation occur as a result of, for example, trauma, surgery, inflammation, infection or ischaemia.

The nociceptors are distributed in the

- somatic structures (skin, muscles, connective tissue, bones, joints); and
- visceral structures (visceral organs such as liver, gastro-intestinal tract).

These are listed in table 4.1.

The C fibres and A-delta fibres are associated with different qualities of pain. The pain stimulus is processed in the brain, which then sends an impulse down the spinal cord, via appropriate nerves which command the body to react, like withdraw the hand from a very hot object such as a cooker top. This is a learned response, which in time will become almost reflexive. At a young age we are told not to touch something which may potentially harm or burn us. However, the body learns this association through the experience of being burnt also.

Perception of the pain stimulus: from the pain receptors to the brain

Pain receptors   Pain receptors are present everywhere in the body, especially the skin, surfaces of the joints, periosteum (the specialised lining around the bone), walls of the arteries and certain structures in the skull. Other organs have fewer pain receptors (gut,

Table 4.1   Characteristics and functions of C fibre and A-delta fibres.

C fibres	A-delta fibres
Characteristics: • Primary afferent fibres • Small diameter • Unmyelinated • Slow conducting	**Characteristics:** • Primary afferent fibres • Large diameter • Myelinated • Fast conducting
Receptor type: • Polymodal respond to more than one type of noxious stimuli: • Mechanical • Thermal • Chemical	**Receptor type:** • High-threshold mechanorecep-tors respond mechanical stimuli over a certain intensity.
Pain quality: • Diffuse • Dull • Burning • Aching • Referred to as 'slow' or second' pain	**Pain quality:** • Well-localised • Sharp • Stinging • Pricking • Referred to as 'fast' or 'first' pain

muscle, deep organs). There are three types of pain receptors: mechanical, thermal and chemical. A mechanical stimulus would be, for example, high pressure or stretch, and a thermal pain stimulus extreme heat or cold.

Chemical pain receptors can be stimulated by chemicals in the outside world (e.g. acids), but also by certain products that are present in the body and locally released in response to trauma or inflammation or other painful stimuli. Examples of these substances are bradykinins, serotonin, potassium ions and acids (such as lactic acid, which causes muscle pain after heavy or prolonged exercise).

Prostaglandins are also mediators that are locally released with painful stimuli and, although they do not directly stimulate pain receptors, they do increase their sensitivity. Paracetamol and non-steroidal anti-inflammatory drugs (NSAIDs), such as Ibuprofen, have an anti-prostaglandin effect; they work as analgesics by inhibiting prostaglandin release and reducing the inflammatory response to the painful stimuli.

Noxious stimuli and responses   There are three categories of noxious stimuli:

- mechanical (pressure, swelling, abscess, incision, tumour growth);
- thermal (burn, scald); and
- chemical (excitatory neurotransmitter, toxic substance, ischaemia, infection such as encephalitis).

The cause of stimulation may be internal, such as pressure exerted by a tumour or external, for example, a burn. This noxious stimulation causes a release of chemical mediators from the damaged cells including:

- prostaglandin;
- bradykinin;
- serotonin;
- substance P;
- potassium; and
- histamine.

These chemical mediators activate and/or sensitise the nociceptors to the noxious stimuli. In order for a pain impulse to be generated, an exchange of sodium and potassium ions (de-polarisation and re-polarisation) occurs at the cell membranes. This results in an action potential and generation of a pain impulse.

Transmission of pain

The transmission process occurs in three stages. The pain impulse is transmitted:

- from the site of transduction along the nociceptor fibres to the dorsal horn in the spinal cord;
- from the spinal cord to the brain stem; and
- through connections between the thalamus, cortex and higher levels of the brain.

The C fibres and A-delta fibres terminate in the dorsal horn of the spinal cord. There is a synaptic cleft between the terminal ends of the C fibres and A-delta fibres and the nociceptive dorsal horn neurones (NDHN). In order for the pain impulses to be transmitted across the synaptic cleft to the NDHN, excitatory neurotransmitters are released, which bind to specific receptors in the NDHN. These neurotransmitters are:

- adenosine triphosphate;
- glutamate;
- calcitonin gene-related peptide;
- bradykinin;
- nitrous oxide; and
- substance P.

The pain impulse is then transmitted from the spinal cord to the brain stem and thalamus via two main nociceptive ascending pathways. These are the spinothalamic pathway and the spinoparabrachial pathway.

The brain does not have a discrete pain centre, so when impulses arrive in the thalamus they are directed to multiple areas in the brain where they are processed.

Perception of pain

Perception of pain is the end result of the neuronal activity of pain transmission and where pain becomes a conscious multidimensional experience. The multidimensional experience of pain has affective-motivational, sensory-discriminative, emotional and behavioural components.

This means that for affective-motivational experience there is an element of anticipation and a knowledge of how a pain will feel before it happens (Melzack & Wall 1965; Meyer et al. 2006). Sensory discrimination means the ability of the body to differentiate the area in which the pain originates from another area of that person's body (Auvray et al. 2008). We are all familiar with the emotional aspects of pain; when a person is bereaved, they talk about their loss of another in terms of feeling physical pain, for example. There are also many different pain behaviours that human beings exhibit when experiencing pain, such as common facial expressions.

When the painful stimuli are transmitted to the brain stem and thalamus, multiple cortical areas are activated and responses are elicited.

These areas are:

- The reticular system: this is responsible for the autonomic and motor response to pain and for warning the individual to do something, for example, automatically removing a hand when it touches a hot saucepan. It also has a role in the affective-motivational response to pain such as looking at and assessing the injury to the hand once it has been removed from the hot saucepan.
- Somatosensory cortex: this is involved with the perception and interpretation of sensations. It identifies the intensity, type and location of the pain sensation and relates the sensation to past experiences, memory and cognitive activities. It identifies the nature of the stimulus before it triggers a response, for example, where the pain is, how strong it is and what it feels like.

- Limbic system: this is responsible for the emotional and behavioural responses to pain for example, attention, mood and motivation, and also with processing pain and past experiences of pain.

Modulation of pain

The modulation of pain involves changing or inhibiting transmission of pain impulses in the spinal cord. The multiple, complex pathways involved in the modulation of pain are referred to as the descending modulatory pain pathways (DMPP) and these can lead to either an increase in the transmission of pain impulses (excitatory) or a decrease in transmission (inhibition).

Descending inhibition involves the release of inhibitory neurotransmitters that block or partially block the transmission of pain impulses, and therefore produce analgesia. Inhibitory neurotransmitters involved with the modulation of pain include:

- endogenous opioids (encephalin and endorphins);
- serotonin (5-HT);
- norepinephirine (noradrenalin);
- gamma-aminobutyric acid (GABA);
- neurotensin;
- acetylcholine; and
- oxytocin.

Endogenous pain modulation helps to explain the wide variations in the perception of pain in different people as individuals produce different amounts of inhibitory neurotransmitters. Endogenous opioids are found throughout the central nervous system (CNS) and prevent the release of some excitatory neurotransmitters, for example, substance P, therefore, inhibiting the transmission.

Pain nerve fibres – fast pain and slow pain

From the pain receptors, the pain stimulus is transmitted through peripheral nerves to the spinal cord and from there to the brain. This happens through two different types of nerve fibres: 'fast pain' and 'slow pain' nerve fibres, (as shown in table 4.2).

What is 'fast pain' and 'slow pain'?

A pain stimulus, e.g. if you cut yourself, consists of two sensations. The first one is the so-called 'fast pain' sensation, and is experienced as sharp. After a few seconds, this goes over into the sensation of 'slow pain', which is more a dull and burning feeling. This slow pain normally lasts a few days or weeks, but if inappropriately processed by the body, it can last several months, and give rise to chronic pain.

Fast pain

Like when you prick yourself with something sharp or touch a burning object, fast pain is mainly related to painful stimuli of the skin, mouth and anus.

Table 4.2 Characteristics of fast and slow pain.

Slow pain	Fast pain
Transmitted by very thin nerve fibres	Transmitted by relatively thicker (and therefore faster conducting) nerve fibres
Poorly localised	Well localised
All internal organs (except the brain)	Mainly skin, mouth, anus
Body wants to be immobile to allow healing (guarding, spasm, rigidity)	Immediate withdrawal on stimulation to avoid further damage
Pain often radiates, or is referred	Pain does not radiate
Good relief by opioids	Little relief by opioids
Examples: labour pain, myocardial infarction, pain starting after fast pain from an injury	Examples: pain from a surgical incision

It is transmitted by comparatively thick nerve fibres, although this is relative, because they are still microscopically thin, with a diameter of 2–5 thousandths of a millimetre. These nerves are called A-delta fibres. Because of their relatively thick size, these nerve fibres allow the pain stimulus to be transferred very fast (at a speed of 5–30 m/second), hence the name. This fast reaction is to make the body withdraw immediately from the painful and harmful stimulus, in order to avoid further damage.

Fast pain is well localised, meaning that a person can normally describe very accurately where exactly the pain is. The pain is described as sharp and 'cutting' or 'stabbing' in nature.

Slow pain

This begins immediately after the fast pain, and slow pain is transmitted by very thin nerve fibres, called C-nerve fibres (their diameter is between 0.2 and 1 thousandth of a millimetre). Because of their small size, the pain impulse can only be transmitted slowly to the brain, at a speed of less than 2 m/second. The response of the body is to hold the affected body part immobile (guarding, spasm or rigidity), so that healing can take place.

Slow pain is poorly localised and, felt more diffusely, unlike pain on the skin, which can be exactly pinpointed. It also often radiates (e.g. gall bladder pain can be felt from the front to the back) or is referred to other parts of the body (e.g. pain from an acute ischaemic cardiac event can be felt in the neck or the left arm).

The opioid analgesics are very effective in treating this slow type of pain. Local anaesthetics block all nerve transmission, so they also easily take this type of pain away, if the appropriate nerves can be blocked.

Pain in labour

Giving birth is a painful process. This applies to all social and ethnic groups and has probably been so since human beings walked upright. The psychological nature of pain and the physiological can sometimes be complex to compare. It is very difficult to measure pain which is recognised via the signals carried through the nervous system and the woman's intellectual response to the stimulus.

Physiology of pain in labour

Labour pain is the result of many complex interactions, physiological and psychological, excitatory as well as inhibitory. Pain during the first stage of labour is due to three factors: distension of the lower uterine segment, mechanical dilatation of the cervix and lastly due to stretching of excitatory nociceptive afferents resulting from the contraction of the uterine muscles which form the myometrium. The childbearing woman would usually describe this pain in terms of a visceral or an abdominal cramping sensation (Melzack & Wall 1996). The severity of pain therefore parallels the duration and intensity of the uterine contraction.

As the woman moves into the second stage, gradually additional factors, such as traction and pressure on the parietal peritoneum, uterine ligaments, urethra, bladder, rectum, lumbosacral plexus, fascia and muscles of the pelvic floor increase the intensity of pain. In the second stage of labour, there is often a sharper and more continuous somatic pain in the perineum. Pressure or nerve entrapment caused by the baby's head can cause severe back or leg pain.

The woman's previous experience of childbirth may affect her sensation of pain. For example, first time mothers generally experience more sensory pain during early labour (Lowe 1992; Scheiner et al. 1998). Multiparous women may experience more intense pain during the late first stage as well as the second stage of labour, as a result of rapid fetal descent (Lowe 1992; Ranta et al. 1996). The woman's previous experience may also affect the extent to which she is able to articulate her pain.

Neural pathway of pain

The uterus and cervix are supplied by afferent nerve fibres accompanying sympathetic nerves in the uterine and cervical plexuses, the inferior, middle and superior hypogastric plexuses and the aortic plexus. The small unmyelinated 'C' visceral fibres transmit nociception through lumbar and lower thoracic sympathetic chains to the posterior nerve roots of the 10th, 11th and 12th thoracic nerves and also to 1st lumbar nerves to synapse in the dorsal horn. The chemical mediators involved are bradykinin, leukotrienes, prostaglandins, serotonin, substance P and lactic acid. As the labour progresses severe pain is referred to the dermatomes supplied by the 10th thoracic and 1st lumbar nerves.

In the second stage, the direct pressure by the presenting part on the lumbosacral plexus causes neuropathic pain, this may be in the form of back pain or even limb pain. The pain is felt as a more nerve related pain, similar to sciatica; for example, stretching of the vagina and perineum results in stimulation of the pudendal nerve (Sacral 2,3,4) via fine, myelinated, rapidly transmitting 'A delta' fibres. This means that the pain is transmitted at a faster rate. From these areas, the impulses pass to dorsal horn cells and finally to the brain via the spinothalamic tract.

The stress response to pain in labour

Segmental and supra-segmental reflex-responses to the pain of labour may affect respiratory, cardiovascular, gastro-intestinal, urinary and neuro-endocrine functions.

Respiratory

Pain in labour initiates hyperventilation, leading to maternal hypocarbia, respiratory alkalosis and subsequent compensatory metabolic acidosis. The oxygen dissociation curve is shifted to the left and, thus, reduces tissue oxygen transfer, which is already compromised by the increased oxygen consumption associated with labour.

Cardiovascular

Labour results in a progressive increase in maternal cardiac output, primarily due to an increase in stroke volume, and, to a lesser extent, maternal heart rate. The greatest increase in cardiac output occurs immediately after the birth, from the increased venous return associated with relief of venocaval compression and the auto transfusion resulting from uterine contraction and involution.

Hormonal

The presence of painful stimuli result in the release of beta-endorphin and ACTH from the anterior pituitary. Associated anxiety also initiates further pituitary response.

Pain also stimulates the increased release of both adrenaline and noradrenaline from the adrenal medulla which may lead to a progressive rise in peripheral resistance and cardiac output. Excessive, sympathetic activity may result in incoordinate uterine action, prolonged labour and abnormal fetal heart-rate patterns. Activation of the autonomic nervous system also delays gastric emptying and reduces intestinal peristalsis.

Metabolic

Maternal

During labour, glucagon, growth hormone, renin and anti-diuretic hormone (ADH) levels increase while insulin and testosterone levels decrease. Circulating free fatty acids and lactate also increase with a peak level at the time of birth.

Fetal

Maternal catecholamines, secreted as a result of labour pain, may cause fetal acidosis due to low placental blood flow.

Severity of labour pain

The woman's perception of the severity of labour pain varies greatly among women in labour. If women are asked during or shortly after birth to score their labour pain, most rate it as severe while few mention little or no pain. Using the McGill Pain Questionnaires

(MPQs), Melzack et al. (1981) found that labour pain usually rated a high score particularly among primiparae, those with a history of dysmenorrhoea and those belonging to low socio-economic groups.

Endorphins, endogenous opioids and the gate control theory

Endorphins (or 'endogenous opiates') were first discovered in 1975 by John Hughes and colleagues in Aberdeen (Hughes et al. 1975). They are natural opiate-like substances, similar to morphine and heroin, but not as potent. Endorphins are manufactured by our bodies in the presence of pain and act as a natural analgesic. There is some evidence to suggest that the pregnant woman's body starts to produce more endorphins just prior to labour (Iverson 1979). Endorphins are released by the ends of the afferent or descending nerve fibres that come down the spinal cord from the brain.

Endorphins counter the stress of birth with their analgesic powers. During the gestation period, the placenta provides the nourishment necessary for the development of the fetus. The placenta also contains the crucial precursor molecule pro-opiomelanocortin from which beta endorphin, met-encephalin and adrenocorticotrophin are all derived (Tortora et al. 2006). In the human placenta, beta-endorphin and met-encephalin are present in the placental tissue and placental blood at higher levels than usual during pregnancy and labour.

When we feel a certain level of pain, the descending nerve fibres release endorphins at the level of the spinal cord, where they meet the sensory nerves carrying the 'pain messages' from our body. This local release of endorphins by the nerves inhibits some or all of the pain messages going up to the brain.

For many women, endorphins will also positively alter the memory of their birth experience and, for some women, induce an amnesic effect (forgetting the pain). Endorphins can therefore have the potential to strengthen the woman's psyche and provide an internal 'protection' against the intensity of labour and giving birth.

The gate control theory

The 'gate control theory' was first proposed by Melzack and Wall in 1965 (Melzack & Wall 1965). They have since refined their theory (in 1988) and it remains one of the most respected understandings of one way our bodies can diminish the perception of pain.

The gate control theory is based on the premise that when the larger A-b (beta) skin nerves (that sense touch, heat, cold and pressure) are stimulated, they are capable of overriding the smaller A-d (delta) and C nerve fibres that sense the sharp, burning or aching pains. The larger fibres carry the sensory message to the spinal cord more rapidly and get priority, closing 'the gate' as it were, to the pain messages being carried by the smaller fibres. If the pain intensifies to a higher level the 'gate' can be pushed back open to a degree, making the pain sensation more intense.

This is presented as the reasoning underpinning the natural instinct to 'rub' or massage the area of the body which has sustained an injury or is in pain. It is also the reason why natural therapies such as massage, water, cold or hot packs being used during labour can alter the conscious pain sensation felt by the woman, changing or modifying the pain she experiences. Other methods of stimulation can consist of changing position, walking, rocking, stomping and pelvic rocking. These will activate receptors in the woman's joints to help diminish pain.

As the labour progresses and intensifies, methods using the 'gate control' can become less effective as the gate is 'pushed back' to some degree. This is particularly so, as the woman reaches the transitional phase, just before the second stage. At this point the pain may become too great for the gate to be closed and the woman's behaviour may undergo a marked change (Mander 1992).

Gate control and physiology of labour pain

The link between what is occurring at physiological level and the understanding of the gate control theory can be seen quite clearly. We have discussed the aspects of 'fast' and 'slow' nerve impulses and this mechanism is demonstrated by this theory. By means of rubbing or massaging an area the woman in childbirth will also be stimulating the release of endorphins to aid in the natural opiate response to the painful stimulus.

Conclusion

In this chapter I have shown that the physiology of labour pain is as complicated as it is significant. While pain is often defined in terms of it being an indication of harm or damage to tissues or surrounding areas (Bonica 1990), the pain of labour may be viewed quite differently. The outcomes ordinarily associated with the birth of a baby mean that labour pain is open to interpretation in other, more positive, ways.

In order that the person involved in the care of the woman giving birth is able to respond to these differing viewpoints, an understanding of the physiological processes is a crucially fundamental requirement. On the basis of this understanding, the carer is further able to provide woman-centred care, which takes into consideration and addresses the woman's view of her experience of labour pain.

Part II

Beginning the Journey

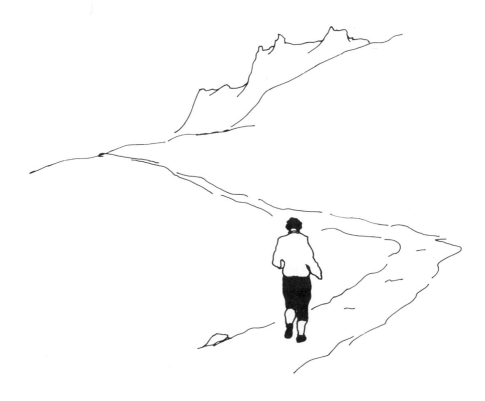

Chapter 5

Childbirth education

The remit of childbirth education is so wide as to be meaningless and the timing is equally variable. For these reasons, in this book I address it before writing about pregnancy (Chapter 6). The 'classes', on the other hand, tend to be provided only during pregnancy and a large proportion of the material is perceived as focussing on labour (Svensson et al. 2007). Thus, I seek to address this topic alongside the material on pain in pregnancy and before labour. In order to demonstrate the close relationship between childbirth education and pain, I discuss first the development of education for childbearing. Approaches to teaching about pain have changed during this development, and I look at these approaches next. Third, this chapter focuses on the effectiveness of childbirth education, particularly in relation to pain, as demonstrated through evaluative research. I then focus down on some specific issues relating to certain groups of clients. Finally, I summarise this chapter by drawing certain comparisons between childbirth education and the woman's experience of labour.

The origins of childbirth education on pain and its control

Childbirth education about pain has been happening through 'women's networks' for almost as long as women have been bearing children (Nolan 1997). The all too familiar tendency of experienced mothers to recount their experiences to new mothers-to-be carries benefits for both, as well as possible risks. The experienced woman's account, however, invariably features the experience of pain (Perkins 1980). While Nolan (1997) argues that childbirth education was a self-help response among isolated middle class women, others relate its development to a range of increasingly complex phenomena in the early twentieth century (Moscucci 2003). Ornella Moscucci's claim that these programmes originally met certain political and religious aspirations contradicts Nolan's emphasis on the programmes simply satisfying the need for preparation for motherhood.

An early example of pain prevention is found in Grantly Dick-Read's pioneering work. His second book 'Revelation of Childbirth' (1933) was later published in its more familiar form as 'Childbirth without fear' (1954). In a context of jingoistic, evangelistic eugenics, Dick-Read introduced the concept of pain being culturally learned and being associated with an escalating vicious cycle of counterproductive

Pain in Childbearing and its Control, Second Edition. By Rosemary Mander. Published 2011 by Blackwell Publishing Ltd. © 1998, 2011 Rosemary Mander.

fear and tension. To break this cycle, in the 1950s he advocated education and developed a programme of classes. The relaxation and breathing exercises were added by his physiotherapist colleagues, although he regarded such 'gymnastics' as 'misguided' (Moscucci 2003: 171). His 'natural childbirth' methods were greeted warmly in North America, but they encountered some degree of resistance in the UK (Arney 1982: 214; Kitzinger 1989).

In contrast, psychoprophylaxis was easily accepted throughout the West, in spite of its Eastern European origins. These techniques were derived from the concepts developed by Pavlov on learning by conditioning (Velvovsky et al. 1960). Because of their French advocate, Ferdinand Lamaze, and group sessions, this approach became known as 'Lamaze classes'. Hence, from its early days, social support, as well as learning about 'preventing' pain, was crucial to childbirth education. Despite the acrimony between the disciples of these two main approaches (Kitzinger 1989), they shared common features, such as their reluctance to admit the reality of labour pain. While I understand that some women experience pain-free childbirth, my personal observation suggests this is not the case for the majority of mothers. The early proponents of prepared or natural childbirth, however, denied that uncomplicated labour is painful; to the extent that Lamaze claimed that his method provided 'complete absence of sensation' (1956). Dick-Read did eventually concede, though, that 'the last few contractions' are possibly painful (Jimenez 1988). The persistence of belief that labour pain is mythological is evident (Langford 1997), but such condescending approaches and their legacy, the euphemistic 'contractions', barely deserve consideration.

Pertinent to the discussion of Dick-Read's approach are questions of the relevance of the pervasive medical orientation of much client, including childbirth, education (Fleming 1992). Similarly, it is necessary to question the role of men, such as Dick-Read, his Russian equivalents and more recently Michel Odent (1994), in defining women's childbirth experience as painless. Valerie Fleming argues against the medical control of childbirth education by describing the ultimate desired outcome. This is not the health of the woman and baby, or even the mother's satisfaction with her birth experience, but (Fleming argues) 'the rewarding of staff with "compliant patients"'. These thoughts are powerfully reminiscent of Mavis Kirkham's authoritative research-based observations (1989). Such medical/antimedical orientations are apparent in different educational approaches and the woman is encouraged to seek the education that fits her view (Monto 1996). This theme of antagonism between medical and childbirth education lobbies continues to feature in the literature on pain control (Simkin & Bolding 2004).

Teaching and learning about labour pain

Even the *possibility* of teaching about pain in childbearing raises a whole raft of issues. Before contemplating what is taught about childbearing pain, though, we must ask whether *anything* is taught about it. There exist textbooks on childbirth education which omit even to index 'pain'! Exceptionally, though, Robertson (2002) devotes a full chapter to issues relating to teaching about pain. The rationale for these omissions may be approached in three ways.

First, we may question whether it is *necessary* to teach about labour pain. Women's innate knowledge has traditionally provided them with what they need to give birth, so any teaching should be superfluous. As Andrea Robertson observes, though, these innate abilities may be inhibited by the woman's upbringing and cultural environment. This may result in the loss of the woman's ability to 'listen to her own body' (2002: 101).

Second, we should further question whether it is actually *feasible* to teach a woman about what pain she should expect in labour. The unpredictability of labour militates against preparing the woman effectively for the type and severity of pain she will experience in labour. Vangie Bergum, on the basis of her qualitative research (1989), attributes this difficulty to the 'horror' of the pain; this may be combined with the limitations of the English language which mean that, for some women, their pain will prove beyond their vocabulary and their 'language runs dry' (Woolf 1867). On the other hand, teaching the reality of birth may be feasible; women who are taught realistically about the anxiety involved experience a less painful birth. Thus, learning about how to control pain, has been linked to an increased likelihood of a positive childbirth experience.

Third, the *P word* involves a long-running argument, which followed the debate about the existence of labour pain, relating to the use of the word pain itself. Margaret Williams and Dorothy Booth (1985) argue that by discussing pain the woman, who has been conditioned to expect that 'labour equals pain', may interpret any 'unusual sensation' as pain. These authors then suggest that the word should be used 'occasionally' (1985: 110). Thus, there is a resistance to the word pain, in that it may be better to avoid a four letter word such as this. It carries the risk of becoming a 'self fulfilling prophecy'. There is a very fine line to be drawn by the childbirth educator in relation to the emphasis attached to pain. It may be necessary to conclude that childbirth involves a positive form of pain which, unlike most pain, does not constitute pathology.

Sheila Kitzinger's well-known aphorism, that labour comprises 'pain with a purpose' (1978), is useful. This view is endorsed by research by Anita Hallgren and her colleagues (1995), which used 'sense of coherence' (SOC), a form of confidence, as the theoretical framework. These Swedish researchers found that a decreased SOC was associated with an increasing need for pharmacological pain control (1995: 134). These findings are clearly very relevant to the childbirth educator.

The issue of teaching about pain is confronted by some midwives, such as Nicky Leap (1997), who discuss pain antenatally in preference to 'pain relief'. This orientation is thought responsible for these midwives', admittedly self-selected, clients' limited use of pharmacological pain control (69% used none).

Teaching approaches

The main approaches to childbirth education are particularly insightful in the context of teaching about pain, as demonstrated by Elizabeth Perkins' classic research (1980). Huge variations emerged in teaching about pain between classes and between teachers. The defining feature in the three different approaches to childbirth education was the teacher's attitude to pain:

- The first, entitled 'old wives' tales', comprises a range of traditional horror stories in which pain invariably predominates.
- The second approach, termed 'new wives' tales', draws on more up-to-date horror stories, usually involving medical technology. These result in iatrogenic pain and further medical interventions to resolve that pain. Thus, the 'cascade of intervention' becomes established.
- The last of Perkins' three approaches is her 'free spirit's tales'. This 'everything in the garden is lovely' idealisation of childbirth seeks to help the woman to cope with pain by redefining it 'as a new, overpowering sensation'. The woman is taught techniques to help her to work with her pain, rather than against it. Despite her criticism of this approach, Perkins admits 'paradoxically, this romantic view of childbirth is the most practical one, in that the woman has something she can do to help fulfil her expectations' (1980: 48).

Although they used different terms from Perkins, Swedish researchers identified the continuing variability in childbirth education approaches (Hallgren et al. 1994). They found obstetric, parent-oriented and mixed perspectives. These potential splits appear resolved in the twin aims of another approach using the 'latest research' and 'understanding the normal birth process' (Robertson 2002).

Recommendations to reform childbirth education (Fleming 1992) built on Perkins' 'free spirit' approach by drawing on critical social theory (Freire & Shor 1987). The traditional didactic and medically orientated format of childbirth education on pain would be replaced by a transformational, negotiated curriculum in which both woman and educator share their experiences and legitimate theoretical standpoints. The resulting joint search for the meaning of the birth experience would facilitate 'personal growth' (Fleming 1992: 162). A more recent North American project with implications for teaching about pain used phenomenology to establish the significance of the childbearing woman's relationships, particularly with her own mother (Savage 2006). By supporting this relationship, the childbirth educator facilitates the childbearing woman's realistic decision-making relating to her birth experience. Thus, rather than supplanting the woman's mother, the educator should seek to increase the confidence of the childbearing woman by enhancing her mother's role with a view to her long term family involvement.

On this basis, it is necessary to conclude that traditional antenatal teaching may not actually teach the woman about labour pain. More liberal approaches, though, are being developed. These, rather than focussing on specific topics, impinge on the woman's attitude to pain by enhancing the mother's wide-ranging education.

Research on the effectiveness of childbirth education

As I mentioned above, since its inception, a major, if not sole, goal of childbirth education has been the alleviation of labour pain. It is unsurprising, therefore, that much childbirth education research has focused on the extent to which it affects pain. Despite the plethora of research projects, evidence demonstrating the effectiveness of childbirth education is still sparse (Nolan 1997). Additionally, the shortcomings in terms of both methodology and applicability of much of the research inevitably mean that 'more research is needed'. Because of the commercial significance of childbirth education in the USA, much of the research has been undertaken there. This leads to the question of the relevance of research undertaken in relatively medicalised, interventionist settings to those countries where intervention may be less institutionalised.

A voice which is infrequently heard in the context of childbirth education evaluation is that of the childbearing woman. This omission is more than corrected by Carine Mardorossian (2003) who drew on her own personal experience to condemn the Bradley method of natural childbirth in general and the provision of childbirth education on pain in particular. Mardorossian denounced the inadequacy of this form of preparation for labour and childbirth as representing a form of 'patriarchal and capitalist power' (2003: 113). The patriarchy operates through the Bradley approach which casts the woman's male partner as 'labor coach'; requiring this ignorant and anxious man to act as the 'team leader' in providing supportive care for the woman in labour. The accusation of capitalism is levelled at the maternity institutions which, effectively, use the partner as an unpaid labour ward employee. While in no way objective, this denunciation of natural childbirth may be recognised by a certain group of women who find that their expectations of their own and their partner's coping abilities have been raised to an unrealistically high level.

Research by Diane Escott and her colleagues (2005) sought to encourage childbearing women to employ their own individual coping strategies in an enhanced form (ESC) during labour. Although the women did employ their chosen techniques, the outcome measures showed no difference between the intervention group and the control group. The researchers argue, however, that childbirth education is shown to be effective in teaching the woman to persist with her chosen strategy.

While more scientific forms of evaluation of childbirth education are more authoritative, they do not necessarily reach very different conclusions. The Cochrane Review by Johanne Gagnon and Jane Sandall (2007) was critical of the generally poor quality of childbirth education evaluations. The reviewers concluded that the resources spent in this way could be used more effectively. This is a damning criticism of what is, in certain countries, a major industry constituting a serious drain on health service finances.

The Clinical Guideline produced by the National Collaborating Centre for Women's and Children's Health considered the effectiveness of many forms of information-giving to childbearing women, including antenatal classes (NICE 2008). The studies on the different aspects of the antenatal classes are, again, inconclusive. The studies were undertaken in various westernised countries and measured different aspects of the couple's experience. Phenomena in the woman which may have been changed by childbirth education include attachment behaviour, fear of childbirth, active input into childbirth, self-care agency and knowledge of health-related behaviour. The studies focusing on pain in labour tended to produce findings which were not clearly significant or with mixed benefits.

The NICE review of the research on the couple's experience of childbirth education produced some unsurprising findings, such as the woman's preference being for information-giving in a one-to-one setting. Similarly, when asked afterwards, the couple would have liked more teaching on postnatal matters. This finding is galling in view of the teachers' perceptions that couples 'won't listen' to such material antenatally, because their focus does not extend beyond the birth and any associated pain (Svensson et al. 2007).

It is clear that teaching methods and evaluation of childbirth education attract considerable attention. Equally, pain is problematical in that this topic is variably taught and constitutes an unsatisfactory measure of the effectiveness of childbirth education. In the same way that effectiveness has been shown to need research attention, the extent to which childbirth education meets women's needs also requires attention.

Specific issues relating to certain groups

While some aspects of research into childbirth education have been shown to be somewhat deficient, certain groups' education deserves to attract particular attention. Although these groups may initially appear to share little in common, the research findings suggest that they share more commonalities than are apparent at first sight.

Men

The anxiety of the father being with his partner in labour is notorious (Mander 2004b). Research into the form of childbirth education most congenial to men is plentiful, suggesting that there are problems still to be resolved (Friedewald 2007, 2008). Despite his presence at the birth having been ubiquitous for at least two decades, the role that childbirth education plays in preventing the father's anxiety or helping him to cope with his partner's pain is uncertain. The existing research, quite serendipitously, shows his feelings of needing to support his partner in coping with her pain at the expense of expressing his own needs:

> You feel quite helpless. You stand by the bed during the delivery … and you can't take over the pain. It is so hard (Premberg & Lundgren 2006: 24)

Although Mardorossian (See 'Research' above) presents her case study in the first person, she occasionally slips into the plural form to include her husband. His inability to fulfil his designated 'husband-as-coach' role was 'pathetic … [as he] felt completely out of his depth in the face of so much pain' (2003: 117). Her decision to seek epidural analgesia was clearly a relief to both; although this decision required him to abandon his assigned role as 'directing' her natural childbirth.

An authoritative study by Rebecca Greenhalgh and her colleagues (2000) investigated the experience of the birth and early fatherhood among men who did or did not attend childbirth education. The researchers found that men who tended to avoid or deny their anxiety had a less fulfilling experience of the birth. On the basis of these findings it is necessary to conclude that childbirth education certainly does not serve as a panacea and that there are many outstanding questions relating to the father's presence at the birth.

Young women

All too often the 'teen mother' is regarded as little more than a problem. For this reason if no other, this young woman's childbirth education should be specifically tailored to address the issues which confront her, of which pain in labour is likely to be but one. Depending on her age and maturity, her social skills may be limited so social support, initially by one person but eventually within a group, is strongly recommended. Such group activity, if it can be achieved, will serve to reduce the isolation which she is more likely to encounter after the birth. With this encouraging background, Karen Cheema reports that the experience of labour is something in which the young mother is likely to 'do well' (2002: S28). Recommendations about the environment in which the support for the teen mother is offered, makes such support both relevant and acceptable (Smith & Nolan 2009: 237).

The plethora of US literature on the topic of teen pregnancy reflects an obsession with one particular ethnic group who are often euphemistically referred to as the 'urban poor'. This orientation emerges in a grounded theory study by Joanne Cox and her colleagues, in which none of the participants was white (2005: 168). Reading it from a UK viewpoint, the sample for this study of 'teen services' was unusual; it comprised participants up to the age of 21 and none under sixteen. The hospital-focussed study by Cox and colleagues demonstrated the desirability of continuity of care and a 'one stop shop' offering health, social and educational advice. The participants valued group activities to reduce isolation, resolve difficult home circumstances and facilitate friendship-building. Thus, this group of young people sought maternity care which provides continuity and is effective in meeting their needs, suggesting that this group may not be very different from other maternity service-users.

While there is a wealth of literature about the 'teen pregnancy problem' and how to prevent and organise services to deal with it, there is little practical advice. An exception to this observation is the useful outline of guidance for practitioners seeking to improve the nutrition of pregnant adolescents (Montgomery 2003). While the recommendations about advice on nutrition make good sense, there is no indication of how or the reasons why adolescents' diets may be anything less than ideally healthy.

Ethnic minority groups

The research on ethnic minority groups' involvement in childbirth education may be the touchstone for how the national health service interacts with minority communities. This is apparent from the sorry picture painted by Perkins in 1980 and the limited change since then (Thorpe-Raghdo 2005). Perkins found that women with an ethnic minority background rarely attended childbirth education for the simple reason that the staff felt it inappropriate to invite them. My observation of little change is supported by one Muslim woman who recently reported:

> I went through my first two pregnancies not knowing about these classes. Luckily in my third I saw ... the classes were brilliant. (Thorpe-Raghdo 2005: 489).

It is clear that the longstanding lack of communication still applies. In the same way, not only is the content problematical, but midwives' lack of cultural competence also makes the social organisation of the classes challenging (Thorpe-Raghdo 2005). Some ethnic minority women, however, really valued the classes that they attended, especially on matters such as breastfeeding. Others, though, were found to prefer to obtain information from their friends and relatives, secure in the knowledge that it would be culturally relevant. This research suggests that a little effort may be necessary for maternity staff to ensure that classes are appropriate to *all* childbearing women, rather than assuming that certain groups' traditional late or non-attendance for antenatal care is also reflected in their low uptake of childbirth education (Rowe & Garcia 2003).

In a Blue Skies Report (2006) the experiences of new migrants into New Zealand showed that in *younger* communities, such extended family support and information-giving may not be available. This makes childbirth education crucially important but its effectiveness may be impeded by language difficulties; the report shows how linguistic difficulties may be overcome by the presence of a more fluent partner. As well as psychosocial benefits, the new migrant mothers in this study recounted being introduced to a wide range of community resources. The childbearing women who attended classes were found to develop more realistic expectations of their care, including being well-informed about pain control. Such a *factual* orientation, though, neglects to address the 'confidence and emotional insights' (2006: 31) which extended family contacts would provide. As found by Beverley Thorpe-Raghdo (2005) in the UK, cultural competence was regarded as essential. Such competence took clinical, organisational and systemic forms, but seeking knowledgeable and consistent care was common to all childbearing women. The Blue Skies Report found, however, that the new migrants' cultural safety was seriously threatened by health care organisations' exclusive focus on the needs of the majority population. Many of the examples in this report relate to fundamental mis-understandings about assumptions widely held but infrequently articulated by the host population and which contradict those held by the new migrants; these include the care providers' assumption that the new mother should wish to quickly 'get back to normal', whereas the new migrant often recognises the importance of rest and sleep in the early days of motherhood.

Lesbian women/couples

In the same way as incorrect assumptions have been shown to be problematical in the care of ethnic minority mothers, the lesbian woman may face a welter of assumptions during the course of her childbearing experience. In a Swedish context, Anna-Karin Larsson and Anna-Karin Dykes found that lesbian women's generally poor experience of the health care system applied particularly to childbirth education (2008). The teaching staff assumed that the parents would be heterosexual, with frequent references to fathers:

> I felt very strongly that that midwife was very unprofessional. She could have said 'couple', then she would have included me as well, and confirmed that she knew who we were.
>
> Larsson & Dykes 2008: 5

The lesbian mothers were not averse to questions about their lifestyle, possibly regarding themselves as having a responsibility for extending the horizons of health care staff. These researchers suggested that, on the other hand, lesbian mothers and single hetero-sexual women may have certain educational needs in common, raising the possibility that shared sessions might be appropriate (2008: 7). The experience of lesbian women in the UK was generally comparable with that of their more recent Swedish counterparts (Wilton & Kaufmann 2001). Similarly, the UK experience of childbirth education 'attracted most negative comment' irrespective of the location of the classes.

The midwives seemed very uncomfortable and unfamiliar with our relationship as lesbians. NCT was a bloody nightmare! My partner ended up with the fathers and felt awful, as I did.

Wilton & Kaufmann 2001: 206

These researchers apply their conclusions about lesbian women's marginalisation to single mothers and members of ethnic minority cultures. The fact that childbirth education tends to be a group or class activity appears to cause difficulty for the teachers in including clients who are something other than an indigenous heterosexual couple. Tamsin Wilton and Tara Kaufmann go on to suggest that there may be a place for women-only childbirth education sessions, which would meet the special needs of single mothers and lesbian mothers as well as some ethnic minority groups. They further recommend that childbirth educators may benefit from specific training to increase their inclusiveness. Additionally, unlike Larsson and Dykes (2008 above) they suggest that lesbian mothers should not be used to act as a teaching aid.

In terms of the duration of their education, Alison McManus and her colleagues argue that the lesbian couple's education begins with their information-gathering around the time of conception; it 'has the potential to shape their birth experience' (2006: 19). A sad reflection on these authors' North American dominant culture, although it features in the UK and Swedish studies, is found in the main thrust of their systematic review comprising a plea for the better education of health care providers.

Conclusion

Preparing the woman to cope with pain has long been childbirth education's major purpose. In this chapter I have sought to address the extent to which it is effective in achieving this aim. The answer, disappointingly, appears to be 'not very'.

Equally disconcerting are the ideas which have been raised relating to the possibility that there may be a different agenda operating. This was first raised in research by Kirkham (1989), when she suggested that the childbirth educator's major goal may be something other than to facilitate the learning of the childbearing woman. She argued that the agenda may comprise the aim of rendering the woman more compliant or receptive to the care and other interventions offered by health care personnel and the system within which they practise.

This point also emerged more recently in an Australian study which proposed that the balance of power in maternity means that childbirth education does not seek to respond to the needs of the woman or couple, but aims to ensure that the couple 'conform to the institution' (Svensson et al. 2007: 14). Learning by the couple is shown to be a relatively low priority for the childbirth educators; they are reluctant to respond to the parents' needs, preferring to ensure that resources and activities are used as instruments to manipulate compliance. This manifested itself in the emphasis on the couple learning about the maternity unit's policies and institutional requirements. Although such material may matter, it is hardly the couple's reason for seeking childbirth education.

Thus, the balance of power seems to be clearly weighted in favour of the educators and against the would-be learners, in order to maintain the organisational *status quo*.

Chapter 6

Pain in pregnancy

As throughout this book, in this chapter I use the broadest possible focus to examine pain as the woman's experience during pregnancy. The model from which my analysis of pain in childbearing begins is the social model of healthy pregnancy. It is from this starting point that this contemplation of pain moves forward.

Healthy pregnancy

Although we are frequently reassured, and reassure others, that pregnancy and childbearing are fundamentally physiological events, perceptions to the contrary have arisen from a number of sources. Historically, our Victorian great-grandparents were embarrassed by pregnancy's sexual connotations, and in their denial referred to it as 'an interesting state'. A well-known example is found in Charles Dickens' novel, Nicholas Nickleby; in which Mrs Lenville is described in these terms (1839). Culturally and possibly for similar reasons, pregnancy is still very much a private matter among certain ethnic groups (Cheung 2000).

A further factor that has contributed to the perception of childbearing as potentially something other than physiological is its medicalisation (Oakley 1980). The extent of the perception of the non-physiological nature of pregnancy was demonstrated by research comparing the views of major actors in the maternity scenario (Schuman & Marteau 1993). Of the three groups of participants, the midwives (n=14) were significantly more likely to view pregnancy as a 'normal' event. The obstetricians (n=15) regarded pregnancy as significantly more risky than any others. Interestingly, the pregnant women (n=136) assumed an only marginally more risk-free stance than the obstetricians. The researchers contemplated whether such differing perceptions affect care adversely.

Thus, the physiological nature of pregnancy is not as obvious as we sometimes assume, and referring to it as 'an altered state of health' may be more accurate. In this chapter I consider some alterations in the woman's health during pregnancy, focusing on those experienced as painful. These alterations vary hugely in their implications for the woman's and the baby's wellbeing. Some alterations have traditionally been described as 'minor disorders' or 'discomforts' (Philipp 1964; Jamieson 1993: 117). Such patronising terminology discounts the woman's experience and I will avoid it here. Similarly, because of

Pain in Childbearing and its Control, Second Edition. By Rosemary Mander. Published 2011 by Blackwell Publishing Ltd. © 1998, 2011 Rosemary Mander.

variations in individuals' perceptions, I avoid categorising the intensity of the pain associated with the different conditions.

To show the close relationship between perinatal pain and women's other experiences of pain, I address the painful conditions in order of their relationship with the actual pregnancy. Thus, conditions associated with or aggravated by pregnancy are followed by those unique to it and, finally, those coincidental to it. Each condition is considered in terms of its pathophysiology, origins of pain and possible remedies. Limited attention is given here to analgesia, except specific types, as pain remedies are discussed in Chapters 8 and 9.

The pregnancy that doesn't happen

While aiming to consider painful conditions associated with the actual pregnancy, it is necessary, at the outset, to think about the pain that may be engendered if the desired pregnancy does not actually happen – that is, if the woman experiences an involuntary form of infertility. Although measurable pain may not feature, the woman is likely to encounter suffering (see the section on 'Suffering' in Chapter 2). This may be aggravated by Western attitudes whose overwhelming focus is on control, that is, prevention, of fertility by contraception. When faced with involuntary infertility, the reality is a shocking contrast to our previous or usual assumptions. The contrast between expectations and reality applies at a fundamental level to all aspects of what has been called 'reproductive failure'. Until problems are encountered, fertility is little more than an, occasionally inconvenient, basic human function. But when we find that the desired level of fertility is beyond our grasp, our integrity as a human being is threatened (Mander 2006).

The suffering arising from the realisation or diagnosis of infertility, unlike other forms of grief which ordinarily involve a specific individual, is relatively unfocussed. This makes such suffering more difficult for others to understand and for the sufferer to explain. For the latter reasons, the infertile person is likely to create two narratives to account for their pain (Kirkman 2001). The first narrative is the reality of the woman's personal experience and remains private; it sits uncomfortably or may even conflict with the other narrative which is essentially for public consumption. This public story is a coping strategy which is one of many (Schmidt et al. 2004) and is for when the small talk turns to family matters; it provides an effective smokescreen for the woman's genuine feelings of painful grief.

While assisted/artificial reproductive technology (ART) is widely represented as a panacea to resolve all of the problems of infertility, this picture may not be entirely accurate. The actual success or 'take home baby' rates tend to remain well-kept secrets. Even prior to conception, the 'roller-coaster' of investigations and interventions brings its own emotional challenges, including suffering in the form of depression and grief; this is clearly long before the ultimate success or otherwise is achieved (Lukse & Vacc 1999).

Our ethnocentric society tends to disregard the even greater significance of children, and hence infertility, in developing countries. Infertility's painful suffering, which is becoming better-recognised in developed settings, is exacerbated in societies in which children are an economic necessity and key to social, and possibly physical, survival. Their absence may lead to ostracism, as the woman in an infertile couple is likely to be blamed as a source of evil or bad luck, or even more desperate outcomes (Daar & Merali 2002).

Suffering in pregnancy

As well as suffering related to regrettable phenomena, women may experience various forms of suffering due to pathological or potentially pathological events. These include suffering caused by intimate partner violence (IPV), abuse by the system of care or suffering associated with sexual discrimination, already addressed in Chapter 2.

Suffering during pregnancy as a long term sequel of childhood sexual abuse (CSA) has received little research or other attention (Leeners et al. 2006). On the basis of what research exists, though, these authors consider that women with a history of CSA tend to experience childbearing as generally more problematical. They are more likely to have mental health problems and during labour may encounter sudden reminiscences of repressed memories. Further, the labour and birth are more physically painful when compared with non-CSA controls. The mental health difficulties continue into the postnatal period with a greater risk of postnatal depression which may be associated with an unsurprising difficulty in breast feeding. Brigitte Leeners and colleagues argue that, if childbearing women with CSA are to be given the help which they both need and deserve, health care providers need to be more proactive in seeking to identify them.

Leeners and her colleagues also show that women with CSA are among those who are vulnerable to another form of suffering in pregnancy; these are the self-harming activities which manifest themselves as risky health behaviours, such as the abuse of nicotine, alcohol and other drugs. Under certain harsh and inequitable circumstances, pregnancy may be construed as a health crisis, which invokes other strategies intended to assist coping. Far from assisting coping, such strategies will serve only to reinforce the severity of the crisis by bringing additional health problems (Singer and Snipes 1992).

Conditions associated with or aggravated by pregnancy

The childbearing woman's body benefits from a number of physiological adjustments during pregnancy. These adjustments are largely hormonally determined and serve many functions, such as ensuring the continuation of the pregnancy or making the labour and birth marginally easier. The bad news, though, is that these adjustments may cause or aggravate painful conditions for which the woman may seek advice or even need treatment. Conditions such as these have long been known as the 'minor disorders', or 'discomforts' in the US, reflecting the inappropriately limited significance attached to them (Lee 1998).

The digestive tract – heartburn

As with some other bodily systems, the activity of the woman's digestive system is slowed during pregnancy under the influence of progesterone produced, initially, by the corpus luteum and later the placenta. This reduced activity may result in symptoms which the woman feels as painful and which may be exacerbated by mechanical or positional changes.

Heartburn's name clearly indicates the nature and site of the pain; likewise, the North American term *pyrosis* suggests its burning nature, which may extend into the throat. Technically, *gastro-oesophageal reflux disease* means that irritation due to regurgitation of acid stomach contents into the oesophagus is responsible. The pain may be accompanied by pharyngeal regurgitation of clear fluid reaching the mouth or throat, causing a bitter/acidic taste. It is estimated that about half of pregnant women develop heartburn, with an increased frequency and severity later in pregnancy (Malfertheiner et al. 2009). Multiparity and older maternal age, as well as pre-existing heartburn, are risk factors. The familiar myth that heartburn is relieved with 'lightening' has been shown to be just that. The research by Peter Malfertheiner and his colleagues is important in that it demonstrates the serious effects of heartburn on the woman's general quality of life, particularly due to sleep deprivation.

The cause of heartburn is partly positional, being associated with stooping or lying down and these effects are exacerbated by changing intra-abdominal pressure due to the growing fetus. Progesterone, in the presence of oestrogen, exerting a relaxing effect on the lower oesophageal sphincter is another contributing factor, as is that hormone's reduction of gastrointestinal motility and delay in gastric emptying (Dowswell & Neilson 2008).

Because the condition is time-limited, suggested remedies tend to be purely symptomatic.

Non-pharmacological remedies include attention to posture, size and timing of meals, and avoidance of fatty, spicy and very cold substances. The recommendation of milky drinks is of uncertain value, as milk may actually irritate the gastric mucosa. Following a survey, it was recommended that at risk groups should adopt preventive measures, such as raising the head of the bed, prior to symptoms appearing, to prevent oesophageal sensitisation (Marrero et al. 1992).

The woman may need pharmacological remedies if simpler ones fail to resolve unacceptable pain. Antacid medications or drugs to reduce the secretion of gastric acids may be recommended. Alternatively proton pump inhibitors (PPIs) serve to inhibit the stomach enzymes involved in acid production. Of course, there are risks involved in taking any drug during pregnancy as well as the known side effects of constipation/diarrhoea, muscle cramps or reduced absorption of nutrients (Dowswell & Neilson 2008). There is also a more serious danger of sodium bicarbonate inducing sodium overload and systemic alkalosis (Bracken et al. 1989). If long term use is considered, the medications based on magnesium salts appear safer than those derived from aluminium salts (Brucker 1988). Therese Dowswell and James Neilson's authoritative systematic review (2008) reaches the all too familiar conclusion that reliable data on the effectiveness and safety of pharmacological interventions is lacking.

Musculo-skeletal pain

Progesterone and related hormones, secreted mainly by the placenta during pregnancy, are usually thought to assist labour and ease birth by allowing the pelvic joints a marginal degree of expansion. As mentioned already, this is the good news. The bad news is that in order to achieve this relatively short term, albeit significant, benefit the woman may find herself suffering months or more of impairment of mobility or other activities. Although the placental hormone, relaxin, has long been given credit for these benefits and impairments, evidence has been found which suggests that the link between relaxin and joint laxity is not entirely straightforward (Björklund et al. 2000).

The bony pelvis

A group of problems that are attracting more attention and more research attention are those which have traditionally been considered to be separate, though related, entities. Because the terminology is in a state of flux, at the time of writing, I will address the newer generic term first and then the more traditional component parts (Wu et al. 2004).

Pregnancy-related pelvic girdle pain   While some may regard medical diagnosis as immutable, the appearance of pregnancy-related pelvic girdle pain (PPGP) is evidence to the contrary (Mander & Smith 2008). A group of epidemiologists, clinical practitioners and physiotherapists in the Netherlands has made a growth industry of this novel term, if not phenomenon (Bastiaenen et al. 2005, 2006). By reviewing the literature on its component parts since the time of Hippocrates, these authors seek to establish the provenance of their newly-invented terminology (Bastiaenen et al. 2005). They show that PPGP is not confined to pregnancy, but may actually begin *after* the birth. This observation clearly calls into question the role of placental relaxin. In spite of this, they condemn previous research on the grounds of the conditions being poorly defined and described, and offer the following definition of PPGP:

> pain during pregnancy in the lower back, the buttocks, the symphyses (sic), groins and/or radiation into the legs. (Bastiaenen et al. 2005: 13).

On the basis of their literature review these researchers undertook an equally novel randomised controlled trial into the treatment of PPGP in the early postnatal period (Bastiaenen et al. 2006). While the control group were given the standard treatment, the intervention group were treated by physiotherapists adopting a negotiated or contracted form of treatment which allowed the affected woman to implement the therapeutic programme at the speed which suited her and her painful condition. The negotiated programme included education, exercise and support. The intervention group were found to experience a statistically significant reduction in the limitation of their activities, suggesting that this novel form of treatment is more effective than standard care.

Low back pain   Often denigrated by being called 'backache', back pain is a feature of labour and the puerperium as well as pregnancy. The prevalence of back pain in pregnancy emerged from Lotta Norén and her colleagues' longitudinal study (2002); their figure of 70% of pregnant women experiencing such pain may be compared with the 23% of non-pregnant women who suffer thus. As usual, relaxin is blamed as the culprit (Kristiansson et al. 1996).

The increasing laxity of the pelvic ligaments and, hence, enlargement of the pelvic diameters is thought to facilitate the birth, but carries the risk of trauma during pregnancy. The sacro-iliac joint is particularly vulnerable to damage because of its relatively greater weight-bearing load; the pain associated with such trauma may radiate around the greater trochanter and down the anterolateral aspect of the woman's thigh.

Further to its effects on pelvic ligaments, relaxin is thought to allow increased spinal mobility, which has been blamed for the vulnerability of the spine to damage during pregnancy. Similarly, greater spinal instability may develop into long term back pain. In spite of this risk, the major effects of relaxin are ordinarily reversed within 3 months of the birth.

Another, less well-researched, explanation of the development of back pain in pregnancy relates to the *strain* imposed by the growing pregnancy. Such strain can only be aggravated by the alteration in posture or lordosis, that is, a 'concavity of the lumbar vertebrae' (Whitcome et al. 2007), which the pregnant woman assumes to maintain her balance. Research, however, refutes this long-accepted assumption, because the incidence of back pain peaks at 24–28 weeks, that is, before abdominal growth reaches its maximum (Kristiansson et al. 1996).

The costs of back pain to the pregnant woman, her family and work place are considerable. So, for these among other reasons, exercise has been recommended as a remedy. In Canada, Genevieve Dumas and her colleagues considered that faulty posture is the key to the problem of back pain (1995). So their photographic research tracked women's changing lumbar and thoracic curvatures and the laxity of knee ligaments. Statistical calculations suggested that the woman's weight gain might affect her posture, but these researchers could find no link between exercise and changes in posture. On this basis they concluded that exercise, as per Canadian government recommendations, has no effect and certainly confers no benefits for posture.

A more recent blinded RCT, though, recruited 107 women in the latter half of pregnancy to undertake exercise for 1 hour three times per week (Garshasbi & Zadeh 2005). The control group comprised 102 women. The benefits to the intervention group were found to include a lowering of the intensity of back pain compared with when they began the exercise programme. In the control group, however, the back pain increased with advancing pregnancy. Interestingly, these researchers found that the women's lordosis was unrelated to their back pain and unaffected by exercise.

Although we have for some time understood how common back pain is in pregnancy, we have not long been able to assess the significance of the so-called 'backache' that women encounter (Kristiansson et al. 1996). These researchers assessed function and identified the 'great difficulties with normal activities' (1996: 703) which back pain causes to 30% of pregnant women. Even more recently it has been possible to build on this picture and show that 8% of pregnant women face severe disability and serious problems persist after the birth for about 7% of women (Wu et al. 2004: 575).

Symphysis pubis diastasis/dysfunction   Together with back pain, symphysis pubis pain is the other main contributor to pregnancy-related pelvic girdle pain (PPGP). The symphysis pubis may separate to differing extents, resulting in different terminology. The less severe degree of separation, symphysis pubis dysfunction (SPD), is present when the joint becomes sufficiently relaxed to cause instability of the joint and, hence, the pelvic girdle. If the symphysis pubis is more seriously separated, there may be some degree of rupture. Where the separation increases to more than 10 mm this is known as diastasis (Jain et al. 2006), an unusual term defined as 'forcible separation of bones without fracture' (Mondofacto 2009).

There are at least three causes of SPD. Postnatal SPD is most likely to be due to traumatic separation during the birth. This may be associated with the second cause, which is the non-infectious inflammation of the symphysis, pubic bones and nearby structures, known as osteitis pubis. Both of these forms of SPD will be addressed in Chapter 10.

The major cause of SPD in pregnancy relates to the physiological changes in the symphysis in preparation for childbirth. The increased laxity of the symphysis, which is regarded as hormonally induced, permits greater mobility of this joint and, presumably, facilitates childbirth. These changes may be hard to envisage as 'forcible separation', so probably better fit the definition of 'dysfunction'.

The gap between the pubic bones outwith pregnancy measures about 4–5 mm, increasing to about 7.7 mm by term, although varying between 3–20 mm. In 24% of women the gap at term is over 9 mm (Jain et al. 2006: 154). Regardless of the timing or the aetiology, the pain of SPD is remarkably similar in quality, if not severity. It begins as well-localised to the symphysis, being shooting, burning or stabbing in nature; particularly disconcerting is the grinding or audible clicking on walking. The pain also radiates up into the woman's lower abdomen, down into her perineum, thigh and leg and round to her back. The pain results in difficulty in walking, especially ascending or descending stairs, and in rising to stand. The pain changes the woman's gait into a waddle. Weight bearing activities are seriously curtailed, such as standing on one leg or lifting/separating the legs. Turning in bed is also problematical.

Caring for the woman in labour involves avoiding abduction of the hips. The posture for the birth may involve the midwife using some ingenuity; she may suggest kneeling or other upright supported positions, or possibly a lateral position. Pain ordinarily disappears soon after the birth, but women may suffer for months afterwards and occasionally pain persists much longer. At 6 months after the birth the reported proportion of affected women still suffering SPD symptoms varies from 0–25%.

Because SPD tends to be unfamiliar, and by its very nature the pain is isolating, the woman may experience psychosocial difficulties. She may find help in a Symphysis Pubis Diastasis Support Group, such as that organised by the National Childbirth Trust (DIWB 2009), the Pelvic Partnership (2009) or the Pelvic Instability Network Scotland (PINS) (Finlayson 2009).

Round ligament pain   Like PPGP (see above) the concept of round ligament pain raises further questions about the scientific nature of medical diagnosis. This form of pain, formerly relatively prominent, has been superseded by PPGP. The result is that it is now rarely mentioned, except in medical textbooks (Kumasaka 2005) and as a last ditch differential diagnosis for that diagnostic minefield – appendicitis in pregnancy (Pastore et al. 2006).

Carpal tunnel syndrome   Like many bodily changes during pregnancy, carpal tunnel syndrome (CTS) is usually assumed to be hormonally caused. Accounts of the incidence of CTS vary with the diagnostic criteria employed, but in a recent study of 259 pregnant women, 72 (28%) women spontaneously reported hand symptoms. Of these, 45 (17.4%) women were diagnosed with CTS using American Academy of Neurology criteria (Mondelli et al. 2007). If CTS happens, its onset is most likely in the last trimester, but rarely it begins soon after birth.

Recognised by the woman as a painful condition of one or both hands, CTS features tingling, numbness and 'pins and needles'. The area affected gradually extends to include the palmar surface of the thumb and three fingers innervated by the median nerve (index, middle and radial half of ring finger). If the condition does not limit itself, by the pregnancy ending at birth, this condition ultimately results in median nerve atrophy (Maldonado & Barger 1995).

CTS is a compression neuropathy, thought to be caused by the entrapment and compression of the median nerve by the surrounding tissues as it passes through the tunnel created by the carpal bones of the wrist. In pregnancy it is assumed that oedematous soft tissues cause pressure. A further aetiological factor is traction on the median nerve due to displacement of the shoulder girdle, attributable to lordosis. There may be other factors involved, however, as menopausal CTS is associated with reduced ligamentous support allowing the carpal tunnel bones to compress the median nerve.

In Mauro Mondelli and colleagues' study (2007), a large majority of those pregnant women whose CTS symptoms required treatment (18 = 40%) were treated conservatively with a back splint. Sometimes unfortunately termed a 'cock up splint', it was worn during pregnancy and for some months afterwards. For those for whom the splint was ineffective (3=7%), steroids and local anaesthetic were injected into carpal tunnel.

Another of the so-called 'minor disorders', CTS deserves to be taken more seriously; not only because of the risk of permanent nerve damage. There is also the disruption which sleepless nights cause to a woman who has multiple obligations, as well as the emotional trauma of being unable to uplift her new baby.

Cramp(s)   A form of pain in pregnancy which appears to be unusual in terms of its unpredictability and severity is the pain of leg cramps, or *systremma* (Ayres 1969). Cramp is a common problem featuring painful spasm of the calf or gastrocnemius muscle. Estimates of incidence vary, but may reach 50% of pregnant women (Young & Jewell 2004).

The nature of cramps may be too familiar to justify being described. It is necessary, though, to differentiate these 'paraphysiological cramps' (Parisi et al. 2003: 178) from those of idiopathic or pathological origin. These researchers define cramps:

- usually foot and/or calf muscles affected;
- associated with muscular tension, local pain and abnormal posture; and
- relief by stretching or massage (2003: 176).

Usually assumed to be nocturnal (Man-Son-Hing & Wells 1995), cramps commonly occur during labour and early post-natal period.

Problems are due not only to the pain of cramps, but to their frequency and the disturbance in lifestyle due to their nocturnal occurrence, as each episode may last for several minutes (El-Tawil et al. 2004). In their study, Lars Dahle and colleagues found that 88% of 73 pregnant sufferers experienced them only nocturnally, but the others experienced them in daytime too (1995). The median frequency was alternate nights, showing high levels of disturbance. Cramps increase towards term but are unrelated to other complications or perinatal morbidity.

An authoritative study of muscular cramps by Parisi and colleagues concluded that 'the causes and mechanisms are not clear' (2003: 178). A systematic review suggested precipitating factors, such as reclining posture due to the gravid uterus compressing nerves supplying the legs; pointing toes when stretching legs or walking is also blamed (Young & Jewell 2004). This review implicates chemical imbalance, especially the build up of lactic and pyruvic acids, necessitating pharmacological intervention.

Whereas the other symptomatic conditions have attracted the attention of, if not researchers, at least clinicians, leg cramps are unusual in the number of remedies that have been proposed. Following a literature review, it was recommend that simple remedies 'are surely worth trying', such as massage of and heat over the affected muscle and stretching the muscle by standing on the affected limb (Bracken et al. 1989). Unfortunately the lack of any known cause has acted as a stimulus rather than a deterrent to pharmacological remedies. Quinine (Brasic 1999), vitamin D (Asvar et al. 1996) and magnesium therapy (Koebnick et al. 2005) are among the many pharmacological preparations that have been recommended and, presumably, administered; although quinine has been incriminated as having oxytocic effects. These remedies indicate the supposed aetiology of leg cramps in pregnancy.

Because the posture of leg cramps appears to resemble hypocalcaemic tetany, the main pharmacological intervention has involved mineral supplementation, including both calcium and magnesium. An authoritative study of magnesium supplementation by Christine Roffe and colleagues (2002), showed no improvement. Thus, not only women's but also their families' lives are likely to continue to be disrupted by this pain of unknown origin.

Pain of cardiovascular origin

Changes in the circulatory system which cause pain during pregnancy include varicosites and thromboembolic conditions. The former is the subject of much non-research-based advice (Quijano & Abalos 2005). Because both of these groups of conditions cause more problems postnatally than during pregnancy and because thromboembolic conditions cause more serious problems postnatally (Drife 2007), I address them in Chapter 10.

Other painful 'minor disorders'

As well as conditions related to the digestive tract and musculo-skeletal system, others also cause pain in pregnancy. Similarly, they attract little research or clinical interest.

Braxton Hicks contractions

Although the myometrium contracts rhythmically and usually painlessly throughout a woman's reproductive life, it is minimally active during pregnancy. The contractions which do happen are named eponymously for John Braxton Hicks who first described them in the nineteenth century (Hicks 1871). Braxton Hicks contractions are weaker than those of labour, peaking at 15 mm/Hg (Llewellyn-Jones 1973; Garfield & Maner 2007). Those nearer 15 mm/Hg are palpable by an attendant, but the woman's awareness of these contractions, however, is uncertain, as is whether or not they are painful.

Braxton Hicks contractions are significant for a number of reasons. First, in my experience, some women feel them as painful throughout pregnancy; for this reason the woman may appreciate being taught coping strategies. Second, these contractions differ only qualitatively from labour, so diagnosing labour may, thus, be confounded; perhaps the transition to labour contractions may only be identified with hindsight (Lauzon & Hodnett 2001), which illustrates the intensity of Braxton Hicks contractions. Third, the purpose of Braxton Hicks contractions is often described in terms of a 'practice' (Kitzinger 1987a: 211), suggesting that the uterus is preparing for labour. Alternatively, as mentioned above, they may present the woman with opportunities to practise coping strategies prior to labour beginning. Fourth, the marked positive correlation between fetal movements and Braxton Hicks contractions indicates their part in the process by which the woman comes to know her fetus as an individual (Mulder & Visser 1987). Fifth, and most significantly physiologically, Braxton Hicks contractions encourage circulation of blood through the placental intervillous spaces. In this way, by intermittently increasing the pressure of blood behind the placenta, fetal oxygenation and nutrition are facilitated (Hytten & Chamberlain 1991).

Thus, Braxton Hicks contractions, though subjected to minimal research attention, may be perceived by the childbearing woman as negative and unexpectedly painful. Alternatively, she may regard them more positively as learning opportunities, as chances to relate to the baby or as fetal growth enhancers.

Pruritis/itching

Perhaps because of its association with socially unacceptable problems, such as sexually transmitted conditions, pruritis (unrelated to liver disease) has received even less attention than other *minor disorders*. Whether it qualifies as *painful* is questionable; I would argue, though, that the unpleasantness of pruritis (Young & Jewell 1997) allows it to be included.

Longstanding work reflects the scientific unpopularity of this topic (Read 1977). This work, although limited in its value, represents the sum total of English language publications on pruritis unrelated to liver disease in pregnancy. It found antihistamines effective in relieving itching in a large majority of women (93%) if it was associated with a rash, but aspirin was ineffective. The reverse situation pertained in the absence of a rash, with 95% of women finding relief in aspirin. There were methodological limitations to this work and there was no attention to fetal/neonatal effects.

Research into the 'minor disorders'

Research and other interest in these conditions has been hampered by the disproportionately low level of concern they cause to carers compared with the effects on the childbearing woman (Lee 1998). Further, as well as being painful, many symptoms are inevitably associated with disruption of the woman's lifestyle (Rodriguez et al. 2001). Thus, the research attention paid to these symptoms continues to be minimal:

> It is surprising how the most prevalent and discomforting symptoms of pregnancy have received such little study in properly controlled trials (Bracken et al. 1989)

What research there has been has tended to focus on interventions to treat the symptoms (NICE 2008) or on single case studies. While, clearly, treatment matters, the significance of these conditions for the woman and her carers also merits attention.

These conditions may conveniently be categorised according to their level of unpleasantness. For example, leucorrhoea is unpleasant and inconvenient, but nausea and vomiting impairs the woman's functioning more seriously (Smith et al. 2000). It may be for this reason, or perhaps because of the potential for medicinal intervention, that nausea and vomiting has been subjected to more research scrutiny than other, more painful, minor disorders.

The general lack of research attention and possible clinical disinterest in the minor disorders may be attributable to one or more of a number of factors. These conditions are clearly not life-threatening to either woman or baby. Thus, they may be seen by maternity care providers as being outwith their field of interest. As the conditions are self-limiting (Everitt et al. 2003), intervention may not be a priority. Alternatively, ignorance of the gravity of these conditions for the pregnant woman, her lifestyle and her family relationships may reduce practitioners' interest in them.

More serious conditions associated with pregnancy

There are certain painful conditions which, though not unique to pregnancy, are likely to cause health problems for the woman and, possibly, the baby.

Urinary tract infection

Just as Braxton Hicks contractions may confound diagnosing the onset of labour, the woman with a painful urinary tract infection (UTI) may have difficulty differentiating the intermittent pain of renal origin from uterine contractions. An accurate diagnosis may prove similarly elusive for her carers, as when distinguishing between the pain of UTI, premature labour and placental abruption. Also, like labour, UTI pain presents in various forms and of varying intensity, depending largely on the location of the infection (Stables & Novak 1999). Additionally, one form of UTI, asymptomatic bacteriuria (ASB/ABU) is, by definition, only diagnosable on urinary microbiological examination (Nicolle 2006).

Even covert UTIs carry the potential for serious maternal and fetal morbidity (Smaill & Vazquez 2007). Through a retrospective cohort analysis of the records of 25, 746 childbearing women, Shieve and colleagues (1994) established the relationship between UTI, hypertension, anaemia and amnionitis. The fetal/neonatal effects, however, of maternal UTI are less clear. While the association between UTI and premature labour/birth is apparent, it is uncertain whether the link is direct or indirect, such as through social class (Cunningham & Lucas 1994). The positive correlation between UTI and low birth weight is better-established (Schultz et al. 1991).

Although a descending route of infection occasionally occurs, ascending infection is more common (Stables & Novak 1999). Perineal commensal organisms, such as *E.Coli*, *Klebsiella pneumoniae* and *Proteus mirabilis*, enter the urethra and proceed to infect the bladder and/or kidney(s). The widely recognised phenomenon of certain women experiencing repeated

UTIs is explained by the adhesive attraction between certain organisms and the woman's uroepithelium. Whereas the adhesins carried by most organisms are weak and washed away by fluid in the urinary tract, certain organisms carried by a minority of people have developed more secure attachments. An example is *P-fimbriated Escherichia coli*, vulnerability to which is associated with certain blood groups (Cunningham & Lucas 1994).

The symptoms of UTI invariably include pain. In cystitis, inflammation of the bladder lining, dysuria presents as stinging when voiding urine as well as suprapubic pain (Higgins 1995). The pain is due to acid urine irritating inflamed tissues. In addition to dysuria the woman with pyelonephritis, infection of the renal pelvis, experiences lumbar pain, which radiates into the abdomen (Vazquez & Villar 2003).

Depending on severity, intravenous fluids, anti-emetics and analgesic medication may be prescribed, with antimicrobial drugs. The woman's pain may be amenable to simple remedies, such as heat over the painful lumbar area, or she may require analgesic drugs, possibly by injection if she is nauseated. The woman may benefit from advice about preventing further UTIs, such as perineal hygiene, avoiding bladder irritants and precautions relating to sex (Olds et al. 1996). For centuries cranberry juice has been justifiably recommended to prevent and limit UTIs (Raz et al. 2004); this acts by reducing pathogens' adhesion to the uroepithelium.

It is necessary to consider the possibility of UTIs being caused iatrogenically. Catheterisation is widely, even routinely, used in labour and birth; this is surprising in view a UTI rate of 3–6%/day post-catheterisation in general hospitals (Moulder 2008). Statistics of post-catheterisation infection among new mothers are unavailable, but such information should be provided to maternity staff, if for no other reason than providing feedback on aseptic technique.

Thus, although UTIs are sometimes regarded as a joke because of their link with sexual activity, their implications for the childbearing woman and her baby are anything but funny. Similarly, their reflection on practice merits serious attention.

Sickle cell disease

The management of pain during a crisis is but one of the major issues raised by sickle cell disease (SCD), a family of blood disorders which, together with the thalassaemias, comprise the haemoglobinopathies (Oteng-Ntim et al. 2008). SCD is inherited through an autosomal recessive gene, making it most common in sub-Saharan Africa and among people who, or whose ancestors, have migrated thence. It also occurs among peoples who originated in the countries surrounding the Mediterranean, and further east in the Indian sub-continent and Albania. In the UK about 0.2% of people of African or Caribbean origin have SCD. This makes the condition more common than cystic fibrosis or haemophilia (Anionwu & Atkin 2001).

Responsible for the transport of oxygen, haemoglobin (Hb) is the iron-rich pigment in red blood cells (RBCs). Ordinarily, in adult blood, the Hb is HbA, but in SCD HbS is present in varying proportions (Singer 1985). Although genetic constitutions vary, people who are homozygous (having two genes or alleles for HbS) present with sickle cell disease. People who are heterozygous (having one gene for HbS and one for HbA) have the less serious sickle cell trait (Pur et al. 2007).

In hypoxic conditions, the RBCs of a person with SCD distort into a crescent or 'sickle' shape (Mueller & Young 1995). This is because in people with SCD a miniscule difference in an amino acid chain causes a unique reaction between the molecules within HbS. Hypoxia causes the molecules to form a rigid structure which produces the 'sickling', although the majority resume their biconcave shape when reoxygenated. It is sickling which causes both the acute and long term problems which the person with SCD faces. First, the RBC's cell membrane is damaged by sickling, leading to faster breakdown and haemolytic anaemia. Second, sickled RBCs are less malleable and block small arteries, depriving tissues of oxygen and leading to infarction and necrosis. Third, the immediate impact of these microscopic areas of infarction in bones and tissues includes pain, and constitutes a sickle cell crisis (Oteng-Ntim et al. 2008).

The painful crisis is the principal cause of morbidity among people with SCD. Crises are unpredictable and vary in severity from mild discomfort for a few minutes to weeks of severe generalised pain; they often require admission for treatment with opioids (Anionwu 1996).

The risks of SCD are no less during pregnancy:

> the majority of women with sickle cell disease in the UK now survive to have children. However, their pregnancies are associated with a high incidence of maternal and perinatal morbidity and mortality. (Oteng-Ntim et al. 2008: 272)

The risks are largely due to the greater frequency of sickle cell crises, which in the UK increases maternal and fetal morbidity and mortality. Research by Richard Howard and his colleagues (1995a) involved 81 pregnant women with SCD and a control group comprising 100 women of similar ethnic background with no haemoglobinopathy. The SCD group experienced two maternal deaths and a perinatal mortality rate of 60/1000. The women in the SCD group were also significantly more likely to develop anaemia and have low birth weight babies.

Although the treatment of SCD in pregnancy is under-researched (Martí-Carvajal et al. 2009), rest, hydration and analgesia are recommended during a pain crisis in pregnancy, together with reassurance of its transience (Koshy 1995). Mabel Koshy, like Howard and colleagues (1995a), discusses the role of exchange transfusion in pregnancy. Koshy links infection in a range of sites with the precipitation of a crisis, as does Felix Konotey-Ahulu (1991), who suggests that UTI, rather than pregnancy, is the precipitating factor.

Personal, political and organisational issues are raised by SCD, which apply particularly during pregnancy. On a personal level, the woman may find difficulty in adjusting to the change in her SCD, which she will have been managing since childhood. She may come to resent the close monitoring of her condition during pregnancy by people who, she may consider, do not know her SCD as well as she does. Thus, 'women should be advised to report ... impending crisis, and not to self-manage (as they might do out of pregnancy)' (Oteng-Ntim et al. 2008: 275).

Staff attitudes to people in sickle cell crisis bring the potential for mutual distrust (Anionwu 1996). This relates to the possibility of opioid analgesia causing addiction or facilitating drug dealing. Anionwu's observations are supported by research into the perceptions of patients and staff about the treatment of crisis pain (Waters & Thomas 1995), which demonstrated staff ignorance as well as the difficulty of translating such knowledge as existed into practice. Unsurprisingly, such uninformed findings lead to accusations of 'individual and institutional racism' (Anionwu & Atkin 2001: 2).

While recognising the risks that maternal SCD carries for the woman and baby, it is necessary to recall that

> women with major sickle haemoglobinopathies can have a good reproductive outcome. This has been achieved through appropriate counselling, aggressive prenatal care and effective intervention by care providers with a high index of suspicion for predisposing factors to untoward outcomes. (Oteng-Ntim et al. 2008: 277)

Abdominal pain of non-uterine origin

Abdominal pain in pregnancy is confused by the huge anatomical changes occurring in the abdomen at this time (Boothby 2005). As well as predisposing to certain conditions, these changes impede the diagnosis of the cause of abdominal pain, such as acute appendicitis, and its treatment. In this section I focus on the frequency and implications of the more significant conditions.

The general impression is that acute appendicitis occurs more frequently during pregnancy than outwith it, in association with the previously mentioned gastrointestinal changes (To et al. 1995). However, pregnancy does not affect the incidence, at about 1 in 5000 pregnancies (Nair 2005). The significance of appendicitis in pregnancy derives, therefore, not from an increased incidence, but from the problems relating to diagnosis and resulting poor maternal/fetal/neonatal prognosis.

Unquestionably the principal diagnostic feature is abdominal pain, which during the first trimester presents in the usual position, McBurney's point, in the right lower abdominal quadrant. This diagnostic indicator becomes less reliable as pregnancy progresses, giving rise to, possibly associated with increasing incidence in the second trimester, increasing mortality. The pain of appendicitis, and the accompanying extreme local tenderness, are located higher in the abdomen in advanced pregnancy. As well as pain and tenderness, the usual picture of abdominal guarding and rigidity may be absent due to enlargement. The other symptoms often accompanying appendicitis, such as nausea, vomiting and urinary frequency, are common in pregnancy, further confounding diagnosis.

In a series of 31 pregnant women with appendicitis, four miscarriages and one neonatal death occurred (To et al. 1995). As well as perinatal risks, ruptured appendix and peritonitis happen at least twice as frequently in pregnant women as in their non-pregnant sisters, probably associated with difficulty in diagnosis and hence delay in treatment (Boothby 2005: 23). Thus, accurate diagnosis of appendicitis is crucial to reduce perinatal and maternal mortality and morbidity. The differential diagnosis of the 'acute abdomen' in pregnancy includes pregnancy-related conditions, for example, abruptio placenta, together with gastrointestinal conditions, for example, biliary tract disease, intestinal obstruction, Crohn's disease or UTI (Boothby 2005). The importance of 'proper assessment' of pregnant women experiencing abdominal pain emerged from a retrospective study, which found that, of women between 20 and 37 weeks' gestation with abdominal pain, in the majority no diagnosis was ever made (Impey & Hughes 1995).

These researchers argue that, in the absence of tenderness, guarding, peritonism or a positive urine culture, hospital admission is unnecessary. Considering the serious implications of hospital admission for the woman's family relationships, caution about admission may be justified.

Serious problems unique to pregnancy

Certain painful conditions occur only during pregnancy. Probably to a greater extent than painful conditions mentioned already, these present a threat, if not to the continuation of the pregnancy, at least to maternal and fetal/neonatal health. For this reason the pain featuring in these conditions is more a diagnostic or prognostic tool than a problem in itself.

Miscarriage

A pregnancy may be accidentally lost before becoming viable which, in the UK, is currently set at 24 weeks gestation. This painful loss may take one of a number of forms, including spontaneous abortion and ectopic pregnancy. While the circumstances differ, the word 'miscarriage' is widely used to include these various forms of loss (SPCERH 2003). The loss of *biological* pregnancies may be much higher, but clinically-recognised miscarriages are estimated to occur in over 10–20% of all pregnancies (SPCERH 2003). The frequency of miscarriage leads some to regard it as a 'normal' event. This information may be used to 'comfort' the woman who has experienced a miscarriage, by telling her that it is 'nature's way' of preventing the birth of a baby with disabilities. Such denigration of her experience may eventually lead to the baby being termed 'product of conception' or 'POC' (Forna & Gülmezoglu 2009).

In the process of miscarriage the woman may seek help at one of a number of stages; that is, when miscarriage threatens, when it becomes inevitable, or when miscarriage becomes either incomplete or complete. When miscarriage seems possible, it is necessary for ectopic pregnancy and hydatidiform mole to be excluded, as both of these conditions bring particularly serious physical implications for the mother in addition to the emotional burden which miscarriage brings (Mander 2006). It is necessary at this point to mention the different types of pain associated with miscarriage. The pain of grief following miscarriage is now widely and appropriately recognised, but its physical pain is regarded as less significant. I discussed the relationship between physical and emotional pain in Chapter 2.

Vaginal bleeding is almost invariably the first symptom when miscarriage threatens and, perhaps for this reason, is regarded as a more significant feature. It may be that the relationship between the appearance of bleeding and the onset of pain indicates an ectopic pregnancy, but this sequence is of little value when suitable diagnostic tools are available. Nevertheless, pain is a more consistent feature of ectopic pregnancy than vaginal bleeding.

The pain of miscarriage has been compared with menstrual pain, being intermittent and cramp-like and intensifying as the uterine contractions strengthen. This information does not help women who have experienced neither menstrual nor labour pain. Because the significance of the pain is widely regarded as more important than its nature (Fleuren et al. 1994), its severity may be disregarded.

Placental abruption

The premature separation of a normally situated placenta or placental abruption (Ananth & Wilcox 2001) is a condition of pregnancy in which the seriousness of the clinical picture and the risk of morbidity and mortality vary hugely. Sometimes referred to as *accidental* antepartum haemorrhage to differentiate it from the *inevitable* haemorrhage of placenta praevia, in only placental abruption may the haemorrhage *not* be revealed vaginally.

In this situation the woman would be likely to experience greater pain because of the retention or concealment of blood in the retroplacental space and its infiltration between the fibres of the myometrium (Stables & Novak 1999). Vaginal bleeding is prevented by their being no escape route for the blood. Such an extreme condition presents as an 'acute abdomen' with profound hypovolaemic shock. There may be severe, continuous abdominal pain and the uterus is wood-hard and tender. There is, however, a range of intensity of pain which the woman may experience, from none, through uterine tenderness, to abdominal pain. The increasing intensity of the pain is due to haemorrhagic episodes, presumably as the retroplacental clot accumulates, increasing in volume within its confined space. The pain is 'sharp, tearing or burning' and 'unrelenting' in nature (Nathan & Huddleston 1995: 57). Labour contractions may be superimposed on the continuous pain, but whether the onset of labour is due to extravasated blood irritating the myometrium into activity or whether there is fetal chemical involvement is uncertain.

Placental abruption is such a significant condition because of its contribution to both perinatal and maternal mortality and morbidity. Perinatal loss is due to that portion of the placenta which has separated being non-functional. Salma Kayani and colleagues' review of severe cases found that one third involved a poor perinatal outcome, meaning that 8 out of 33 babies died and three suffered brain damage (2003). This series, unusually, encountered no maternal morbidity or mortality.

Diagnosis is a major clinical problem, being made in 0.6–1.0% of births (Ananth & Wilcox 2001). As mentioned at the beginning of this section, the severity of abruption varies hugely, as changes indicating abruption were found in up to 4.5% of placentae (Fox 1978). For these reasons, the treatment is problematical due to uncertainty about whether to initiate surgery, for the baby's sake, which may jeopardise the woman's life (Kayani et al. 2003). The intensity of the woman's pain, which aggravates her shock, means that maternal resuscitation and analgesia are clearly priorities. Opioids are indicated, despite their hypotensive effects.

Unlike most painful conditions of pregnancy, the problems for the woman with placental abruption do not end with the birth. The coagulation defects and anaemia, which began antenatally, will have been corrected effectively by blood transfusion; however, coagulopathies may actually be aggravated postnatally due to myometrial damage and reduced contractility, caused by extravasated blood. Thus, the woman who has experienced placental abruption, and its dreadful sequelae, is also vulnerable to postpartum haemorrhage and further morbidity.

Severe or fulminating pre-eclampsia

Although the condition that precedes it has changed its name, eclampsia remains the state of having or having had an eclamptic convulsion. Eclampsia is usually preceded by pre-eclampsia (PE), which is associated with pregnancy induced hypertension (PIH) featuring rising blood pressure during pregnancy. Proteinuria confirms the diagnosis of pre-eclampsia. In both PE and PIH, only signs appear, so the woman feels well. It is only when pre-eclampsia becomes severe and eclampsia threatens that the woman complains of symptoms and feels unwell, in the form of pain and visual disturbances. She typically reports headache and 'epigastric' pain, felt in the right upper abdominal quadrant due to the oedematous liver stretching its capsule (Nair 2005).

There is a danger that this pain may be overlooked, which happens if a woman is admitted in advanced labour and, with no time to check her blood pressure, syntometrine is administered with dire consequences (Neilson 2007: 76). The UK Confidential Enquiries into Maternal Deaths report that headache may similarly be overlooked, as happened when a new mother attended Accident & Emergency with headache and epigastric pain. Her blood pressure was 155/95 mm/Hg, having previously been around 90–120/50–60 mm/Hg. Her urine was not tested. An obstetric SHO was contacted, but did not attend the woman. Discharged home, she collapsed and died of intracranial haemorrhage (Neilson 2007: 76).

These forms of pain herald an eclamptic fit. The headache of fulminating pre-eclampsia is severe, persistent, frontal/occipital and accompanied by visual disturbances, caused by retinal oedema. A woman recently described her fulminating pre-eclamptic headache to me as 'like a migraine only ten times worse'. The onset of eclamptic convulsions is attributed to cerebral vasospasm, yielding ischaemic areas causing abnormal electrical activity (Stables & Novak 1999).

The significance of severe pre-eclampsia lies in its unpredictable nature combined with its dire prognosis for woman and baby. That most practitioners in developed countries have never witnessed eclampsia only serves to aggravate these problems. In the UK 18 women died of eclampsia or pre-eclampsia between 2003 and 2005 (CEMACH 2007). Of the estimated 50 000 women who die annually from eclampsia, 99% die in low and middle income countries (Aaserud et al. 2005).

Thus, the international significance of eclampsia and its treatment is unquestionable. The MAGPIE trial (2002) established magnesium sulphate as the appropriate treatment, rather than other anticonvulsants (Duley et al. 2008). Although widely disseminated, the efficacy of this safe and disconcertingly cheap remedy has yet to impact on maternal mortality and morbidity in low-income countries. The study of this problem reached the heartrending conclusion that policy makers need more than information if practice is to change (Aaserud 2005).

Our limited knowledge of eclampsia remains; further, little is known of the woman's experience of this devastating condition, especially relating to her disappointed expectations of healthy childbearing. Additionally, knowledge is lacking concerning how health care personnel cope with the possibility of conditions such as eclampsia which appear like 'a bolt from the blue'. It is not only their unpredictability which may be hard for staff, but also the possibility that they may incur maternal and perinatal loss.

Incidental (non-childbearing) pain

There are a number of painful conditions which may coincide with pregnancy and child-bearing. The extent to which the conditions affect the pregnancy or the pregnancy affects the condition is variable.

Cancer

Because we live in a pronatalist society in which cancerophobia prevails, the pregnant woman with cancer encounters diametrically conflicting responses both in herself and others. While pregnancy engenders optimistic pleasure, cancer brings pessimistic horror. In terms of its numerical significance, North American literature suggests that cancer complicates 1 in 1000 pregnancies (Leslie 2005). Drawing on a UK perspective, Gwyneth Lewis et al. (2007) translate this into one case per 6000 live births. These latter authors warn, though, that this figure may be misleadingly lowered by difficulties in diagnosing certain cancers during pregnancy.

A number of sites may be affected; tissues most commonly involved include the breast, the cervix, the skin and the thyroid, where tumours are reported as being painless. On the other hand, in pregnancy cancer of the gastrointestinal tract, the lung, the ovary, the brain and bony tissue does tend to cause pain of variable intensity. Although rarely seen in pregnancy, bony tumours, such as sarcoma, are *very painful* because of myelitis affecting nerve roots.

The issues around this topic are many and complex and mean that the pregnant woman with cancer and those near her will face hard decisions. The literature suggests that these decisions focus on the relative interests of the mother and baby, with a particular emphasis on the continuation or duration of the pregnancy (Leslie et al. 2005; Oduncu et al. 2003). Pain associated with cancer during pregnancy, attracts little attention in comparison with these life and death issues. Wen and colleagues (1996) address this problem to a limited extent, in that they consider the risks of long term opioid therapy, but only to the fetus. This brings physical dependence on the drug, causing acute withdrawal symptoms and growth retardation neonatally. The woman's experience of the pain directly attributable to the tumour and its effect on nearby structures is neglected. In addition to this direct pain, there is that caused by investigations and therapeutic interventions. Additionally, the inevitable emotional pain should not be underestimated (Mander in press).

Rheumatoid arthritis

Rheumatoid arthritis, an autoimmune condition involving long term inflammation of synovial joints, such as knees, interphalangeal and metacarpophalangeal joints, presents with morning stiffness pain, joint tenderness and pain on movement. Vulnerability to rheumatoid arthritis is genetically determined, and women are more at risk than men.

For a majority of pregnant women with rheumatoid arthritis, pregnancy alleviates painful symptoms (Østensen & Villiger 2002). The bad news manifests itself in the first trimester as *overwhelming* fatigue and postnatally as an exacerbation or 'flare up' of the condition. The pregnant woman with rheumatoid arthritis is said to have a fine line to tread between sufficient exercise to maintain mobility and excessive activity aggravating fatigue (Carty et al. 1986). This line becomes even more difficult to identify postnatally with the demands of a new baby.

Medication is the mainstay of treatment, and the regime is modified prior to conception to reduce the risk of drug-induced fetal damage. In the event, however, of unplanned conception the woman may be up to 8 weeks pregnant before the regime is modified. Opinions differ on the teratogenicity of medication used to treat rheumatoid arthritis, and this prevents reassurance being offered to the woman with an unplanned pregnancy (Carty et al. 1986). This point should be discussed with the woman with rheumatoid arthritis during family planning counselling. The questionable medications include non-steroidal anti-inflammatory drugs (NSAIDs) like indomethacin as well as immunosuppressants, penicillamine and gold. Corticosteroids in low doses are considered safe, but the risk of neonatal adrenocortical insufficiency persists. Because of their link with platelet dysfunction, low birth weight and stillbirth, salicylates are avoided in pregnancy (Carty et al. 1986).

Thus, the woman with rheumatoid arthritis would benefit from counselling about the risks of childbearing before the conception, both for her own sake and her child's. Canadian research into childbirth education for the woman with rheumatoid arthritis suggests that neither counselling nor information relating to sexuality or contraception is available (Carty & Conine 1983). While recognising the importance of midwifery intervention, researchers suggest that women who have personal experience of this condition are ideally placed to assist others (Lipson & Rogers 2000).

Systemic lupus erythematosus

Like rheumatoid arthritis (see above) systemic lupus erythematosus (SLE or 'lupus') is an autoimmune condition presenting as a collagen tissue disease. Unlike rheumatoid arthritis, which is tissue specific, SLE affects various body systems. These two important conditions are further similar in their likelihood of causing joint pain during pregnancy, although the related issues differ markedly.

SLE is a complex disease, influenced by hormonal, genetic/racial and environmental factors; it involves production of antiphospholipid autoantibodies causing inflammation and tissue damage in varied sites, resulting in typically varied features (Khamashta & Hughes 1996). The feature making SLE relevant in the present context is the arthritic joint pain experienced by virtually all people with this condition. Other characteristic features are splenomegaly, thrombocytopaenia, nephritis, thrombosis and skin changes.

During pregnancy the progress of the disease is not affected; similarly the maternal risks are limited to pre-eclampsia, unless there is gross renal or vascular impairment (Khamashta & Hughes 1996). Like rheumatoid arthritis, SLE goes into remission or at least stabilises during pregnancy, although antibodies survive in the woman's circulation; the tendency for a postnatal exacerbation bears comparison with rheumatoid arthritis. The treatment of SLE depends largely on corticosteroids and immunosuppressive therapy, and during pregnancy prednisolone, azathioprine, cyclosporin A and hydroxychloroquin are regarded as safe (Khamashta 2006). Paracetamol and codeine-based analgesia may be used, and are preferred for pain control.

The preconceptual advice given in a multidisciplinary 'lupus clinic' focuses on the exacerbations (flares); in pregnancy these most frequently involve musculoskeletal and/or cutaneous symptoms, confirming the importance of pain for this woman during pregnancy (Ruiz-Irastorza et al. 1996). These researchers concluded that pregnancy aggravates SLE significantly, activity being worst in the second trimester, and that exacerbations are unaffected by prednisolone.

Unlike other conditions which we have considered, the serious significance of SLE lies not in its effect on the mother's health, nor in the adverse effects of medication on the fetus, but in the effect of the disease, that is maternal antibodies, on the fetus. While the maternal-fetal passage of antibodies in the form of immunoglobulin G (IgG) may be beneficial to the neonate in conferring passive immunity, it may also be harmful. The transplacental passage of autoantibodies in the circulation of the mother with SLE have the potential to adversely affect the fetus/neonate.

Obviously these antibodies eventually disappear from the neonate's circulation, hopefully having caused no permanent damage. Unfortunately, in SLE such damage is a distinct possibility. This damage is likely to take the form of neonatal lupus erythematosus (Khamashta 2006), which varies hugely in the extent of the harm that it causes. The neonatal effects of the pathogenic maternal autoantibodies may be as benign as discoid lupus, which is brief and harmless. On the other hand, at the opposite extreme there may be hepatosplenomegaly, blood dyscrasias, skin changes and congenital complete heart block (CCHB). The extent of the problem is that CCHB occurs in 2% of babies of women with SLE; 24% of these babies die.

The childbearing decision by a woman with SLE needs particularly serious consideration. Preconception counselling and contraceptive advice facilitate the most appropriate timing of pregnancy. Munther Khamashta, though, is positive about current outcomes, rendering questions about termination of pregnancy less significant.

Conclusion

It is clear from this chapter that, as throughout a woman's life, pain in pregnancy is not uncommon. We have also seen that that pain is variable in both its intensity and significance. It is necessary to teach the woman to recognise when her own coping strategies are adequate and when others' interventions are likely to help. It has become apparent that on certain topics there is little research or education; this may be because the attraction of researching or teaching about non-life-threatening conditions is limited. The result is that many untested remedies have been introduced:

> the most prevalent and discomforting symptoms of pregnancy have received such little study in properly controlled trials (Bracken et al. 1989).

What has also emerged from this chapter is that the pain *per se* tends to be regarded by researchers and medical attendants as of limited significance. Because, through medicalisation, pregnancy has been transformed from an 'altered state of health' into a 'medical problem', those who provide care accept that, as with any health problems, some discomfort or pain is inevitable. My own unsystematic observation leads me to suspect that, for some women, this view prevails and a 'mustn't grumble' ethos is widespread.

Pain in pregnancy tends only to be taken seriously when it indicates a condition threatening the life of either the woman or baby. Even then, with the exception of placental abruption, the pain itself is not considered sufficiently important to deserve treatment, but rather it is hoped that it resolves as the underlying condition is treated.

Part III

The Journey

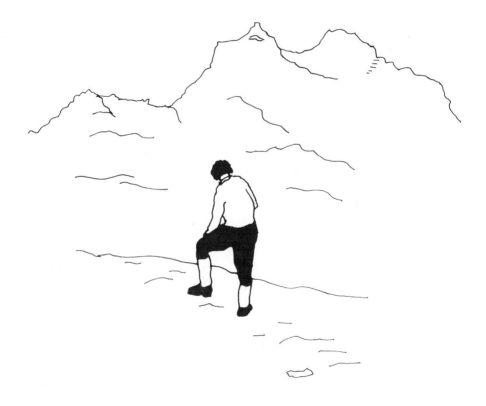

Chapter 7

Labour pain

While supposedly more tenuous as interventive pain control becomes more prevalent, links between labour and pain remain strong. A perceived inevitability about labour pain persists; if nothing more, this encourages the woman to contemplate her preferred coping strategies and pain control alternatives. Before considering childbearing as a journey (Halldorsdottir & Karlsdottir 1996), in which labour is a major component including 'pain and hard work', I contemplate pain. Together with influences on attitudes to labour pain, I take this opportunity to scrutinise ideas about the origins of labour pain.

Realities

In contemplating labour pain, questioning its existence seems quite unjustifiable. Despite this, questions emerge, endorsing persistent 'misunderstandings' between some medical practitioners and the women they attend. 'Proponents of natural childbirth' (Bonica 1990a: 1314) have been condemned for arguing the cultural component of labour pain, which is then demolished, along with criticisms of obstetric anaesthetic intervention, utilising unpublished data. The proponents, or labour-pain deniers, to whom John Bonica referred include, crucially, Grantly Dick-Read, who wrote:

> Pain of labour must therefore be accepted as a psychic stimulus, reproduced from misconceptions (1933: 52).

While accepting that labour pain exists, the role of such severe pain deserves attention, because pain is widely assumed to indicate real or potential damage (Chapter 2). Nancy Lowe unconvincingly envisages labour's role as alerting the woman to the impending birth in preparation for childcare (2002). Hardly less unlikely is Kate Niven's explanation when writing for Linda Jauncey:

> I have been known to remark facetiously that the real purpose of labour pain is to prepare women for the much greater pain of childrearing! (2008: 80).

More plausible is the likelihood that an evolutionary balance has been reached between the minimum viable size/maturity of the human fetus and the most intense endurable pain

Pain in Childbearing and its Control, Second Edition. By Rosemary Mander. Published 2011 by Blackwell Publishing Ltd.   © 1998, 2011 Rosemary Mander.

(Niven & Gijsbers 1996a). These researchers further incriminated human cerebral development relative to bipedal posture's reduced pelvic capacity.

As mentioned already, the link between pain and pathology is pervasive (Melzack & Wall 1991); this is counterproductive in labour, because this sociophysiological process becomes labelled 'illness'. Such labels bring with them the demand for intervention by illness experts – medical practitioners. These experts use objective measurements of intensity of labour pain (Melzack & Wall 1991; Niven 1992) which, when compared with common syndromes, as measured by a Pain Rating Index (PRI), exceeds disease conditions (Niven & Gijsbers 1984). These longstanding authoritative findings have been endorsed in 'grand multiparas', ordinarily assumed to experience less pain (Ranta et al. 1996).

This evidence matters because, like others, labour pain is fundamentally personal, private, unshared and unshareable. Although a woman makes assumptions about how her pain corresponds with others', this is unknowable, establishing the relevance of the cliché:

> Pain is whatever the experiencing person says it is, existing whenever [s]he says it does.
>
> McCaffery 1979

Certain physiological factors have been linked with variations in the severity of labour pain (Niven 1992; Lowe 2002). These factors include fetal size, primiparity, maternal stature, pain sensitivity and posture. The latter aspect and other interventions, such as amniotomy, raise the spectre of iatrogenesis. The impact of factors such as duration of labour are of less certain significance.

The significance of labour pain

Despite conundrums about the reality, purpose and intensity of labour pain, what remains unquestionable is that it matters. Its significance relates not only to the unpleasantness of pain at an otherwise joyful time. Pain matters further for its personal long term implications, about how the woman considers that she did or didn't handle her experience of giving birth.

Whether the woman 'handles' labour as she wishes has attracted much research attention under numerous guises. One of these is 'control', which was one of the 'Three Cs', alongside choice and continuity, intended to transform maternity care (DoH 1993). The variety of forms of control proved a source of confusion, unpicked by Jo Green and Helen Baston (2003). These researchers focussed on the woman's perception of external control (staff behaviour towards her) and her feelings of internal control (her own behaviour, including during contractions) in order to relate them to the positive or negative nature of the birth. All three forms of control were important to the woman in achieving a satisfying birth experience. External control while most significant, was least frequently achieved.

Not completely unrelated to control is the concept of self-efficacy (SE) (Bandura 1977); it comprises the belief that one can perform necessary behaviours to influence the outcome of an experience, in this context a satisfying birth. Lowe (2002) reports that higher SE correlates strongly with decreased pain perception and decreased medication/ analgesia use in labour. The relationship between SE and confidence is complex, as both are enhanced by experience of labour and by childbirth education. SE is associated with the woman having confidence to draw on various coping strategies which, clearly, allow her to assume greater control over the birth.

A further phenomenon which affects the woman's experience of labour pain is her 'fitness' (Gross et al. 2005; see section on 'Pain assessment tools in labour' in Chapter 2); the importance of which emerged in a study undertaken in Hanover, Germany. The researchers defined fitness as 'both physical and psychological strength (2005: 123). While Mechthild Gross and her colleagues recognise that fitness as a specific concept has not been studied previously, they also identify its significance in terms of being involved and assuming some control (2005: 127). They go on to relate such active involvement in labour as being positively associated with satisfaction with the birth.

Although I have discussed the meaning of pain in general (see section on 'Meanings' in Chapter 1), this research on control, self-efficacy and fitness lends new meanings to pain in labour (Vague 2003). Drawing on previous research, Stephanie Vague identifies the traditional medical assumption of the totally negative nature of labour pain. An important contributor to the rethink on labour pain is Nicky Leap, who espouses the transformatory nature of labour pain for the childbearing woman. Writing that labour pain is infinitely more than the expulsion of the baby from its intrauterine world:

> Pain marks an important transition, musters support, develops altruistic behaviour in mothers, triggers beneficial neuro-hormonal cascades and empowers women through an ensuing sense of achievement (1996: 67).

The sense of achievement brought by coping with labour pain carries with it personal growth. Through the fitness, self-efficacy and sense of control which the woman employs during labour, she is convinced that she has grown into a fully mature person (Leap & Anderson 2004). Hence, knowing that she can work though the pain of birth, she is likely to be able to summon up sufficient resources to mother this new human being to whom she has given birth. In this way the woman's ability to handle labour pain may correctly be regarded as life-changing or transformatory.

Tocophobia

While midwives emphasise the personal benefit of physiological childbirth, others achieve the reverse by accentuating fear of childbirth; this is not new, but shores up the burgeoning caesarean industry (Mander 2007). Tocophobia may derive from fear of labour pain, but other fears, such as hospitals, self-exposure, losing control or severing the bond with the 'inside baby', may also feature.

Tocophobia is defined as 'an unreasoning dread of childbirth ... so intense that childbirth is avoided whenever possible' (Hofberg & Brockington 2000: 83). These researchers identified women who had never been pregnant manifesting 'primary tocophobia'. The pain of labour appears to be the focus of their fears, on the grounds that an elective caesarean is presented as the solution to their phobia. 'Secondary tocophobia' is associated with a previous traumatising experience, such as instrumental/operative birth. This research attributes tocophobia to mental health problems following sexual abuse; it discusses the motivation for pregnancy as the 'overwhelming desire to be a mother [which was] their *raison d'être*' (2000: 83). Despite having been able to overcome fear sufficiently to conceive, some tocophobic women still resorted to termination of pregnancy when the reality of the possibility of childbirth dawned. Thus, these researchers demonstrate the *unreasoning* nature and *intensity* of this dread.

Clearly, a morbid and incapacitating fear of childbirth is all too real for some women. That this diagnosis, though, may be used by both women and their attendants to justify unnecessary caesareans, is a possibility. The question of who should be 'blamed' for this sorry state arises. Without actually naming it, Gian Carlo Di Renzo raises the potential for an unholy alliance; on one side is the pregnant woman seeking to avoid 'nature's obligations', while on the other side is the

> condescending obstetrician [avoiding attending] a labour while gaining more income and at the same time giving his patient the illusion of happiness (Di Renzo 2003: 217).

Clearly, the reality of tocophobia and the mis/use to which this term is put, are in need of serious research attention.

Stages of uncomplicated labour

Our understanding of the physiological factors that cause labour to be painful is less than adequate and tends to rely on the variably authoritative work of Bonica (1990a), which is echoed in Lowe (2002). As the cervix dilates and the lower segment forms, visceral pain predominates and, simultaneously, myometrial contractions cause some degree of ischaemic pain (Trout 2004). As the presenting part descends through the pelvis and reaches the pelvic floor and the perineum, somatic pain results from the associated stretching, pulling and, possibly, tearing. While describing pain according to 'stages' of labour is very convenient, Tricia Anderson (2007) argued that stages are no more than artificial constructs. She considered that such artifices serve only to impose an unnatural aura of science on women's unscientific labours. While accepting that shoehorning their labours into unrealistic categories does not benefit women, the experienced midwife is able to recognise changes in the woman's vocalisation and behaviour which indicate that birth may be imminent. Such changes are familiar during the transition phase, when the woman feels that her labour has become interminable and her resources are totally depleted. The creation of the 'transition', as it is sometimes known, supports Anderson's argument in that it serves as the signal to call the obstetrician to 'catch' the baby. The 'total pain' of transition (see section on 'Total pain' in Chapter 2), though, is also an opportunity for the midwife who recognises it to encourage the woman to persevere to achieve a satisfying birth.

Complicated labour

The idea of pain in 'complicated' labour begs many questions. These relate partly to the pain and whether it is due to the complication or due to the intervention introduced to resolve that complication. The questions also relate to the complicated labour itself and how this concept is defined. UK midwives are now effectively cornering the market in 'normality' (Downe 2004), but this USP (unique selling point) has developed without defining what this term or its antonyms, complicated or abnormal labour, mean. The demarcation between normal and complicated is not a fixed point, as it has been manipulated by experts in the abnormal to the disadvantage of the 'normality expert'. Such manipulation is recorded as having begun in 1902 in England, but the manipulation is now being exercised by midwives (Cronk 2005; Beech 2001/2). Thus, 'complicated' is coming to mean something other than merely outwith the midwife's province.

In this section, I consider certain conditions in which labour pain is different in terms of its significance and, possibly, its nature.

OP labour

The pain of an OP (occipito-posterior position) labour is part of midwifery folklore. This is because the care of this woman challenges all of the midwife's skills, as well as constituting an even greater challenge to the woman's endurance. OP labour, or back labour in North America, is due to the most common fetal malposition, occurring in up to 20% of labours (Ridley 2007). Calculating incidence is complicated by the problems of diagnosing OP position in early labour, compounded by anterior rotation of the head having started when labour becomes established.

Occurrence of OP labour is interestingly related to the pain control method often used by the woman. Epidural analgesia may be very suitable for a woman with an OP labour, as I learned in the 1960s when caring for a frightened young woman whose baby was lying posteriorly. After it was suggested, she agreed to an epidural and became able to appreciate and learn about becoming a mother. While epidural analgesia is appropriately used to control the pain of OP labour, it also contributes to such malpositions developing (Yancey et al. 2001). This scenario has been identified as part of the 'cascade of intervention' (Jouppila et al. 1980; Williams et al. 1985).

This phenomenon may be associated with epidural-induced neurological changes which cause pelvic floor relaxation and fetal head malposition. Oxytocic drugs, administered to overcome delay, cause fetal hypoxia, manifested as fetal distress (Keirse & Chalmers 1989), for which interventions to expedite the birth are regarded as necessary. Thus, the solution to the problem may also be its cause, as well as the cause of further morbidity.

A symptomatic remedy, similar to acupuncture, for the low back pain of OP labour is intracutaneous or intradermal injection of sterile water (Fogarty 2008). This unlikely-sounding form of analgesia has been over-researched, and statistically significant effects have been found, which last up to 2 hours. These injections or 'blisters' bring the potential to decrease or delay the use of epidural analgesia.

The challenging nature of the OP labour complication lies, first, in the pain's character, which is 'unremitting' (El Halta 1996), precluding respite. The constant pain is blamed on the fetal occiput pressing against the maternal sacrum. Second, the duration of labour, if the head rotates anteriorly, is markedly increased. Because of the duration of this unremitting pain, the woman's physical condition may deteriorate and dehydration and ketosis develop.

Problems for the woman experiencing OP labour do not end with the birth (Pearl et al. 1993). Morbidity for the mother, in the form of perineal trauma associated with instrumental birth and/or large presenting diameters, is increased. Instrumental intervention also increases neonatal morbidity, manifesting itself as facial (Bell's) palsy or Erb's palsy.

On the basis of this poor prognosis, a new challenge has developed for midwives, which only indirectly influences the woman's pain. It comprises the midwife preventing or correcting this malposition by encouraging maternal action which facilitates rotation of the presenting part. This intervention, utilising the principle of the fetal back being heavier, encourages rotation anteriorly if the woman adopts a lateral position (Stremler et al. 2006). Thus, we observe that the woman and the midwife working together may prevent or resolve a problem caused or aggravated by other practitioners.

Uterine rupture

Although concentrating here on complications which present with or prominently feature pain in labour, uterine rupture or dehiscence constitutes an exception. This is because it infrequently occurs antenatally.

The pain of uterine rupture is variable and its prominence depends on the severity of the clinical picture, which in turn is due largely to the extent of the rupture. The pain of uterine rupture, including tenderness, is characteristically persistent, continuing suprapubically, between contractions. The degree of maternal shock and fetal morbidity depend on the timing, suddenness and extent of the rupture. The increasing use of more interventive methods of pain control, though, mean that the pain of uterine rupture may no longer be the most significant symptom and it may be necessary to rely on sudden and severe changes in the fetal heart rate.

Factors predisposing to uterine rupture include excessive uterine activity and previous myometrial damage and traumatic birth. Currently, active management of labour and the frequency of uterine surgery, such as caesarean or hysterotomy, may combine to increase the incidence of this complication. It is the potential for uterine rupture that produced the, then dire, warning to obstetricians 'Once a caesarean, always a caesarean' (Craigin 1916). Risk of rupture of the uterus features in the debate on vaginal birth after caesarean (VBAC), which rages more acrimoniously in North America due to the higher caesarean rates there (Macones 2008).

Uterine inversion

Like rupture, uterine inversion is a catastrophe of labour which puts the woman's life in jeopardy. Unlike uterine rupture, inversion is most likely during the third stage (Beringer & Patteril 2004). There are a number of predisposing factors, including various forms of mismanagement, such as 'improper fundal pressure and traction on the cord' (Oxorn 1986: 547).

As with uterine rupture, inversion varies in its severity and, hence, in the degree of pain. The woman's pain is due to pulling on the uterine ligaments, which provide support through their attachment of the uterine cornua to the pelvic walls. The pain is serious, not only in itself, but also in its aggravation of the hypovolaemic shock which supervenes if the placenta has separated. Thus, the degree of the woman's shock is disproportionately severe relative to the haemorrhage.

The pain of disappointed expectations

I have mentioned already (see Chapter 2) the suffering which the woman may encounter due to being let down by the system of 'care'. I make no apology for returning here to a not dissimilar problem which may follow the woman's experience of labour. Recent escalating caesarean rates have coincided with changes in women's attitudes to birth. Rising expectations have been linked to the information now widely available regarding the choices facing the woman (Hillan 2000) and have been fuelled by statements from, for example, governmental bodies (DoH 1993). Obviously, the reaction of the woman if her expectations of childbirth are not fulfilled varies according to many factors, including her attitudes and aspirations, not to mention her birth experience. Variations will apply to the timing as well as to the nature and occurrence of her emotional pain.

The inability of childbearing women to engage with their carers results in expectations and aspirations being dashed (Green & Baston 2003; McCourt & Pearce 2000: 151). Thus, if a woman's expectations of healthy, satisfying childbearing deteriorate into a complicated and/or traumatic and/or surgical birth, the pain is different again. The role of the woman's culture in building up her expectations is crucial. Hence, the importance of culturally sensitive care in achieving a satisfying birth experience should not be underestimated (Adewuya et al. 2006).

If the woman's expectations fail to be fulfilled by her birth experience, a form of loss ensues. In this event a number of painful emotional reactions emerge, of which post traumatic stress disorder (PTSD) is but one. Early work in this area was brought together by a ground-breaking research project by Janet Menage (1993). Although this research involved a volunteer sample, Menage identified the obstetric and gynaecological procedures likely to be sufficiently traumatic to engender PTSD. The procedures may appear relatively trivial to a professional health care provider, including cervical smear, induction of labour and removing an intrauterine contraceptive device (IUCD). Perhaps more importantly, Menage identified factors aggravating perceptions of trauma, such as the attendant being male and a sexual component. This research found that the woman's perception of control of the situation is fundamentally important. Her control may be as basic as knowing that the attendant will stop the painful intervention if and when asked.

Menage concluded that she was unable to ascertain whether the painful trauma of the procedure was due to the intervention itself, or whether the woman had been sensitised by previous experience. This dilemma was later addressed in a questionnaire survey of 289 women (Ayers & Pickering 2001). The existence/level of PTSD were ascertained and measured at 36 weeks gestation and 6 weeks and 6 months postnatally.

Seven new cases of PTSD were identified at 6 weeks, suggesting that the experience of birth is a trigger factor for PTSD. For the majority of women with PTSD the condition persisted for at least 6 months after the birth. These quantitative studies have been criticised for the instruments being designed for use following large-scale armed conflicts, predominantly involving men and major disasters affecting large numbers (Moyzakitis 2004). This critique identified vulnerable women and painful interventions in childbearing traumatising the mother. Such trauma is doubly significant, not only affecting the woman's emotional state, but also threatening developing family relationships (Beech 1998/9).

Although the significance of the trauma to the new mother appears clear, research into her care is not. 'Debriefing' has been widely embraced as solving postnatal problems (Steele & Beadle 2003); its precise nature and aims, though, are unclear. The midwife's role has been demonstrated in reducing postnatal depression (Lavender & Walkinshaw 1998; Small et al. 2000), but these interventions have not yet been applied to mothers with PTSD (Joseph & Bailham 2004).

In an examination of the emotional repercussions of traumatic or surgical birth, grief reactions were considered appropriate (Lowdon 1995). While the mother grieving the loss of her hoped-for experience of uncomplicated childbearing (Mander 2006) may be regarded as 'selfish', Gina Lowdon considered it to be a coping strategy. She argued, though, that such coping is fragile and may be threatened by any possibility that the intervention was not 'absolutely necessary' (1995: 14). On the basis of these emotional aftershocks, Lowdon pleaded that space and time be made for the woman to articulate her doubts and confusion.

This picture of perplexity and traumatisation following an interventive birth is supported by research (Clement 2001). The situation regarding postnatal depression after a challenging birth, though, is less straightforward (Robinson 2007). The conclusion is that the type of birth has some, albeit small, effect. Other factors have been shown to exert marked effects, including a lack of social support, a personal psychiatric history and a stressful life.

With regard to the effect of caesarean the picture is even less clear; emergency, rather than elective caesarean, carries a poorer psychological prognosis. Lack of preparation time for the emergency surgery has been blamed for adverse psychological outcomes (Clement 2001). Similarly, and possibly for similar reasons, suffering is less likely if regional, rather than general anaesthesia, is used. Swedish research demonstrated the extent of psychological suffering following emergency caesarean under general anaesthesia (Ryding et al. 1998). The emotional trauma of emergency caesarean under general anaesthesia fulfilled the stressor criteria for PTSD. The women experienced painful feelings of guilt, anger, ignorance and abuse.

Some women responding to Sarah Clement's questionnaire on caesarean experiences reported feelings of 'overwhelming' loss (Clement 2001: 117). The focus of the woman's loss related to (i) not experiencing the planned, hoped-for birth, (ii) not being able to give birth and (iii) not actually 'being there' if the caesarean involved general anaesthesia. Thus, loss of the birthing experience causes painful regret and is linked to fear of loss of the baby and even her own life. This applied most to women undergoing emergency caesarean.

Clement's respondents also felt that their relationships with their babies had been damaged due to the interruption by, for example, general anaesthesia. Some of the informants perceived that the caesarean had adversely affected their identity. For this woman there was a conviction that she had failed to achieve what may be regarded as the basic female function of giving birth. Thus, the woman's feelings about herself as a woman had been damaged. In slightly more concrete terms the women reported that their body image had been spoiled by the surgery and words such as 'mutilated', 'butchered' or 'a piece of meat' were used to recount the woman's feelings of painful violation.

Memory

Clearly, the memories of an unsatisfactory birth experience are obviously associated with painful suffering postnatally, and possibly beyond. This is in spite of the old adage that labour pain is forgotten with the birth:

> The moment of birth is indescribable! The feeling of happiness and new found strength were wonderful. All the work and pain were quickly forgotten.
>
> Niven & Murphy Black 2000: 246

This truism has been used to encourage mothers to tolerate treatment that might otherwise be intolerable and I never cease to be surprised that so many endorse this platitude. In logical terms, it may be surmised that this aphorism came about because of the impossibility of recalling the precise nature of such extreme sensation (Erskine et al. 1990).

An authoritative literature review suggested that this adage is in fact a fallacy (Niven & Murphy Black 2000), although it is beyond these researchers' remit to propose how it came about or for what purpose. This review found that women do not completely forget their labour pain, but that the accuracy of their recall is uncertain. Unsurprisingly, the authors, being researchers, warn of the implications of these findings for other researchers collecting data on labour pain postnatally. They also provide another warning which is relevant to childbearing families keen to record the birth; it is likely that viewing recordings of the birth will resurrect memories of the pain experienced at the time of the birth, which the woman may find challenging if she is not well-supported while viewing.

Because of the possibility of memory of labour pain giving rise to tocophobia (see above), Ulla Waldenström and Erica Schytt undertook a longitudinal prospective research project to assess whether and how any memory of labour pain changed over a 5-year period (2009). These researchers are appropriately cautious about the interpretation of their findings; but they are confident in reaching an interesting conclusion. This is that the woman's memory for the intensity or severity of labour pain was linked to the woman's initial view of the quality of her childbirth experience. Thus, if the woman reported a good birth, she was likely to report lower and declining intensity/severity of labour pain. On the other hand a woman reporting an unsatisfactory or negative birth experience would be more likely to report pain of a high intensity/severity, which remained high over the 5-year study period. A midwife would tend to conclude that these findings further indicate the importance of ensuring a good birthing experience for the woman for whom she cares. Giving rise to particular concern in Waldenström and Schytt's research is the tendency of women who used epidural analgesia to recall their most severe pain and associate this with the quality of their entire birth experience.

Approaching pain

Throughout this book I seek the widest possible interpretation of childbearing-related pain. Despite this broad approach, it is necessary to accept the link, mentioned already, between labour and pain. Thus, in examining the pain remedies in Chapters 8 and 9, I focus mainly on labour pain in terms of who or what accompanies or helps the woman on her childbearing journey. Additionally, other (non-labour) pain in childbearing may be pathological; this requires resolution of the pathology while dealing with the pain engendered. This in no way reduces the relevance of the approaches mentioned in the following chapters to non-labour pain. Many of these remedies are likely to be used by the mother and by her carers in non-labour situations, but I discuss specific interventions when considering the various causes of such pain.

Because of the range of methods available to assist the mother in coping with the pain of labour it is helpful to categorise them using a theoretical framework. Medical writers tend to use objective frameworks; examples are the pharmacological/non-pharmacological divide (Chalmers et al. 1989), or mode of action (Simkin 1989) or frequency of use (Steer 1993). Other frameworks may be chosen, such as according to who controls the method or the extent to which maternal choice features (Mander 1997c).

In the following chapters, however, I have chosen to draw loosely on Nicky Leap's terminology, because it situates the woman at the centre of pain decision-making (Leap & Anderson 2004). Thus, in Chapter 8 I address the 'working with pain' paradigm. Although Leap strenuously avoids equating this paradigm with non-pharmacological methods, I take the liberty of making this connection. After this initial distinction, I then subdivide these methods according to Penny Simkin and April Bolding's literature-based categorisation (2004). The 'pain relief' paradigm is addressed in the form of the pharmacological methods in Chapter 9.

For each method I maintain my woman-centred approach by considering the mother's input, describing the mode of action and then the application in childbearing. Next, drawing on research data, I identify the relevant issues for those involved in the utilisation of each method; this will include the mother, the fetus/neonate (or 'baby' when differentiation is unnecessary), the midwife, and any others making contributions or being affected.

Chapter 8

'Working with pain': non-pharmacological methods

It is fitting to adopt Nicky Leap's terminology to entitle these two 'methods' chapters, having referred already to her work (1996). Leap provides a model of pain control reflecting her midwife respondents' rejection of bio-medical paradigms. At the same time, though, she was moving away from reductionist models emphasising the midwife/doctor divide and the home/hospital divides. Although Leap did not relate the 'Working with Pain' paradigm purely to non-pharmacological approaches, I am taking the liberty of making this connection. This paradigm, even though the title overlooks the pain being the *woman's*, correctly situates the woman at the centre of pain control decisions. The paradigm accentuates the physiological nature of labour pain together with woman's innate ability to bear it. The role of the midwife features in this paradigm (Leap & Anderson 2004:34) as, first, facilitating physiological endorphin secretion, second, attending to the woman's vocalisation and, third, addressing her personal concerns about labour pain. Crucial to this paradigm is the midwife's ability to distinguish 'normal' from 'abnormal' pain. This distinction is less easy in settings, like hospital labour rooms, where a web of intervening variables complicates the woman's perception and expression of pain, and the midwife's interpretation of that expression.

After Leap's initial distinction between the two major paradigms, I use a literature-based categorisation according to effectiveness in reducing pain and preventing suffering as outlined by Penny Simkin and April Bolding (2004). These authors' backgrounds as physical therapists, may be the reason for their neglect of specialised approaches, such as biofeedback, therapeutic touch, guided imagery and homeopathy. Sylvia Brown and colleagues' (2001) analysis of women's evaluation of the effectiveness of non-pharmacological methods would have been a more appropriate framework in this woman-centred context, but their data are even less complete. A medically focussed categorisation by a European anaesthetist, brought its own shortcomings (O'Sullivan 2004). The importance of cultural factors in pain control cannot be ignored, as none of the classifications included the 'environment'; thus, for completeness' sake and to maintain my broad interpretation, I address these other methods.

My woman-centred approach to discussing the methods considers her place relative to the mode of action and applications to childbearing. I then use research to identify relevant issues for all involved, including mother, baby, midwife and others affected.

Pain in Childbearing and its Control, Second Edition. By Rosemary Mander. Published 2011 by Blackwell Publishing Ltd. © 1998, 2011 Rosemary Mander.

A number of phenomena have fuelled interest in non-pharmacological approaches to pain in childbearing. First is disillusionment resulting from medication's adverse side-effects. These are perceived differently by different contributors to childbirth; for example, one of chloroform's side-effects, uterine inertia, historically provided obstetricians with opportunities to intervene to remedy iatrogenically slowed labour (Mander 2004a). Second, women are assuming more responsibility for managing their childbirth pain, which particularly features non-drug pain control. Women's attempts to assume autonomy in many aspects of childbearing are reflected in avoidance of professional control over pain (Simkin 1989). Thus, spin-offs from self-care constitute an important influence.

As becomes apparent in my scrutiny of methods, research into non-pharmacological pain control is plentiful. The quality and authority of this research is, however, another matter (Simkin & O'Hara 2002). That there is 'little interest from funders to finance research on these seemingly simple, safe, and innocuous measures' (Simkin & Bolding 2004) should be no surprise, in view of the limited 'marketable' products.

Labour support

Since the serendipitous finding by Roberto Sosa and colleagues (1980) of the improved birthing outcomes in the presence of a companion, research into support in labour has assumed the proportions of a veritable growth industry. At the last count, 16 RCTs had been undertaken, all endorsing the 1980 findings (Hodnett et al. 2007). Labour support, being largely psychosocial, involves emotional help, basic physical comforts, information-giving and representing the woman's views to care providers (Mander 2001).

The role of the woman in physiological labour is thought to be encouraged by support, to the extent that Ellen Hodnett and colleagues regard this as the 'mode of action':

> [Support enhances] normal labour processes as well as women's feelings of control and competence, and thus reduces the need for obstetric intervention (2007).

This plethora of RCTs endorses support's effectiveness, first, in terms of the type of birth, which is more likely to be unassisted by instruments or surgery. Second, the supported woman is less likely to receive analgesic or oxytocic drugs, is more likely to be satisfied with her experience of birth and new motherhood, and may have a marginally shorter labour. The woman's satisfaction with the birth experience serves as her evaluation of this pain control approach. In terms of neonatal effects, support causes either 'no difference' or an improvement in neonatal condition and NNU admissions (Simkin & Bolding 2004).

Thus, published RCTs have clearly established the benefits of support to the woman. The implications for the midwife, though, are less clear. Those RCTs which have involved support by hospital staff have included a range of personnel, such as student midwives, nurses and midwives. The settings vary similarly; countries studied have very different health systems, such as Belgium, France, Greece, Finland and Canada (Hodnett et al. 2007). The education, practice and cultural orientation of midwives obviously varies between settings, so it is unsurprising that:

the results indicated greater benefit if the labor support provider was not a member of the hospital staff with clinical care responsibilities, and whose only task was to provide continuous support to one laboring woman throughout her labor. (Simkin & Bolding 2004: 490)

Based on unfounded claims of deriving from ancient Greek practice (Mander 2001) the North American doula industry has become established globally (DONA 2005). This development emerged from early RCTs showing that untrained and unqualified women could produce statistically significant improvements in maternal outcomes. The doula's USP (unique selling point) lies in her sole focus on one woman/couple in labour. This focus allows her to provide continuous support, which is a luxury rarely available to NHS-employed midwives.

In view of the origin of the doula being through an RCT, her functioning is surprisingly *under*-researched. Particularly relating to the doula's entry into the birthing room bringing the potential for 'turf wars', her relationship with other staff is disconcertingly disregarded (Papagni & Buckner 2006). Similarly, Simkin and Bolding highlight the paradox of this attendant's creation being through research, but her practice 'has never been studied in RCTs' (2004: 482).

The importance of research to the advent of the doula should not be underestimated, especially because her continuing existence may serve to enhance the research credentials of those medicalised maternity systems in which she functions. The maternity systems in which the original, and some subsequent RCTs, were undertaken serve to further illuminate the doula's research base. The locations of these studies were largely either in third world settings or settings in developed countries reminiscent of the third world, due to their focus on minority ethnic groups. Thus, these research projects certainly improved the experience of the childbearing women; but that improvement was from a base so low as to be beyond the belief of Western practitioners. The plethora of RCTs, therefore, does little more than demonstrate how a hostile birthing system is ameliorated by a research intervention rendering it marginally more humane. The underlying brutality of the maternity system, though, is left unscathed by the introduction of this new attendant who is, effectively, bolstering an iniquitous regime.

Hydrotherapy and temperature modulation

Water has long and commonly been used to comfort and heal; using water during childbearing, however, is more recent. Birth in water (waterbirth) has attracted publicity, not to say notoriety, but here I focus on water to help the woman cope with the pain of labour, or 'hydrotherapy'. Although water may be applied externally in various ways, immersion baths have become widely available and more researched since being recommended in 'Changing Childbirth' (DoH 1993). Using showers, for example, has been disregarded; similarly, the woman's experience of using water had attracted little research attention until Robyn Maude and Marlyn Foureur undertook their qualitative study (2007). These researchers clearly demonstrated the extent to which using water empowers the woman to assume control over her birth experience. This empowerment manifested itself in the form of 'sanctuary', when the water served as a barrier with which the woman protected herself from unwelcome contact:

> they couldn't reach me – when I didn't need them, there was no way they could have touched me because I was over the other side of the pool (2007: 22)

Hydrotherapy benefits the woman in labour in a number of ways. Increased buoyancy helps the woman adopt more comfortable positions and reduces pressure on the pelvis and other structures, while encouraging fetal flexion. Further, the water's warmth acts as a heat conductor to release muscle spasm and, hence, relieve pain.

Assumptions about the effectiveness of hydrotherapy resulted in its widespread use. These assumptions have now been strengthened by a systematic review, although some research lacks authority (Cluett & Burns 2009). Regional anaesthesia was shown to be significantly less needed when hydrotherapy is used; additionally no increase in assisted or operative births was found, nor any increase in perineal damage. Because of its inherent appeal, the practice of hydrotherapy has overtaken research. This ubiquity means that experimental studies may no longer be feasible, and practice remains based on less than authoritative observational studies (Cluett & Burns 2009: 2).

The evaluation of hydrotherapy has focused largely on its safety, after considerable early medical opposition to 'aquatic fanatics' (Loeffler, cited in Beech 1995b: 1). Beverley Beech argued that our medical colleagues attempted to limit the availability of hydrotherapy on the grounds of risk to the baby; the basis of these attempts has now been questioned. Medical practitioners' concerns about fetal/neonatal dangers were based on certain over-publicised cases and the water temperature causing hyperthermia became a bone of contention. The risk of the baby breathing prematurely and, effectively, drowning was also raised, following a small number of unfortunate outcomes. Third, neonatal infection has been blamed on the possibility of contamination, but the risks are no greater than birth in air. Elizabeth Cluett and Ethel Burns' systematic review shows that when hydrotherapy is used Apgar scores are no different and neonatal infection rates and NNU admissions are no higher (2009).

While the advantages to the woman of using water are becoming clearer, the implications for the midwife are widely disregarded. Clearly the welfare of the woman should be the midwife's prime concern, but there may be other factors, such as the midwife's exposure to contaminated fluids or her posture relative to the bath. Dianne Garland considered the midwife's position in terms of the legislative framework controlling or limiting midwifery practice (2000). Maude and Foureur briefly contemplated the role of the midwife in developing a shared philosophy of birthing (2007). These researchers relate how the harmony of physical, emotional and philosophical attunement develops when water is used. In this way, midwifery knowledge and the meaning of 'evidence' are extended. It may be necessary to consider whether the empowerment which hydrotherapy offers women has any similar effects for the midwife.

As mentioned above one of the possible reasons for the benefits of hydrotherapy relates to the warmth of the water. Thus, hydrotherapy may simultaneously be a method of temperature modulation. Because of the importance of ensuring that the woman does not become overheated while immersed during labour, I seek to differentiate these two approaches to pain control. Rather like massage (see below), heat and cold have long been used as a comfort measure. According to Simkin and Bolding, this history means that these interventions are now seriously under-researched relative to the ubiquity of their use (2004). Because of this deficiency, these researchers find themselves recommending 'common sense' (2004: 499) to prevent any untoward side effects. Various modes of applying heat and cold are mentioned, including ice and frozen peas, but the cold hands which are required of midwives are neglected! Bette Waters and Jeanne Raisler's study (2003), a major exception to the lack of research, involved massage with ice on an acupuncture point on the hand during contractions. The researchers confidently asserted the effectiveness of this intervention, although they ignored the deprived nature of the sample and the possibility of the Hawthorne effect at least contributing to the women's appreciation of this intervention. A retrospective study by Sylvia Brown and colleagues (2001) included heat and cold therapy as one of the battery of complementary interventions; while virtually all respondents had been taught about the use of temperature modulation, it was one of the four least used approaches, ranking lower than guided imagery (see below). For those women who used this technique, it was found to be largely effective. Whether this positive outcome was linked to the tendency for it to be used by women already using pharmacological analgesia is difficult to assess.

Injections of sterile water

The injection of plain water is probably the most counter-intuitive of pain control methods. Perhaps for this reason, and unlike other methods, it has been heavily and authoritatively researched. Water injections are more specific than other pain control methods in their aim; the intention is to relieve the back pain of labour, associated with occipito-posterior position (see section on 'OP labour' in Chapter 7), asynclitism or the pain of contractions.

The woman's role is minimal, although the discomfort of the injection and the burning sensation lasting up to two minutes afterwards demands a high level of tolerance (Fogarty 2008). This 'discomfort' has been shown to be sufficiently severe for women to decide to decline this effective treatment for back pain in future labours (Labrecque et al. 1999).

Injection of sterile water (ISW) involves it being injected either intradermally as a very superficial injection or subdermally at a deeper level, with the former attracting more research attention. The injections are sited over the sacrum at the angles of the rhomboid of Michaelis, although precision does not determine effectiveness.

The mode of action is uncertain, despite having been used in general surgery for over a century (Mårtensson et al. 2008); but at least one of three factors may be operating (Simkin & O'Hara 2002). The injection may act as a counterirritant, causing pain at a different site to be relieved; additionally, the initial stinging may activate the gate control mechanism and the 'needling' may cause the release of endogenous pain modulators, such as beta endorphins, into the cerebrospinal fluid.

A systematic review of intradermal ISW, based on six studies of acceptable scientific merit (Fogarty 2008), found this technique to be rapidly effective and without side-effects. ISW carries many advantages, such as potentially decreasing the need for epidural analgesia and caesarean and being appropriate for use in rural/remote/developing situations where low-tech low-cost interventions are needed.

These evidence-based findings clearly make this method of controlling low back pain ideal for use by midwives. The study by Lena Mårtensson and colleagues, though, suggests that midwives may not share this enthusiasm (2008). The researchers focussed on certified nurse midwives, comparable with many UK midwives, and obtained a response rate of only 29%, yet confidently state that 'More midwives chose sterile water injections than any other method for managing back pain in labour' (2008: 119). Unfortunately these researchers cannot make assumptions about the ISW use of the 71% of the population who did not reply; their non-response might have indicated indifference, ignorance or even suspicion. Although Sweden is widely considered to be more familiar with ISW, a comparable study there produced similarly disappointing findings, despite a healthier response rate of 59% (Mårtensson & Wallin 2006). These results suggest that the multiple benefits of ISW identified by Fogarty may not yet have been recognised, even less implemented, by practitioners. The reasons for this disregard urgently need research attention.

Maternal position, posture and ambulation

Although the benefits of the woman changing her posture have been recognised since the days of William Smellie (McLintock 1876), they have related more to the progress of labour than the woman's comfort. In addition to the effects of gravity, the benefits of a non-recumbent or upright posture in labour are associated with enlargement of pelvic dimensions. Radiological evidence has long shown that squatting increases the diameters of the pelvic outlet by up to 30% or 2 cm (Russell 1969).

While 'Optimal Fetal Positioning' (Sutton & Scott 1994) is thought, by adopting a cross-legged sitting position, to relieve back pain, it is also thought that upright positions, like ambulation, permit better alignment of the fetal head with the woman's pelvis. Such strategies are particularly appropriate if the woman experiences back pain due to an occipito-posterior position; then the woman's upright posture facilitates rotation of the fetal occiput anteriorly. Thus, it becomes apparent that alterations in posture which encourage the progress of labour may also help alleviate pain.

Research focusing on the pain-controlling effects of posture and ambulation is seriously limited. The effects of posture on the woman's pain has, however, been addressed indirectly through studies on the progress of her labour. It was a classic, though flawed, study by Mendez-Bauer and colleagues (1975) that originally stimulated interest in posture in labour. These researchers found that, in terms of uterine efficiency, standing produces the most favourable outcomes. In their sample of 20 women, however, each acted as her own control and, as well as changing her position half-hourly, was subjected to a vaginal examination at the same time. It is possible that these examinations affected, that is accelerated, the progress of labour. This less than satisfactory study persuaded McManus and Calder to replicate Mendez-Bauer's research and refute the benefits claimed, by demonstrating no difference between upright and recumbent groups (1978). The replication recruited women having labour induced and, unsurprisingly, the maternal response to induction varied hugely and probably influenced the findings. Additionally, minimal information is provided about the postures and positions in which the women *actually* laboured.

Researching posture and ambulation is still more problematic than researching other 'complementary' therapies. The difficulties relate to the impossibility of concealing the treatment/intervention group to which a subject is allocated, preventing 'blinding' either carers or researchers to the experimental/control groups. Unsurprisingly all involved have their own feelings about particular positions, so the potential for inadvertent, or even deliberate, bias is massive. Additionally, the individual woman may find difficulty maintaining the allocated position/posture, which is more likely if the woman becomes sleepy due to medication or tired as labour advances.

Posture and ambulation in labour are influenced, even determined, by prevailing culture; thus the domination of the hospital birthing room by the bed sends very clear messages to the woman about where she should be and what position she should adopt. Further, non-recumbent postures have been associated with 'primitive peoples all over the world' (Dening 1982: 440). The cultural implications and benefits of posture and ambulation became apparent to me when a labouring woman chose to practise her belly dancing. This involved complex pelvic movements, which in other circumstances would have been erotic, but for her assisted achieving realignment of the fetal head.

The recumbent posture has been attributed to the advent of male midwives in Western Europe. A hegemonic analogy links the woman's recumbency as it denotes her 'weakness, inferiority and submission', compared with the 'strong superior obstetrician … who stands before her' (Banks 1992: 43). The issue of power is further elaborated in this historical account of posture in labour, when observed that the upright woman is able to develop a 'better relationship' with carers, presumably because she is, at least physically, on their level.

As noted by Penny Simkin and Mary-Anne O'Hara (2002) maternal recumbency is convenient for carers, to the extent that other positions may threaten their comfort and control; this is associated with recumbent postures also facilitating a range of interventions. A systematic review (Lawrence et al. 2009) found the only significant difference to be labour being shorter for non-recumbent women and their use of regional analgesia reduced. While shorter labour and less regional analgesia may indicate less pain, this is not a safe assumption. More importantly, this systematic review indicates that women's views about labour positions have still to be investigated. Thus, while positioning and ambulation are widely used and thought beneficial, their effect on the woman's pain remains uncertain.

Manual, quasi-manual and related therapies

Massage/effleurage and aromatherapy

Like hypnotherapy (below), the reputation of massage has suffered salaciously adverse publicity, leading to the seedy and erotic applications of this intervention. A further issue, highlighted in research, lies in the uncertain nature of massage. Philip Steer (1993) found that while 19.3% of women reported having been massaged to relieve childbirth pain, only 5% of midwives reported having used it. This discrepancy contrasts with the administration of medications like pethidine, which was reported by 37.8% of midwives and 36.9% of women. The discrepancy lies in the intervention, identified as massage by the woman, being regarded as mere 'back rubbing' by the midwife.

The potential for confusion about what massage involves makes a definition useful, so I here define massage by combining Haldeman's (1994: 1252) and Mobily et al.'s (1994: 39–40) definitions:

> Massage is the application of hand pressure to soft tissues, usually muscles, tendons or ligaments, without causing movement or change in position of a joint in order to decrease pain, produce relaxation, and/or improve circulation.

Although this definition fits perineal massage, I give it no further attention here. Massage is claimed to be the 'most primitive pain remedy' (Lee et al. 1990: 1777), utilising an innate human reflex to hold, rub or squeeze a hurt body part. Such self-administered massage is less relevant to labour, thus marginally reducing the mother's contribution. The five basic components of massage comprise: effleurage, petrissage, tapotement, friction and vibration (Radnovich 2005). Each is characterised by differing pressure, direction, speed, movement and hand position to differentially affect underlying tissues.

In the context of pain, massage 'closes the gate' to inhibit the passage of pain stimuli to the higher centres of the central nervous system and stimulates the local release of endorphins (Chang et al. 2002). Further, the benefits of massage are reinforced by the relaxation response which the experience engenders. Tactile stimulation and positive feelings, developed when caring and empathetic touch is applied, serve to enhance the pain-controlling effects of massage, while massage also alleviates pain by reducing anxiety, which both aggravates and is aggravated by pain.

The beneficial effects last only as long as the massage continues and, when discontinued, the pain increases (Simkin 1989). This disadvantage is due to the process of adaptation, by which the nervous system accustoms itself to stimuli and sense organs cease to respond. The result in this context is diminution of the pain-relieving effects of massage. Thus, it is recommended that massage during labour be intermittent, like back rubbing which is only applied during contractions, or varied in the type of touch and the location.

As mentioned already, the benefits of massage are claimed to extend beyond purely physiological changes, and psychological effects may also ensue. The RCT by Mei-Yueh Chang and colleagues (2002) examined this association by applying massage, and teaching partners the technique, during labour. Pain and anxiety were measured using the PBI (present behavioural intensity) and VASA (visual analogue scale for anxiety) respectively. The massaged group reported significantly lower pain reactions throughout labour, whereas anxiety was only lower during the latent phase. The psychological support inherent in the massage was appreciated, even though anxiety was hardly affected. A larger study comprising three arms (Kimber et al. 2008) produced generally similar findings in the UK.

The major contraindications to massage relate to its stimulating effect on the circulatory system. For this reason people with health problems such as thrombophlebitic, arteriosclerotic or cardiovascular conditions may be unsuitable subjects. Apart from this, local skin conditions may contraindicate massage; examples are acute inflammation, burns, dermatitis or wounds. Despite the frequency with which Steer (1993) reported that women receive massage during labour, research into its effectiveness is notable by its absence

(Simkin & O'Hara 2002). This is partly due to the confusion already mentioned about what constitutes massage. As well as 'basic' massage, specialised forms, like reflexology and shiatsu, may be used. The theoretical bases of both of these therapies relate to traditional Chinese medicine (TCM), but poor knowledge limits their use in childbearing.

A pain control technique frequently combined with massage is aromatherapy. The choice of mode of administration of essential oils is determined by the time available, meaning that bath/footbath, taper, inhalation or compress could be preferred (Dhany 2008). A large evaluative study using a convenience sample has suggested that benefits are derived from aromatherapy in labour, although any pain controlling effects are indirect (Burns et al. 2000). This study suggested that aromatherapy relieved anxiety and stress and encouraged feelings of well-being. Both mothers and midwives were satisfied with this intervention. Burns and colleagues also found a reduction in pharmacological analgesia use, such as pethidine, in the experiment group and the need for augmentation was also reduced.

Rather different findings emerged from a more recent non-randomised controlled trial of aromatherapy in labour (Myung et al. 2005). This trial suggested only minimal differences between intervention and control groups, although labour tended to be marginally shorter in the former. It may be, therefore, that aromatherapy is another intervention which indirectly benefits the woman by facilitating relaxation to reduce pain perception.

Therapeutic touch

The name of this intervention serves to disguise the complex theoretical background underpinning it, leading to misunderstandings (Tournaire & Theau-Yonneau 2007). It may be that any form of touch is therapeutic, but therapeutic touch (TT) is unusual in that it does not actually involve physical touching; rather the hands are employed in a less than orthodox approach to achieve 'transpersonal healing' (Kreiger & Kunz 2004: 2). Like specialised forms of massage, TT is a healing intervention which may be used to alleviate pain and derives its theoretical framework from American nursing practice (Krieger 1979).

Although much of the literature on TT suggests a more spiritual than physical action (Krieger 1979), some argue that the spiritual aspect is of limited significance (Mackey 1995). Others deny that any religious input or professed faith or belief by either practitioner or client is needed and, additionally, the action of TT in no way involves sensory modulation. This is because, first, no physical contact between the practitioner and client is involved, hence the 'non-contact' principle (Grabowska 2001). Second, practitioners claim that TT corrects energy fields, rather than neurological activity.

According to its originators, TT's action relies on the energy field, of which Rogers' Theory of Integrality (1980) states all living things are a part. This concept is similar to the Eastern concept of *prana*, which relates to factors organising life processes, including physiological ones (Krieger 1979). Health is associated with an abundance of *prana*, whereas a deficit causes illness. A characteristic of *prana* or energy which is crucial to TT is its transferability. Thus, the healthy practitioner's abundance is transferred to correct the recipient's deficit. TT utilises the two-way energy flow which comprises each individual's energy field and through the practitioner's hands energy is directly transferred, rather like a conduit (Grabowska 2001).

Four stages feature in the application of TT, although variations exist. To prepare, the practitioner focuses the mind by 'centring' to silence irrelevant activity, although there are similarities with meditation or trances. Next, 'assessment' involves sensing differences in energy flow by a non-touch technique, known as 'clearing', in which the hands are moved along the clothed body of the client, 5–15 cm away from the body. The initial assessment is rapid and may be followed by a recheck. The intervention stage comprises 'unruffling' and redirecting energy. The practitioner aims for a uniform and flowing energy field for the patient to induce relaxation and accelerate healing. The practitioner, finally, 'evaluates' the patient's energy field to ensure that flows are balanced. The contraindications to and side-effects of TT tend not to be mentioned, but Simkin (1989) concludes that TT is 'apparently a harmless intervention'. The therapeutic touch literature does mention its application during labour, but the basis of these recommendations is unclear; for example Lothian (1988) maintains that TT may be used to ease anxiety and pain in childbearing, especially for couples who are 'uncomfortable with physical touch'. TT carries the advantages that it may be acceptable to labouring women and is easily discontinued if necessary. Although research of varying quality has been undertaken on the effects of TT, research in childbearing is lacking. Concerns have been raised about effects on people with mental health problems, based on which psychosis is a contraindication (Booth 1993b).

While there is no evidence that TT is widely used by midwives or nurses in the UK, the situation differs in North America. The limited research into TT has contributed to the American debate regarding nurses' use of TT. Another factor is the enthusiasm with which TT has been accepted by American nurses, as demonstrated by its endorsement by the National League for Nursing. Thus, TT became a standard curriculum component in many nurse education institutions. These two factors have combined to cause concern, aggravated by a third factor: that TT may constitute spiritual or faith healing. Such suspicions carry the aura of 'charlatanry' (Booth 1993b), from which nurse TT practitioners seek to dissociate themselves. These three factors have created an acrimonious debate about the nature and use of nursing knowledge. Nurses cautious about the limited evidence on which TT is based are resentful of its media exposure, exposure which reflects adversely on a profession aspiring to become research-based, and augurs badly for the generation of research funds. Thus, it must be asked whether this situation could have been avoided had TT been adequately researched prior to endorsement. This only reinforces Simkin's observation (1989) that 'careful scientific investigations' are needed.

Acupressure and acupuncture

Having considered the place of massage (above) in controlling childbirth pain, it is appropriate to examine the role of *acupressure* (also known as shiatsu massage) before discussing its more invasive counterpart, acupuncture. Acupressure comprises fingertip massage over the acupuncture points (see below; Kao et al. 2006). Like acupuncture, acupressure's mode of action remains uncertain, but three possible explanations are suggested (Tournaire & Theau-Yonneau 2007): first, local endorphin production is stimulated, second, acupressure enhances the circulation or, third, the harmony of the *yin* and *yang* is enhanced (see below). Research on both the action and effectiveness of acupressure are lacking, although any benefits may derive not only from its specific analgesic effects, but also from counter-irritation and social reinforcement (Conduit 1995). Acupressure is preferred to acupuncture in labour, because it is easily self-administered and has particular benefits for back pain (Chung et al. 2003).

Many non-maternal inputs affect the pain control of the woman choosing *acupuncture*. They include the needles themselves, the acupuncturist positioning them and teaching the woman to stimulate them, but perhaps most significant is the woman's need to accept acupuncture's ideological basis. Classical acupuncture derives its theoretical basis from 3000-year-old TCM (Unruh & Harman 2002). The crucial concept is that health depends on a balance between opposing energy forces; thus, ill-health/disease is due to energy imbalance. This energy takes two forms: a negative female passive form, known as *yin*, and the positive male active *yang*. Collectively this 'energy' is known as *Chi, ki* or *qi*. These various names illustrate the problems of communication in this context, due to different nomenclature, dialects, pronunciation and translation.

A person's vital energy is thought to flow through 12 paired interconnected body channels or meridians (Chapman & Gunn 1990; Grabowska 2000). Although the symbolic names of the meridians relate to organs of the body, such as gallbladder, they do not correspond to Western anatomy. The 365 acupuncture points are sited along the meridians and are recognisable as areas of low electrical resistance. The meridians have been shown to correspond to areas of rapid cell death. Each acupuncture point represents a diseased organ, and puncture there is to allow noxious air to escape from it and the blood to be cleansed (Bond 1979).

The conditions for which acupuncture is applied vary with the training and experience of the practitioner. There are also variations between practitioners in applying this intervention. The length of the needles used depends on the tissue that is being punctured, shorter needles being used for bonier areas. The individuality of therapists' approaches also becomes apparent in the metal of the needles which, classically, are gold or silver. The insertion of the needle, in terms of speed, force and direction, affects the success of treatment and, once inserted, they are manipulated by moving, twirling or vibrating them, perhaps electrically.

While aiming to rebalance the *yin* and *yang*, the action of acupuncture has been hypothesised as taking one or more of three forms (Tournaire & Theau-Yonneau 2007). First, psychological effects have been identified, which are associated with cultural components and the required preparation for acupuncture, comparable to prepared childbirth. These psychological effects are described as 'cultural susceptibility rather than individual suggestibility' (Arthurs 1994: 496); the mode of action, however, is not only psychological, as evidenced by its effectiveness on dogs (Conduit 1995). Second, the conviction that acupuncture will work causes the higher centres to 'close the gate' to the passage of pain impulses (Melzack 1975b). Third, the needles assist pain-inhibiting mechanisms in the central nervous system, such as endogenous opioid production in the pituitary or brain stem being enhanced by acupuncture (Unruh & Harman 2002). This is supported by observations of sedation that ordinarily occur 1 hour after the acupuncture session, suggesting that naturally occurring opioids are being stimulated. Fourth, the closure of the gate to pain impulses may be by the presynaptic inhibition of sensory fibres at the level of the dorsal horn due to the stimulation of large diameter sensory fibres.

In a classic study of the use of electroacupuncture in labour, differing perceptions emerged (Abouleish & Depp 1975). Nine out of twelve women were happy with it, despite about eight needles being inserted. In contrast, the obstetricians thought that the insertion of the needles was complicated and 'time consuming', interfered with fetal monitoring and caused immobility for the woman. Such inconvenience to obstetricians begs many questions, but explains acupuncture's limitations, making acupressure the more acceptable.

Acupuncture's effectiveness has been well-researched and a Norwegian RCT, using genuine and 'sham' acupuncture for women in labour, is particularly relevant (Skilnand et al. 2002). A linear VAS was applied at 30, 60 and 120 minutes after treatment. Each recording showed significantly lower pain scores in the genuine acupuncture group and the use of both epidural and systemic analgesia were significantly lower. The existence of psychological benefits of acupuncture has been supported by observations of analgesia lasting only as long as stimulation was maintained. By comparison the emotional response, that is, not being upset by the pain, has been longer lasting.

A limitation of acupuncture is that the pregnant woman should not have needles inserted below the waist, because of an association with starting contractions (Arthurs 1994). This prohibition does not apply during labour, as needles are inserted during the second stage 'in the perineal body, behind the anus and beside the vagina' (Abouleish & Depp 1975), although ear points may be used. Michel Tournaire and Anne Theau-Yonneau (2007) warn that the long induction period of immobility may be unacceptable in labour. Side-effects of acupuncture include infection due to dirty needles and damage to nearby anatomical structures associated with inadequate anatomical knowledge; although these problems are rarer than those caused by pharmacological iatrogenesis.

Inevitably, medical authors have raised the possibility of symptoms remaining undiagnosed by non-medical practitioners. Such defensive medical attitudes remind us of the ongoing power struggle to control acupuncture practice. Arthur O'Neill (1994) explored physicians' double standard when arguing:

> on the one hand acupuncture is unscientific and should not be used but, on the other hand, if it is used it should be only by physicians.

He compares the medical use of science with the wearing of a phylactery, and the safety or otherwise of interventions, for example, acupuncture, as being more related to the status of the practitioner than to the practice itself. Since then a number of organisations have become established with the stated aim of regulating the practice of acupuncture in the public interest. The extent to which regulation would assist the professionalisation of acupuncturists tends to be disregarded, though (Thorne 2009; Price & White 2004). Meanwhile acupuncture is becoming more accepted in maternity care (Hope-Allan et al. 2004; Münstedt et al. 2009). Unfortunately, despite the success of a midwifery acupuncture service, its future is jeopardised by funding difficulties (Lythgoe & Metcalfe 2008).

Transcutaneous electrical nerve stimulation

A crucial difference between transcutaneous electrical nerve stimulation (TENS) and other pain control methods derives from its origins. While most methods have evolved over hundreds, even thousands, of years, TENS was invented relatively recently in a laboratory (Wall & Sweet 1967) following the development of the gate control theory. This intervention may, however, relate to electric fish, used in Socrates' era, on which the sufferer stood to reduce pain. TENS' action probably exploits the woman's in-built neurobiological control mechanisms (Woolf & Thompson 1994). Thus, in physiological terms at least, TENS permits the woman a large degree of control.

The main action of TENS comprises closing the gate to the passage of pain impulses, which results from a below-pain-threshold barrage of impulses produced by a current generator (Dowswell et al. 2009). The other action of TENS is to stimulate the release of endorphins which modulate the transmission of pain perceptions and raise the pain threshold to produce sedation and euphoria (Lechner et al. 1991). Thus, TENS' action is less debated than is its effectiveness.

The equipment needed to administer TENS comprises a pulse generator and amplifier. This hand-held unit combines an on/off switch, intensity (amplitude) control and continuous/pulse control. This TENS unit is attached by insulated wires to electrodes, which are made of rubber impregnated with carbon and are applied to the skin, using saline gel for contact, and fixed with tape. The siting of the electrodes is recommended to be at the location of the pain, contrasting with acupuncture and acupressure, which are applied distantly along the lines of the relevant meridians. Contradicting this recommendation, the siting of TENS on acupuncture points has been found to increase TENS' effectiveness (Chao et al. 2007). In labour the TENS unit is set just below the woman's pain threshold and maintained there between contractions. The woman increases the intensity of electrical stimuli during contractions to compete with her pain.

Contraindications to using TENS in labour are few. Localised phenomena, such as skin reactions to adhesive tape and interference with cardiotocograph recordings appear to be the most serious side-effects (Dowswell et al. 2009). In assessing TENS' effectiveness, like other complementary methods, research is fraught with methodological weaknesses (Vander Spank et al. 2000). The result is considerable uncertainty about the effectiveness of TENS in childbirth. An example of the problems frequently encountered in TENS research materialises in a planned RCT (Hardy 1991), but recruitment problems prevented the trial's completion. Based on 80 women using TENS and 67 controls, and disregarding Entonox use, more (albeit not significantly) women using TENS were found to have used no additional analgesia. Whereas the originators of TENS claim that it is beneficial for back pain (Melzack & Wall 1991) Hardy's work did not support this. The midwives' tendency to assess the TENS users' pain as more severe than the women's assessment and more severe than the controls' pain leads Hardy to contemplate midwives' preference for caring for narcotised women.

A further benefit of TENS was identified postnatally, as TENS users were significantly more likely than those who used pharmacological methods to be breast feeding at 6 weeks (Rajan 1994). It may be that this was due to the 'type of woman' who uses TENS; alternatively, as Linda Rajan argues, these babies' behaviour may not have been negatively affected in the way that, as she also identified, the babies of women who have received systemic analgesics are affected.

Women's use of TENS raises many issues for midwives as, if adequately instructed, they are permitted to 'encourage, advise on and use TENS equipment to relieve labour pain' (Ralph 1991). Whether any practitioner should be *encouraging* the use of any analgesic, even less one based on such inconclusive research evidence, is questionable.

Other midwife-related issues include staff training, uncertain availability of TENS units and organisation of TENS services – all of which constitute challenges to midwives.

Thus, TENS is non-invasive, cheap and portable, with few side-effects. Its favourable reception by women may compensate for persistent doubts about TENS' effectiveness. The consensus appears to be that TENS is appropriately regarded as one of a repertoire of pain control methods for established labour, one or more of which any woman may consider using. As Therese Dowswell and colleagues observe, however, existing research has focused on labour in hospital; homebirth and the situation before any admission may be different and need attention (2009). In view of questions about effectiveness, Judith Van der Spank and colleagues' conclusion is appropriate:

> It is not possible to predict which women may benefit from TENS. But if TENS appears to be ineffective, no time is lost, no harm has been done and no drugs remain to be eliminated.
>
> 2000: 136

Reflexology

This quasi-manual therapy employs gentle manipulation or pressure on reflex points on (usually) the foot to effect change in distant organs, possibly by improving the general circulation (Botting 1997). Reflexology is increasingly used in maternity, courtesy largely of Denise Tiran (1996; 2003), despite relatively weak research evidence. This criticism applies particularly to reflexology for labour pain, although Edzard Ernst and Kerstin Köder found that pressure applied to the feet resulted in an anaesthetising effect on other parts of the body (1997). An attempt was made to study the effects of reflexology on labour outcome (Motha & McGrath 1994), but the high attrition from the already small sample prevented significant conclusions; although, again, the duration of labour appeared to be reduced.

Mind-body techniques

According to Ronald Melzack and Patrick Wall (1991), the use of psychological methods for relaxation to counteract pain derives from research showing the significance of the psychological contribution to pain. The introduction, however, of psychological methods such as natural childbirth and psychoprophylaxis long pre-dated such research. The interconnectedness of the various psychological methods is clear. For example, relaxation constitutes a basic component of many methods, such as hypnosis, biofeedback and guided imagery. Thus, the distinctions may be academic, but, as they probably exist in the mind of the woman user, examining them separately is worthwhile.

Relaxation

Relaxation is the pain control method allowing the woman most input. Her contribution is necessary in deciding to use this method, whether and where to learn the chosen technique and whether and for how long to continue its use in labour. The only non-maternal inputs comprise her teaching during pregnancy and reinforcement from her birth companion/attendant.

According to Steer (1993: 49), relaxation was the most frequently used non-pharmaco-logical method of pain control in the UK, with 34% of women practising it (Chamberlain et al. 1993). This frequency lags some way behind the use of Entonox (60%), but not far behind the second most frequently used method, pethidine (36.9%). In a more recent US survey Eugene Declercq and his colleagues (2002: 19) found that breathing tech-niques was the most frequently used drug-free method, being used by 61% of women. This method was second only to epidural, which 63% of women used. That breathing, relaxation and childbirth education are closely interdependent is attested by Simkin and Bolding (2004) and the three have been cornerstones of prepared childbirth since Grantly Dick-Read introduced it (1933). The theory underpinning the use of relaxation during childbirth lies in the physiology of the autonomic nervous system (ANS). The ANS is that part of the peripheral nervous system which maintains homeostasis within the individual's internal environment; thus, these functions rarely reach consciousness-level and there is little, if any, voluntary control. In potentially stressful situations the sympathetic component of the ANS swings into action by increasing the blood supply, and hence oxygenation and function, of those organs likely to be needed, as well as increasing the functioning of other crucial structures. This reaction has become known by the unfortunately memorable title of 'fight or flight' (Cannon 1932). The relevant organs are dually innervated and, in more vegetative circumstances, the parasympa-thetic component increases the body's restorative functions.

During childbirth education, the woman learns to minimise functioning of the sympa-thetic and to increase activity of the parasympathetic component. This breaks the escalating fear-tension-pain cycle first described by Dick-Read and subsequently generally accepted, but scientifically unproven. Thus, the woman may reduce her pain by diminishing the sen-sation of pain and by controlling the intensity of her reaction to it. The technique which the woman learns may involve focused, or progressive, relaxation or more meditative relaxa-tion techniques. Other forms of relaxation bear the name of the originator, such as Wolpe or Bradley and Lamaze's name is firmly linked to psychoprophylaxis. Childbirth educators recommend practising relaxation during classes and at other times, preferably with the intended labour companion.

Research probing the effectiveness of relaxation is confounded by the multiplicity of other educational inputs during pregnancy. As mentioned already, relaxation is not taught without breathing and other potentially helpful activities. Thus, authoritative research has not focused purely on relaxation, but has ranged broadly. It may be that research projects on childbirth education omitting such wide-ranging topics would not be ethically permis-sible. Relaxation alone has, however, been researched in other conditions, which have invariably been chronic and pathological, such as insomnia and hypertension. Relaxation techniques to control pain appear to have been shown to be effective, but, as is usually the case with complementary therapies, methodological criticisms have emerged (Vickers & Zollman 1999). The aggravating effect of anxiety, however, has been shown to have been reduced by relaxation, authoritatively supporting Dick-Read's longstanding but otherwise unsubstantiated hypothesis.

In terms of effectiveness, Declercq and colleagues found that the majority (69%) of women using relaxation techniques regarded them as 'very' or 'somewhat' helpful, while 30% of women considered them 'not very' or 'not at all' helpful (2002). As Simkin and

Bolding observe, though, employing these techniques usually ceases when pain medication is administered. A further advantage of relaxation techniques taught by childbirth education is their social function, which may be indirectly beneficial.

While difficult to imagine that relaxation techniques have any adverse side-effects, it may be that the method not reaching the woman's expectations is sufficiently disconcerting to justify this description. Writing for medical personnel, the possibility of unrecognised psychological trauma being reactivated is raised by Andrew Vickers and Catherine Zollman (1999).

Hypnotherapy

The centuries-long, high media profile of hypnosis contrasts with its infrequent use in labour. According to Steer, only 0.07% of women chose this technique (1993: 50). Although distinctive in its induction, hypnosis is just another route to relaxation. Further confusion arises from the unclear distinction between hypnotherapy and hypnosis, but hypnotherapy is defined as hypnosis inducing compliance and suggestibility in a trance-like state to treat conditions with significant psychological components (Booth 1993b). Despite being poorly-authenticated, reports indicate that hypnosis has existed since time immemorial; modern hypnotherapy, and the bad press bedevilling it, date from Anton Mesmer's (1734–1815) meteoric yet fateful career (Nash 2001).

The mode of action of hypnosis remains uncertain. Advocates compare it with the mesmerising effects of boring activities such as motorway driving or 'highway hypnosis' (Booth 1993b). Explaining hypnosis, Ernest Hilgard (1973) suggests that an individual's consciousness comprises several levels of awareness, permitting functioning at levels other than that at which pain is perceived and resulting in no pain. Simultaneously, a 'hidden observer' maintains awareness of all activities and permits total recall, and the perception of pain, when the hypnotic trance ceases. Alternatively, according to the gate control theory, hypnosis closes the gate comprising the inhibitory interneurons in the substantia gelatinosa of the dorsal horn (Melzack & Wall 1965). Detractors, however, regard hypnosis as a conspiracy resulting in the subject's 'exaggerated role-play in compliance with the hypnotist's suggestion' (Conduit 1995: 253).

That hypnosis acts to enhance the placebo effect of other remedies is still propounded (Melzack & Wall 1991: 248). It is argued, however, that hypnotherapy's mode of action matters less than 'that the individual believes in his experience' (Woods 1989: 38). This is influenced by the individual's 'hypnotisability' or susceptibility, which arouses concern and stimulates research about hypnotherapy in childbirth. David Baram (1995) states that only 15% of the general population are 'highly suggestible and easy to hypnotize'. Perhaps because of increased susceptibility during pregnancy, Allan Cyna and colleagues suggest that nearer 25% of childbearing women find pain controllable by hypnosis (2004).

Involuntary aspects of pain, such as tachycardia and rising blood pressure, were found to be unaltered, even during deep hypnosis, by Hilgard and Hilgard (1986); but they observed that more voluntary components of pain, such as crying or facial expression, are reduced. In childbirth, self-hypnosis is the method of choice, rather than post-hypnotic suggestion. If used then, like relaxation, the only non-maternal input is the hypnotist. Unlike relaxation, however, learning self-hypnosis during pregnancy is time-consuming and militates against its use.

During childbearing, hypnosis aims to allow the woman to reinterpret the pain of contractions as benign sensations. In this way the gates in the substantia gelatinosa are prevented by descending impulses from opening and allowing the perception of pain. As with relaxation (see below) the autonomic stress response is reduced and stress hormones, which ordinarily increase pain perception in labour, are not secreted.

A systematic review indicates that hypnosis controls labour pain effectively (Cyna et al. 2004), if reduction in pharmacological analgesia use is accepted to indicate effectiveness. This effectiveness, though, may not be directly due to hypnosis, but to women using hypnosis experiencing significantly shorter labours, resulting in them having less augmentation (Harmon et al. 1990). The heterogeneity of the trials, however, limits the value of research evidence as techniques and timing of induction varied. As with other non-pharmacological methods, blinding women and staff in the control group is invariably problematical. While some claim that hypnosis is risk-free for woman and baby, it has been argued that women with mental health problems may become disturbed by induction of hypnosis.

As mentioned already, hypnosis has always been vulnerable to a bad press; hence allegations of sexual improprieties may be a further deterrent. Hypnosis, however, is compared with 'a gun – it's not the tool, but the operator who makes it dangerous' (Olsen 1991).

Yoga

Yoga represents another technique for achieving relaxation to assist pain control, as mentioned above. Again, preparation by childbirth education is necessary, although years of practice are recommended for maximum benefit. Through breathing and relaxation, yoga seeks to change the level of consciousness and awareness of internal and external phenomena (Tournaire & Theau-Yonneau 2007). An RCT of yoga in labour (Chuntharapat et al. 2008) suggested that learning yoga in pregnancy is good preparation for using it in labour. While the experiment group underwent yoga training, the control group made casual conversation. These researchers, though, found no difference between the experiment and control groups in objectively measured pethidine use, Apgar score and augmentation. Interestingly, though, the experiment group experienced significantly shorter labours. In this study, pethidine use was blamed for the lack of improvement in the experiment group's Apgar scores.

Music

Although often heard in the labour ward, I doubt if music is anything more than aural wallpaper. If it has a purpose, it is uncertain who benefits or it is used, as I have occasionally found necessary, to disguise other less congenial sounds. Audioanalgesia includes both music and other forms of purposeful sound, such as white sound, but the latter has attracted little attention since its 1960s' heyday. Music therapy is used to treat chronic conditions that feature emotional disturbance, but its use in childbirth is little-publicised. The action by which music may help the woman to cope with her labour pain may lie in its distraction and its timelessness; although it may also relax and close the gate (Phumdoung & Good 2003: 55). Of course, the uplifting effects of music should be borne in mind.

As well as these rather general environmental effects, perhaps more usefully in this context, the rhythm of music may bring a sense of order; thus music of an appropriate tempo assists the woman to regulate her breathing to facilitate relaxation. Additionally, it may encourage rhythmic movement, or even dancing, to enhance progress in labour.

In a different context, music therapy's benefits were established in the care of depressed elderly people (Hanser & Thompson 1994). This controlled study involved 30 community-based volunteers. The two intervention groups' depression, anxiety, self-esteem and mood showed significant improvement, which continued over a 9 month follow-up. Similar beneficial results have been demonstrated in the care of cancer patients as well as women experiencing acute obstetric/gynaecological pain (Locsin 1981; Sammons 1984; Durham & Collins 1986). Inevitably, these long standing studies feature some methodological weaknesses.

More recent research has shown that, although infrequently used, women who chose music found it largely effective (Brown et al. 2001). An RCT focusing on the pain of active labour for a small sample of women applied soft music of the woman's choice without lyrics (Phumdoung & Good 2003). The women, rather onerously, completed VAS scores on four occasions. The music group reported experiencing significantly less pain and also being significantly less distressed by the pain which they did experience. The sample comprised primigravid women, but those who experienced a speedier labour derived less benefit from the music. The literature suggests that this harm-free intervention has the potential for enjoyment by all who hear the music. The general acceptance of music into the labour room, though, has been poorly thought-through and may constitute an example of a potentially helpful intervention being introduced, despite the evidence. The result is that women and midwives find themselves listening to local commercial radio stations whose output satisfies no-one. Accurate information should be available based on authoritative research; this could change the role of music in labour from environmentally polluting to therapeutic.

Biofeedback

Like TENS, biofeedback is a recent addition to the pain control repertoire, having first been reported in 1970 (Blanchard & Ahles 1990). Like relaxation, however, much of the biofeedback research has focused on the treatment of headache.

Biofeedback comprises learning to influence physiological responses of which the person is ordinarily unaware through controlling autonomic functions (Tournaire & Theau-Yonneau 2007). This learning comprises two stages utilising classical conditioning (Conduit 1995), and is facilitated by equipment measuring the effectiveness of that conditioning, such as a sphygmomanometer. The training involves 'weaning' the individual off the equipment to rely on perceptions of their bodily responses. Women who used biofeedback in labour, though, did continue to rely on their equipment, which was intrusive (Bernat et al. 1992). Despite such obstacles a systematic review of biofeedback in labour is progressing (Barragán Loayza & Gonzales 2006).

Guided imagery

Guided imagery involves the woman using imagination to control her pain by creating images which either decrease the severity of her pain or comprise a more acceptable, painless substitute; these techniques are comparable with hypnosis (Vickers & Zollman 1999). Because of the woman's crucially active involvement, she feels in control of her pain which, in turn, facilitates relaxation. Just as hypnosis is compared with the trance-like states associated with boring activities, imagery is compared with day-dreaming. Such similarities resulted in the name 'oneirotherapy', from the Greek for dream, and has been termed 'waking-dream therapy' (Sheikh & Jordan 1983). The essential difference, however, relates to guided imagery's *purposeful* creation of an image by the person herself for specific purposes, such as pain control.

In the US, a large majority of childbearing women were taught to use imagery, one third did so, and only a small proportion (2.2%) was dissatisfied with their experience (Brown et al. 2001).

Homeopathy

UK data showed that only 0.4% of women use homeopathic remedies to control labour pain (Steer 1993). More recently in Germany, however, homeopathy was found to be widely available (95.7% of 138 maternity units) for physiological and pathological situations (Münstedt et al. 2009). Homeopathy developed from observations by Hahnemann (1755–1843) that 'like cures like'. Thus, substances causing symptoms may reduce those symptoms when part of a disease (Smith et al. 2006). Homeopathic remedies work not by curing the disease, but by stimulating the body to heal itself. Homeopathic remedies are thought to assist coping with the emotional challenges of childbirth, such as aconite to relieve anxiety, fear and panic and to facilitate relaxation (Smith et al. 2006). Additionally remedies such as kali carbonicum may relieve back pain in labour. Although some women choose homeopathy to help with the pain of labour, research evidence is lacking.

Other interventions and strategies

My account of non-pharmacological pain control methods is in no way exhaustive, because some methods are used less frequently, such as 'sophrology' and 'haptonomy' (Tournaire & Theau-Yonneau 2007: 4). Others have yet to be published including the 'idiosyncratic strategies' (Niven & Gijsbers 1996); these pain control strategies, which could not be categorised using orthodox frameworks, included reversal of affect and 'time limiting' to persuade that 'it will all be over by tomorrow'.

One widely neglected coping strategy is 'shouting' (McCrea 1996), which may alternatively manifest itself as crying or moaning. Midwives' attitudes to the woman articulating her pain are mentioned elsewhere (Chapter 12). McCrea found that midwives discourage 'making a noise' by condemning it as a waste of energy (1996) or that women nearby would be upset. Despite these arguments, a feeling persists that staff face difficulty with pain vocalisation. Perhaps because many women seem to find it helpful, McCrea concludes that the 'value of moaning or shouting should be investigated'.

Pain control methods are constantly developing and attitudes changing, making methods more or less significant. This dynamic situation may cause difficulties for the practitioner trying to keep abreast of new approaches to pain as well as for the writer describing them, but such dynamism can only benefit the woman, who is able to choose methods best attuned to her view of labour.

Labour environment

In considering the link between the woman's environment and her pain control I interpret 'environment' broadly. Thus, I include the physical environment or place where she labours as well as the emotional environment, particularly the woman's relationships with attendants, such as formal and informal care providers. Clearly, support (see above) is crucial, although support may merely modify the alien physical environment which the labouring woman all-too-frequently encounters (Kitzinger 1992a). Marc Keirse and colleagues (1989) contemplate the woman's physical environment in terms of its unfamiliarity and its isolation, not to mention invasive practices. The debate on the place of birth often mentions Dutch women giving birth at home and links this with their decreased use of analgesic medication (Mander 1995), but no causal relationship between these phenomena has yet been shown. A Danish study, which examined pethidine use in labour, showed the moderating effect of an alternative birthing centre (ABC) (Skibsted & Lange 1992). The researchers studied 295 women who chose to give birth in either an ABC or an obstetric ward. While 18% of the women in the ward used pethidine, only 4.8% of the women in the ABC did so. This difference is partly explained by the differences in the women themselves, as the women in the ABC were older and of higher socio-economic status and parity. The influence of the environment is clear, however, in the 24 women refused ABC care due to lack of 'accommodation' who gave birth in the ward. These women shared the characteristics of the ABC women but the pethidine use of the ward women.

Although the physical environment of labour influences her pain, this is another aspect over which the woman may experience little control.

Conclusion

In this chapter it has become clear that many non-pharmacological methods of pain control are inadequately researched or incompletely understood. It is necessary to question whether, in pursuit of the holy grail of evidence-based practice, abandoning interventions satisfactory to women is justified. The effectiveness of some of these techniques in controlling pain clearly remains uncertain. This uncertainty, though, applies to only one aspect of their action. Many of these techniques, while limited in analgesic properties, appear to address the woman's suffering (Simkin & Bolding 2004) which may constitute an equally significant requirement.

Additionally, the question emerges of whether a double standard is operating in regard to non-pharmacological interventions – with particularly rigorous criteria being applied to less orthodox methods, which are not applied to medical interventions. The answer to the latter question may be clarified in the next chapter on the pharmacological methods of pain control.

Chapter 9

Pain relief: pharmacological methods

For the title of this chapter, as with the preceding chapter on non-pharmacological methods of pain control, I have taken the liberty of borrowing Nicky Leap's woman-centred terminology (1996). While Leap did not tie the concept of 'pain relief' to pharmacological approaches, I consider that these methods of pain control approximate closely to her theoretical framework. Her concept of relieving pain involves the well-meant, possibly altruistic, offering of a 'menu' of pain control methods to the woman early on in her childbearing experience. This may happen during childbirth education or else at the beginning of labour. While the midwife certainly has no intention of doing so, this menu has the effect of convincing the woman that she will need these medications and techniques. In this way, a self-fulfilling prophecy begins to unfold, due to the insidiously subliminal messages carried by this menu. Such a humanitarian approach transmogrifies to become increasingly directive, so that pressure may be exerted to encourage the woman in labour to accept hi-tech forms of pain control. Such pressure may be exerted by staff who, the woman had hoped, would be sympathetic to her goals and ideals. In this way, the woman becomes doubly vulnerable to external pressure, having been let down by those in whom she hoped to find support.

Similar disillusionment may also lie in wait for those who, as in other aspects of health care, seek a 'magic bullet' to 'solve' the problem of labour pain. A panacea or single-action remedy would be universally welcomed. Our knowledge of the disadvantageous side-effects of the current analgesic repertoire is constantly increasing, with iatrogenesis proving to be both short and long term. The plethora of interventions which pharmacological analgesia brings with it should not be underestimated; the onus for even the simplest actions is removed from the woman into the professional remit. As Penny Simkin and April Bolding astutely observe, this includes:

> highly skilled personnel to control the accompanying undesirable side effects (2004: 489).

The existence of some iatrogenic effects, is disputed; hence, this chapter shows the extent to which those administering these interventions accept and convey relevant information.

Pain in Childbearing and its Control, Second Edition. By Rosemary Mander. Published 2011 by Blackwell Publishing Ltd. © 1998, 2011 Rosemary Mander.

Before examining its various pharmacological forms, we should recall the meaning of 'analgesia'. Defined as 'a decreased or absent sensation of pain' (Anderson 1994), analgesia is sought through various pharmacological and other techniques. We should distinguish this reduction or removal of pain from the intervention with which it is closely pharmacologically linked; anaesthesia is 'the absence of normal sensation' (Anderson 1994) and is ordinarily achieved by medication. The distinction between analgesia and anaesthesia is significant in childbearing for two reasons.

The first reason relates to the pharmacological effects of the agents themselves. Certain drugs, such as nitrous oxide, at one dosage or concentration produce analgesia, whereas at a higher dosage or concentration anaesthesia results. Second, the intent underpinning administration may appear too obvious for words, but may become blurred in the minds of those involved (Mander 1998b). Whereas certain techniques may be administered initially to achieve analgesia, they may later in the labour be used for anaesthesia. An example is epidural analgesia, which may be established or 'sited' for a woman with difficulty coping with painful contractions, but it also increases her risk of an interventive birth (Torvaldsen et al. 2004). So, although the woman requests, consents to and has administered epidural analgesia, the ultimate intention, unbeknown to her, is that it will be in position in the increasingly likely event of anaesthesia being required. The increasing use of 'neuraxial block' represents a source of pride to anesthesiologists who regard their input as 'one of the major growth areas in health care' (Crowhurst & Plaat 2000: 164); these authors continue by emphasising the need for 'marketing' their services, for which anaesthetists seem to have been striving for decades (Mander 1993).

Inhalational analgesia

Analgesics have been inhaled for as long as human beings have been able to create and breathe fumes from naturally occurring substances, such as opium poppies. James Young Simpson's introduction of anaesthesia/analgesia into childbearing took the form of first ether, then in 1847 chloroform, administered by inhalation. Various inhaled analgesics have been or are used in childbearing, including methoxyflurane (0.35%), trichlorethylene (0.25–1%) and different concentrations/combinations of nitrous oxide (Rosen 2002). In the UK premixed nitrous oxide and oxygen (50% N_2O and 50% O_2) delivered by the Entonox apparatus, which in common usage gives its name to the gas, is currently permitted for use by a labouring woman supervised by a midwife. A major principle, which enhances inhalational analgesia's safety, is self-administration. The woman is prevented from excessively high intake leading to overdosage, by causing sleepiness and the face mask or mouthpiece falling away, thus preventing further inhalation. The woman learns, ideally during pregnancy with reinforcement in labour, the principles of self-administration to maximise pain control.

Nitrous oxide achieves analgesia, or anaesthesia, by limiting neuronal and synaptic transmission in the central nervous system (CNS), by increasing the threshold for the firing of the action potential (Trevor & Miller 1992). The popularity of Entonox derives from it being moderately effective without causing significant maternal or fetal/neonatal side-effects (Rooks 2007). The potential for fetal hypoxia exists if the woman hyperventilates to control her pain while using Entonox, highlighting the importance of education and supervision.

Due to its low lipid solubility, nitrous oxide quickly reaches analgesic levels in the maternal circulation (Rosen 2002), and analgesia ends equally quickly when inhalation ceases. A slight delay in nitrous oxide taking effect means that the woman should begin self-administration before the most painful part of each contraction. This regime provides at least 50% of women with significant analgesia and a further 30% with partial analgesia (Rosen 2002).

Being self-administered, Entonox allows the woman to control its administration. Its effectiveness, however, is less controllable, dependent as it is on her having been given and being able to follow instructions about self-administration. Another advantage of nitrous oxide and oxygen, also relating to its administration, lies in its low cost, as no medical involvement is necessary and supervision by the midwife is minimal following initial instruction and direction.

Entonox has been found to be the most widely available agent used for controlling labour pain in the UK, being provided in 99% of maternity units (Chamberlain et al. 1993). Judith Rooks reports that 62% of women in labour in the UK use Entonox, possibly in combination with other techniques or medication (2007). Rooks emphasises the crucial role of Entonox in achieving and maintaining physiological birth experiences for childbearing women, hence her clarion call for its rejection in the US to be reversed.

Despite its widespread use and anecdotal reports, research-based evidence about the effectiveness of nitrous oxide and oxygen is scarce. A large study of childbirth pain led Ann Wraight (1993) to conclude that 85% of women users were satisfied with this agent. She notes, however, that their satisfaction did not necessarily derive from the pharmacological effects, which were impeded by the woman's difficulty in implementing the regime of administration. Wraight maintains that women's satisfaction derives from Entonox 'as a distraction and an activity which assisted in relaxation and breathing exercises' (1993: 80). Perhaps the pharmacological effect is further enhanced by the woman's feeling of control over this agent. The 15% of women in Wraight's sample who were not satisfied with nitrous oxide and oxygen is likely to have included those who disliked either the 'mask' or the psychotropic effects of this drug; these latter effects gave it its original name 'laughing gas' which, I have occasionally found, may actually be appreciated by the woman in labour.

Although it is relatively safe for the baby and satisfactory to the woman, concerns have emerged relating to nitrous oxide's potential for harming staff. Teratogenic and other pathological effects on reproductive performance have been reported among staff frequently exposed to nitrous oxide, such as dentists and midwives (Newton 1992; Ahlborg et al. 1996). A study of 14 midwives showed that their exposure levels to nitrous oxide greatly exceeded those stipulated in countries where legislation controls upper limits. This finding is endorsed by a more authoritative study of 242 midwife shifts (Mills et al. 1996). Newton concludes that midwives should take 'personal responsibility' for their safety when supervising Entonox administration. Rosen observes, however, that these studies predated the general installation of scavenging systems and good ventilation in birthing rooms, reducing the validity of such concerns (2002).

Systemic opioid analgesia

Although often used interchangeably (Melzack & Wall 1991), the terms 'opioids' and 'narcotics' are subtly different. Opioids are derived, naturally or synthetically, from the opium poppy, but narcotics include all drugs that cause sleepiness or ultimately narcosis, that is insensibility. Thus, opioids used in labour are also narcotics. Narcotics have become associated with illegal drug use, especially in the US. Partly for this reason and partly because of its imprecision, the term is best avoided; it has been replaced with opioids when referring to the legal therapeutic use of these drugs, to which Controlled Drugs regulations apply.

It took women's campaigns in Germany and then America, according to Donald Caton (1995), to entice medical practitioners away from their inherent dread of opioids. Although initially reluctant, the regime of 'twilight sleep' took hold in the US in the second quarter of the twentieth century. This regime offered some analgesia through morphine, together with scopolamine to ensure amnesia.

Frequency of use

Their powerful pain-controlling action may make the strong opioids appropriate during labour. The weak opioids, such as codeine, have no place in childbirth. In a UK-wide study of 6093 labouring women in 1993, 2247 (36.9%) women received pethidine, 128 (2.1%) received diamorphine and 107 (1.8%) received meptazinol (Steer 1993). Thus, 41% of women were administered opioids during labour. This proportion, though a minority, is significant because opioids were second only to nitrous oxide and oxygen in frequency of use. A recent picture of opioid use in America shows that it is the second favourite, after regional analgesia (Declercq et al. 2002). Even more recently in England, one third of women (34.1%) used systemic opioid analgesia, second only to nitrous oxide and oxygen (80.7%) (Healthcare Commission 2007).

Actions

The actions of the opioids result from their ability to bind with receptor sites in the CNS. Physiologically these receptors respond to endogenous opioids, sometimes known as 'endorphins'. The receptor sites include the mu, kappa, sigma and delta sites and their heterogeneity reflects the range of effects of these substances; the kappa receptors, however, are primarily responsible for analgesia (Wright et al. 2002). The receptor sites where the opioids are active are located in two main areas in the CNS. First, in the substantia gelatinosa of the dorsal horn of the spinal cord, there are high concentrations of opioid receptors. Second, in the midbrain a system of periaqueductal grey matter, together with thalamic and hypothalamic nuclei, indirectly inhibit the transmission of pain impulses to the cerebral hemispheres. These two groups of receptor sites enhance each other's activity in limiting the transmission of pain impulses to the higher centres (Melzack & Wall 1991).

The role of the higher centres is less clear than that of the areas in the cord, brain stem and thalamus. Perception of pain in the cerebral hemispheres is assumed to occur in the functional areas of the frontal cortex. This assumption arose from similarities observed between the action of opioids in reducing concern with pain and responses following psychosurgery.

While opioid activity is initiated at various receptor sites, the action at cell level is to reduce the release of neurotransmitters by affecting the presynaptic neurone. Neurotransmitter release, involving serotonin, acetylcholine and noradrenaline among others, is inhibited. In the same way as the variety of receptor sites is partly responsible for opioids' wide ranging effects, the variety of neurotransmitters affected may be similarly responsible.

Effects

Because few interventions produce only one single effect, we should consider their main and side-effects. The main effect, or reason for the intervention, is invariably regarded as beneficial. The side-effects or by-products, however, are variably advantageous and less significant, even disregarded. Here I first consider the main effect and then the side-effects.

Main effect

Systemic opioids are administered in labour for analgesia, which derives from two sources: alteration of, first, the perception of pain and, second, the reaction to it. Opioids raise the pain threshold and personal accounts show the effect on the woman's reaction to pain:

> I felt pethidine helped relaxation ... [but it] made me mentally dopey and out of control and less concerned with the pain (Steer 1993: 51).

The woman planning to use opioids should also be aware that this main effect is incomplete, as pain will not be *totally* removed (BCPHP 2007: 11).

Side-effects

Whereas the main effects of interventions are supposedly beneficial, the side-effects may be less so, inasmuch as they range from being appreciated to being life-threatening. Despite this, rather than classifying them as beneficial or harmful, the individual woman should decide whether a side-effect is acceptable to her. The actions of the systemic opioids, including side-effects, are either depressant or excitatory. In humans the depressant effects tend to predominate, as evidenced by the usual sedation. The side-effects which feature excitation are caused by opioid-induced depression of inhibitory pathways (Cox 1990).

Considering the use of opioids in controlling cancer pain, Twycross (1994) distinguishes clinical pharmacological problems from those relating to laboratory-based investigations. While we may safely assume that the experience of cancer pain is essentially different from childbearing pain, the intensity of these forms of pain is comparable (Melzack & Wall 1991). It may be, therefore, that the methods of controlling each of these forms of pain are also comparable; thus, research into the side-effects may be transferable.

Respiratory depression   Systemic opioids have been shown experimentally to induce respiratory depression through inhibition of the brain stem respiratory centre (Way & Way 1992). The main feature of this depression comprises inhibiting the response to rising CO_2 levels. Knowledge of respiratory depression is significant for two reasons: first, the woman in labour is protected from opioid-induced respiratory depression because 'pain acts as a physiological antagonist to the central depressant effects of morphine' (Regnard & Badger 1987). Second, risks of neonatal respiratory depression are aggravated by easy transplacental transfer. While the mature blood–brain barrier limits opioid transport into brain tissue, its perinatal effectiveness is reduced by immaturity, even in term babies. Thus, opioid-induced respiratory depression threatens a baby whose mother has recently been administered opioids and this threat determines their use (BCPHP 2007: 11).

Euphoria/dysphoria   The psychotropic or mind-altering effects of opioids probably explain their longstanding popularity as drugs of abuse. The more congenial aspects of these effects are described as 'a pleasant floating sensation and freedom from anxiety and distress' (Way & Way 1992: 425). Sedation may also result from the depressant effects of the opioids and, while sedation may be welcomed in labour, the dizziness, dysphoria and drowsiness accompanying it are not. Dysphoria is defined as a 'disquieted state ... and a feeling of malaise' (Way & Way 1992: 425). Such unwelcome side-effects have serious consequences for the woman (Kitzinger 1987a) as they 'cause confusion and can make a woman feel powerless to cope actively with labour', thus reducing her control. As examples, two psychotropic reactions are recounted by Wraight's respondents (1993: 81):

> I had pethidine for the birth of my first baby and felt relaxed and happy during the birth.

> I was very disappointed with the pethidine as I could not think straight and could not do as I was told. This was because the pethidine made me very sleepy.

Gastrointestinal effects   The excitatory effects of the systemic opioids on the chemoreceptors in the brain stem result in the all too familiar nausea and vomiting. These symptoms may be further aggravated by movement or ambulation, due to opioids' effects on the vestibular apparatus. Because of this side-effect, it is usual to administer a prophylactic anti-emetic with the opioid. More sinister is the opioid-aggravated delay in gastric emptying (Walldén et al. 2004), which underlies Mendelson's syndrome (acute pneumonia due to maternal acid aspiration, see 'General anaesthesia' below).

Cardiovascular effects   While not exerting any direct effect on the heart, the opioids engender mild hypotension in a cardiovascular system that is already stressed. While the reason for this hypotensive effect is uncertain, it may be used to the woman's advantage.

Tolerance and addiction   Staff anxiety about the possibility of engendering opioid dependence has resulted in the under-prescription and under-administration of therapeutic opioid analgesics and has caused immeasurable unnecessary suffering (Twycross

1994: 947; Chapter 2). While caution is necessary in comparing childbirth pain with that which nurses treat patients for, it may be that midwives who have been nurses bring these anxieties with them. Tolerance of a drug or intervention comprises a decreased response, in the desired or main effect, requiring greater doses (Hollister 1992). Research involving 1000 patients with advanced cancer showed that only 5% developed any degree of tolerance to long term opioids (Twycross 1994); this suggests that in childbearing this phenomenon is irrelevant.

Addiction, or more correctly drug dependence, has been shown to constitute a rare side-effect of cancer patients' opioid therapy. A study of 12 000 hospital patients being treated with strong opioids showed that only one person developed dependence on these drugs (Porter & Jick 1980). Like tolerance, addiction is irrelevant in childbearing pain control decisions.

The place of systemic opioids in childbearing

Having examined some general issues relating to their use, we now consider what opioid drugs currently offer to the woman in labour. As with most medical and other interventions, the woman needs information to help her to judge the costs and benefits. Increasing knowledge is giving rise to concern about the opioids' effects on more general outcomes, as well as longer term neonatal, infant and even adolescent behaviour.

Effectiveness.

Authoritative research into the analgesic effectiveness of opioids began by focusing on pethidine. A prospective randomised double-blind trial involving 1100 labouring women showed pain scores falling for only 90–120 minutes following intramuscular injection of pethidine (Morrison et al. 1987). The researchers were appropriately critical of its poor effect.

These concerns about the effectiveness of opioids resulted in a Swedish study of morphine and pethidine (Olofsson et al. 1996). Unfortunately this small study provides a rallying point for those advocating other pain control methods (Reynolds 1997). Olofsson and colleagues recruited and randomly allocated 20 nulliparous women in labour, each of whom was given three doses of either pethidine or morphine intravenously (IV). Each woman received weight-related doses of opioid over the duration of three contractions. Pain intensity and sedation were assessed using visual analogue scales. Data presentation is crude with little detail except to claim 'no significant change' (p. 969) and the researchers conclude that opioids have no analgesic effect, just sedation. Thus, even the analgesic effectiveness of opioids is uncertain.

Breastfeeding

The benefits of breastfeeding and particularly early breastfeeding are clearly apparent, but the possibility of problems when opioids have been administered has emerged (Freeborn et al. 1980). Researchers measured opioid (pethidine) levels in the neonatal circulation and saliva and, unsurprisingly, found that the opioid had been transferred transplacentally. Babies given infant formula excreted the opioid rapidly, resulting in an elimination half-life of approximately 30 hours. In a stark and disconcerting contrast, breast-fed babies demonstrated a significant *increase* in salivary opioid in the first day, followed by a gradual reduction in the second 24 hours. The conclusion was that the opioid was also transferred during breastfeeding, and the woman who receives an opioid in labour and breastfeeds puts her baby in double jeopardy.

Canadian research utilised a specially designed Infant Breast Feeding Assessment Tool (IBFAT) to identify the woman's perceptions of her baby's breastfeeding at each feed (Matthews 1989). The sample comprised multiparous women, 18 of whom had received no opioid in labour and 20 who had. The data collection ascertained when effective breastfeeding became established. Babies in the medicated group were found to initiate effective breastfeeding hours, or even days, later than those in the unmedicated group.

A further attempt was made to compare the effects of opioids on breastfeeding using IBFAT in a small sample incorporating new and experienced mothers (Crowell et al. 1994). These researchers also showed the unhelpful effects of opioids on the initiation of breastfeeding. Their conclusions, however, are confounded by differences in reactions to labour pain and medication use as well as previous infant feeding experience. Kathryn Crowell and colleagues did find, though, that the breastfeeding of babies whose mothers received an opioid within an hour prior to the birth was less affected by the drug than those who had it administered 1–3 hours before birth, findings which were supported by a more recent study (Nissen et al. 1997). It may be that the babies with the shortest dose-delivery time interval were given a narcotic antagonist to counteract respiratory depression; this may also have lessened more general opioid-induced depression, thus facilitating the initiation of breastfeeding. On the basis of their findings, Crowell and colleagues suggest that better support in labour and postnatally prevents the need for opioids and the ensuing neonatal problems, respectively, and encourages perseverance with breastfeeding. Crowell and colleagues' mention of perseverance with breastfeeding reminds us of the limited research attention given to the effects of opioids administered in labour on the woman's continuation, or all too frequently discontinuation, of breastfeeding.

Effects in adolescence

The long term effects of opioids may also give rise to concern (Robinson 1995). Swedish research suggests that diamorphine given during labour is associated with a greater risk of drug addiction when the 'baby' reaches adulthood. Thus, not only are the woman's control and neonatal well-being jeopardised when opioids are administered, but also the autonomy of the one to whom she gives birth.

Dystocia

The effects of opioids on the progress of labour have been assumed to be beneficial (De Voe et al. 1969), but a pilot RCT on directed versus spontaneous second stage pushing produced unexpected findings. It identified a positive correlation between the length of the first and second stage of labour and the amount of pethidine that had been administered (Thomson & Hillier 1994). In the sample of 32 women, 14 had not received pethidine and 18 had, in doses totalling up to 250 mg. There were no differences in ethnic origin, gestation, haemoglobin, other drug use or baby details. Significant differences were identified between the two groups' duration of the first and second stage. For the unmedicated women the mean length of the first stage was 7.7 hours, whereas for the medicated women it was 11.7 hours. The difference in the length of the second stage was similarly significant. That pethidine interferes with efficient uterine contraction is further supported by the observation of increased third stage haemorrhage. The authors admit, though, that this may be associated with the increased incidence of instrumental assistance for the birth in the medicated group. The researchers' literature review found no evidence to contradict their findings. They are critical of the low-quality data on the effects of this frequently used drug, stating that the side-effects have been inadequately assessed. Contemplating further research, the authors discuss the ethics of an RCT which would deprive some women of their chosen method of pain control. It is necessary to further question, though, the ethical basis of widespread administration of a drug whose effects are inadequately researched and whether the woman should be expected to make decisions about pain control based on incomplete information (Mander 1993a).

Opioid drugs

I now outline the main aspects of the opioids used most commonly in labour in the UK.

Diamorphine

Due to its chemical structure, diamorphine has greater lipid solubility than morphine, allowing faster penetration into cerebral tissue. This rapid diffusion permits an equally rapid conversion into morphine, the active agent. Diamorphine is less likely to cause gastrointestinal upsets than morphine and the psychological benefits are more intense. Intramuscular (IM) administration of diamorphine results in the drug taking effect within 5–10 minutes and lasting for up to 3 hours. The recommended dosage varies between 2.5 and 7.5 mg, although whether this is adequate for a woman in labour is uncertain.

Pethidine

A synthetic analgesic, pethidine is metabolised in the liver; this is significant because the neonatal liver is immature, thus prolonging pethidine's neonatal effects (see 'Breastfeeding'). With IM administration the analgesic effect begins within 15 minutes and is supposed to continue for 2 hours. The recommended IM dosage is 50–150 mg.

Meptazinol

Meptazinol may be preferred to pethidine because neonatal respiratory depression is less marked. The analgesic action begins within 15 minutes and continues for about 4 hours. The recommended IM dosage is 75–100 mg.

Remifentanil

Although not widely used in the UK, this opioid has attracted some attention because of its ultra short action. For this reason it has been recommended for administration via patient controlled analgesia (PCA), although respiratory depression continues to cause concern (Blair et al. 2004).

Summary

In attempting to describe the opioids' place in the control of labour pain, the woman and her attendants must take account of the disadvantages of these agents as well as their benefits. In this section I have shown that the costs may be medium and long term as well as immediate and that although any benefits accrue mainly to the woman, the baby carries the burden of costs through respiratory depression and breastfeeding difficulties. The woman's control over these drugs is clearly non-existent once she has agreed to accept them and they have been administered. However, even before she agrees, her input may be limited by the lack of information available to her, which in turn is limited by the lack of research about issues that concern her, such as the effect of these drugs on her labour.

Before the question of opioids' relevance may be answered definitively, though, it is necessary to contemplate the alternative. When considering pharmacological approaches to controlling labour pain, the only effective alternative to opioids is regional or epidural analgesia, which I examine next.

Regional analgesia/anaesthesia

Methods of regional analgesia/anaesthesia which have been used during childbearing are legion, varying hugely in extent but usually involving the administration of a local anaesthetic, opioid or combination. Opioids' mode of action has been described already. Local anaesthetics act by altering the plasma membranes of excitable cells, that is, neurones. The resting potential of the cell membrane is unaffected by these drugs, but they prevent transmission of the action potential. This inhibition is due to the interruption of the first part of the action potential, the rapid inflow of sodium ions, by the displacement of membrane-bound calcium and the constriction of the sodium channels. Receptors for local anaesthetics, which are sited on either the neuronal membrane or within the sodium channel, initiate this response (Steinberg et al. 1996). Additionally, there is a decrease in the rate and degree of the depolarisation phase of the action potential, resulting in failure to reach the threshold potential. Thus, a blockade of conduction is achieved.

Regional analgesia/anaesthesia varies in extent from the patch sometimes applied prior to IV cannulation (Needham & Strehle 2008) to the spinal block which engenders 'not only numbness but also paralysis of the lower limbs' (Bonica 1990a: 1336). While epidural analgesia is the regional approach widely used to control labour pain, I refer briefly to spinal anaesthesia for completeness' sake.

Spinal anaesthesia

Sometimes indicated because it carries certain advantages over other anaesthetic or analgesic approaches, spinal anaesthesia bears some similarities to the epidural approach. The advantages include easier introduction, lower dosage, speedier onset and shorter action. These advantages, though, must be balanced against the greater risk of hypotension. Additionally, because the subarachnoid space is accessed, the likelihood of cerebrospinal fluid (CSF) leakage is increased, resulting in headache (Warwick & Neal 2007). These considerations result in spinal anaesthesia being used to facilitate specific interventions, such as caesarean. Despite its widespread use, the effectiveness of spinal anaesthesia still arouses some concerns (Krishnan 2002).

Epidural analgesia (and combined)

A surgical technique, like lumbar puncture, facilitates the injection of slow-acting local anaesthetics, such as bupivicaine, or other analgesic medications into the lumbar epidural space. The cannula, for delivering the drug, is sited and the initial injection administered by an obstetric anaesthetist. The administration may be on an intermittent or 'top up' basis, by a suitably trained midwife with written instructions from an anaesthetist. Alternatively a PCA delivery system or continuous infusion may be used. A shorter-acting local anaesthetic, such as lignocaine, is injected as a test dose in view of the potential complications, or opioids may be administered epidurally.

Effects

Epidural analgesia blocks the transmission of pain impulses via the afferent spinal nerves that traverse the epidural space and transmit pain impulses from organs, such as the uterus, to the CNS. The efficient binding of bupivicaine with maternal plasma proteins prevents more than 20% being transferred transplacentally.

Incidence

Because of the serious maternal risks associated with this form of pain control (Lieberman 1999; Kinsella et al. 2007), the maternity units offering it were limited. The widespread closure of smaller units, though, has changed this picture. Steer found that epidural block was used to control pain in 19.3% of labours in the UK in 1993. The use of this intervention has increased markedly since then; its use in England averages 33%, with a range from 5% to 'over 45%', suggesting that the upper end of the range is not for public consumption (Richardson & Mmata 2007). In Stockholm, an epidural rate of 52% was reported among first time mothers in 2009 (Bergström et al. 2009), while in the US, Eugene Declercq and colleagues identified an epidural rate of 63% (2002).

Issues

When first introduced, epidural analgesia in labour provided effective pain control in well-defined and potentially pathological situations, such as a woman experiencing incoordinate uterine action (Moir 1973). The realisation that epidural anaesthesia could also remedy the abysmal contribution of obstetric anaesthesia to maternal mortality provided the obstetric anaesthetist's excuse for entering the birthing room (Doughty 1987; Morgan 1987). In this way our anaesthetic colleagues established a power base, from which they could expand their role and professional status (Mander 1993). This expansion involved epidural analgesia in uncomplicated labour being 'fostered directly or indirectly by the professionals' (Hibbard & Scott 1990). Such 'fostering', 'encouragement' or 'hard selling' has been reported anecdotally (Wilshin & Wilson 1991; Machover 1995), but that such 'marketing' still persists is evident in the writing of John Crowhurst and Felicity Plaat (2000: 165).

Effectiveness

An effective epidural unquestionably eradicates the pain of uterine contractions more completely than any other method (Simmons et al. 2007). The proportion of epidural blocks that are effective, though, is difficult to estimate as data are not readily available. The success rate of epidural analgesia varies between 67% and 90% (Simkin 1989); this is supported by one of the few, albeit shaky, studies to even mention the risk of epidural failure (Kitzinger 1987b).

Other problems

Unfortunately, as well as pain impulses, non-pain efferent impulses may also be blocked (Pursey 1994), causing immobility and the woman to be bedfast for at least the duration of the epidural block. Additionally, sympathetic nerve fibres are blocked, resulting in vasodilatation in the lower body, which causes sudden and potentially life-threatening hypotension. To prevent this, a rapid IV infusion is established prior to siting the epidural and a supine posture discouraged. In 2% of women receiving epidural analgesia the hypotensive episode is sufficiently severe to require stimulation using ephedrine (Van de Velde et al. 2007). Together with pain, bladder sensation is removed resulting, due to the IV fluids, in the bladder becoming distended in up to 18% of women. Without urinary catheterisation, and attendant infection risks, labour becomes further prolonged (Evron et al. 2003).

The tendency of epidural analgesia to cause dystocia and lengthen labour, especially the second stage, is long-recognised (Williams et al. 1985), although a more recent systematic review has questioned this finding (Zhang et al. 1999). While these reviewers refuted the lengthening of labour, they clearly identified the increased use of augmentation associated with epidural analgesia. Williams' classic study, involving 85 women of whom 38 chose epidural analgesia, demonstrated the increased incidence of a series of obstetric procedures, recognised as the 'cascade of intervention'. This has been identified in obstetric practice and may have been facilitated or aggravated by the introduction of effective pain control (Varney Burst 1983). The 'cascade' may be associated with neurological changes mentioned above in 'Other problems' which cause pelvic floor relaxation, malposition of the fetal head, incomplete rotation and second stage delay. Oxytocic drugs which correct the delay are associated with fetal hypoxia. Thus, interventions to expedite the birth, for example forceps or caesarean, become necessary.

Obstetric anaesthetists have worked long and hard against the perception that epidural analgesia is associated with interventive birth (Zhang et al. 1999). These strenuous efforts, if nothing else, suggest that this perception is founded in reality.

Problems associated with epidurals, such as immobility, difficulty bearing down, motor block, malrotation and deflexion, have long been recognised; for a similar time there has been confidence that 'variations in anaesthetic technique' will resolve them (Scottish Home and Health Department 1985: 4). An example is the combination spinal/epidurals, introduced to overcome some of the hazards associated with traditional epidural techniques. A systematic review suggests that the problems are not remedied by this novel approach (Scott et al. 2007).

After-effects

The problems that the woman encounters after epidural analgesia have been similarly widely investigated. The occurrence of headache varies in intensity, duration and, hence, treatment. 'Spinal axis syndrome', involving subclinical neurological and orthopaedic damage, has been suggested to explain the symptoms that women experience after an epidural (MacArthur et al. 1991). Of the epidural users in their retrospective sample, 18.9% developed back pain, compared with 10.5% in those women using other analgesia. In a study with a better response rate (MacLeod et al. 1995), those with back pain increased to 26.2%. On the basis of a volunteer sample, these claims have been dismissed as 'amnesia', because some women's back pain preceded their labour (Russell et al. 1996).

Perinatal and woman-oriented issues

The lack of authoritative data on neonatal and long term maternal effects has been highlighted. The rise in maternal temperature associated with the administration of epidural analgesia (Lieberman 1999) inevitably causes fetal changes. If the woman's epidural has been ongoing for over 8 hours fetal tachycardia may result and be misdiagnosed as fetal distress, leading to supposedly appropriate intervention in the labour and subsequently.

The paucity of research into woman-oriented aspects of epidural analgesia has been noted repeatedly (Mander 1994), as has the need for suitably timed strong research (Chalmers 1993; Oakley 1993). This omission has been applied particularly to women's poor knowledge about the multitude of potentially serious side effects (Declercq et al. 2002). The care of the woman in labour involves supporting her in a series of decisions, which are impossible without comprehensive research-based information. Those caring for the woman are responsible for ensuring that the information which exists is available to her.

Methods of administration

Because certain developments in drug administration relate particularly to epidural analgesia, I discuss them here. As mentioned in Chapter 8, the woman's control over her use of non-pharmacological methods of pain control tends to be great but variable. Traditionally, there has been less maternal control over the administration of pharmacological methods, because they are prescribed and (generally) administered by professionals; inhalational analgesia is the exception to this observation. Feelings of powerlessness inherent in any pain experience are aggravated by dependence on others for analgesia and by uncertainty about its availability and effect. The delayed onset of some drugs' effects together with the large doses needed to prolong their effects has long been recognised as 'roller coaster analgesia' (Sechzer 1971; Reynolds 1990), which comprises huge swings in pain control between peaks of sedation and troughs of agony.

To overcome these problems in acute pain situations, PCA ('patient controlled analgesia' or 'parturient controlled analgesia') systems may be used to administer drugs either IV or epidurally (Schlug & Watson 2002). The pumps employed to administer the drug may permit a background infusion and/or a patient-triggered bolus. The rate of the infusion, the size of the bolus and the lockout period (during which no bolus is obtainable) are programmed by the physician setting up the PCA.

Research undertaken in non-maternity postoperative situations indicates widespread user-satisfaction with opioid PCA systems despite severe pain (Lebovits et al. 2001). There is considerable variation in drug intake between users, suggesting that PCA does individualise doses; however, this variation tends towards higher drug intake (Rogers et al. 1990). More recent research, though, suggests that other outcomes, such as ambulation, may not be improved or may even be impaired by PCA use (Snell et al. 1997). Snell's study raises the issue of postoperative nausea and vomiting among PCA users which, in my experience, is more prevalent and causes greater upset than among women receiving intermittent opioids. A study of the addition of a prophylactic anti-emetic suggests that this problem is not easily remediable (Cherian & Smith 2001).

Patient controlled epidural analgesia (PCEA) has been compared with a continuous epidural infusion for women in labour (Ledin Eriksson et al. 2003). For both groups the 'study solution' comprised the same opioid and local anaesthetic combination. A large majority of the women were well-satisfied with their pain control; the exception being the women's displeasure with their feelings of pressure during the second stage. The side effects of pruritis and hypotension are reported as not being serious and the women's mobility was variably affected.

The implications of these method of drug administration for midwifery staffing and practice are clearly immense, but appear to be unresearched.

General anaesthesia

While not a conventional form of pain control, general anaesthesia (GA) is included here because it is used in maternity care to permit interventions that would otherwise be too painful to contemplate; and also because it raises important pain-related issues. GA is used to facilitate the birth of the baby by caesarean, or only the placenta, in emergencies. It is appropriate when there is insufficient time and/or expertise for establishing regional anaesthesia.

General, or whole body, anaesthesia involves the patient's loss of consciousness as the brain is exposed to controlled concentrations of reversible medications, which would otherwise be poisonous. The crucial characteristics of GA include amnesia and freedom from pain (Boswell & Hameroff 1996: 457). These writers admit ignorance of the action of the agents used; such ignorance applies to the mechanism as well as the site of action.

Incidence

A number of accounts show how infrequently GA is used in maternity; in one series only 238 women out of 6459 (3.9%) were administered GA during labour (Steer 1993). More recently this figure has been confirmed at 'about 3% of women' in labour, with antenatal and postnatal interventions superimposed (Scott & Wee 2007: 48). This small number is probably due to the increasing availability of regional anaesthesia and GA's risk of serious harm, and possibly death, for the childbearing woman. The absolute *number* of caesarean operations performed under GA may not have changed, because the falling proportion of GAs is compensated by the increasing number of caesareans (Banks & Levy 2007). Disconcertingly paradoxically, GA is used relatively frequently in small and very small maternity units (<2000 births per annum) (Scottish Office Home and Health Department 1996). As I discuss below, the frequency of obstetric GAs matters because it has implications for their safety.

General anaesthesia and maternal death

Barbara Morgan (1987) relates the dreadful history of the contribution of obstetric GA to maternal mortality. The number of maternal deaths due to or associated with GA peaked during 1964–69 (in which time 100 women died thus); however, of greater significance is the *proportion* of maternal deaths that were due to or associated with GA. Despite the rising birth rate then, the number of maternal deaths due to other causes was falling markedly; this resulted from various factors including higher living standards, smaller families, better antenatal care and the availability of antibiotics and blood transfusion.

The number of direct maternal deaths attributed to anaesthesia is now relatively stable, and it is estimated that anaesthesia currently features in approximately one half of maternal deaths (Cooper & McClure 2007: 107).

A large proportion of maternal deaths due to or associated with GA have traditionally been caused by the aspiration of acid stomach contents into the woman's lungs during the induction of GA in labour (Mendelson's syndrome; Banks & Levy 2007). Although this condition does not feature in the most recent *Confidential Enquiries* (Cooper & McClure 2007), it is addressed at suitable length in *Crises in Childbirth – Why Mothers Survive* (Scott & Wee 2007). The death of a mother in association with anaesthesia is currently more likely to be blamed, at least in part, on her obesity (Cooper & McClure 2007); according to Stacey obesity causes death by impeding ventilation (2007: 19). Such technical difficulties have been shown to lead to tragedies, which are frequently ascribed to the 'trainee' status of the anaesthetist (Cooper & McClure 2007: 107). Clearly trainee anaesthetists need sufficient experience and 'hours of work' to make them competent in an area as challenging as obstetric anaesthesia. The difficulty of providing trainees with suitable experience in GA is well-recognised (Banks & Levy 2007: 319). Similarly, such junior staff need to be encouraged to accept other disciplines' advice and to call on their senior colleagues when in doubt.

Awareness

Unsurprisingly, the possibility of maternal death is not included in the information given to the woman preparing for a GA, but the risk of the woman being 'aware' during GA has attracted attention among consumer groups (Beech 1995a). This 'awareness' results from the likelihood of a light GA being administered to minimise transplacental passage of anaesthetic drugs, which would cause neonatal respiratory depression (Banks & Levy 2007: 318). This precaution clearly benefits the neonate. It may mean, however, that the woman is less than adequately anaesthetised, causing her to remain conscious but unable to communicate her consciousness. I first realised the existence of this problem when, as a student midwife 'running' for a caesarean, the woman's hand sought to push away the scalpel as the skin incision was made.

The extent of this problem becomes apparent in Beverley Beech's quotation of Selwyn Crawford's estimate of 1% of women being aware during GA; she converted this into 400 women every year (1995a). In the absence of research on this topic, we have to rely on anecdotal evidence to indicate the traumatic nature of such an experience. These accounts lead us to question whether the woman should be informed of the possibility of awareness, as she should be informed of the potential for other adverse outcomes.

The father's presence

In their discussion of women's experiences of caesarean delivery, Anne Oakley and Martin Richards (1990) recounted the benefits to all involved of the father's presence during the operation. In the event of a GA, they explained how the father, having been in the operating room, is able to give the woman an account of the birth. These researchers implied that this 'account' is helpful to the woman who was unconscious for the birth. Is the father ordinarily permitted to be present in this situation? My observation is that the father is excluded on the grounds that the couple are unable to 'share' the birth. It has been suggested that his presence, far from being unnecessary, matters more than ever if the woman undergoes a caesarean (Koppel & Kaiser 2001).

Cannabis

Anecdotal reports have suggested that cannabis (marijuana) may carry beneficial psychotropic and pain controlling effects for the woman in labour (Beil-Hildebrand 1999). This should come as no surprise, as it has been 'used for the treatment of … dysmenorrhea' by Queen Victoria among others (Baker et al. 2003: 291). Research has shown, though, that cannabinoids have a limited place in the control of pain which is long term (Hosking & Zajicek 2008; Campbell et al. 2001). In the context of more acute pain, a major research project showing some benefits was ended prematurely because of an untoward incident; despite the major input of an anaesthetist with a special interest in pain in women, this report made no mention of childbearing women (Holdcroft et al. 2006). Thus, research evidence to support the anecdotal reports is lacking.

Conclusion

In this chapter I have drawn on Nicky Leap's pain relief model to scrutinise the options available to the woman who selects pharmacological methods of pain control. The reliance on these methods depends on the perception that labour pain is inevitably associated with suffering; the basis of which may be linked to a medical orientation to labour and childbearing. This orientation brings with it the panoply of interventions which are widely referred to as the 'cascade'. Such an orientation removes autonomy from the woman, and allows it to be assumed by her professional carers. This means that they 'take the lead and dictate such basic human actions as eating, drinking, using the toilet, even rolling over in bed' (Simkin & Bolding 2004: 489). As these researchers identify, pharmacological analgesia may relieve pain, but it also carries the risk of aggravating the woman's suffering through increasing her dependence on others. Being more dependent may be less than appropriate at a time when she needs to be confident enough to rely on her own ability to become a mother.

Through the medium of this chapter I have shown that, while our knowledge of the effects of pharmacological pain control methods is more extensive than of their non-pharmacological counterparts, great gaps in our knowledge still persist. These gaps apply particularly to the 'softer', more woman-oriented effects.

For these reasons, I would argue that it may not be justifiable for the midwife to dismiss a woman's concerns about pharmacological analgesia in terms as familiar as:

You don't get a medal for being a martyr (Langford 1997).

Part IV

The Journey's End

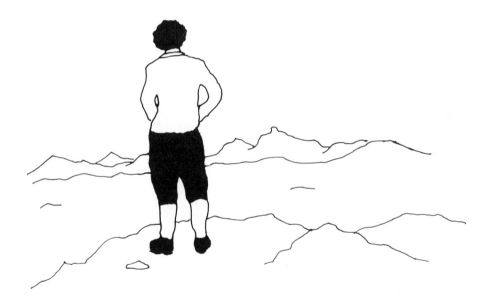

Chapter 10

Postnatal pain

Postnatal care is currently held in low regard. One of the reasons for this relates to a general perception that care postnatally is the 'Cinderella' of maternity (i.e. it is undervalued and under-funded), despite the fact that it traditionally consumes over half of available midwifery resources (Schmied & Everitt 1996; Ball 1991). Is this because it lacks the pregnancy's exciting anticipation or the glamorous uncertainty of intrapartum care? Or is it because postnatal care relies so heavily on interpersonal skills, probably the most fundamentally important in the midwife's repertoire?

A further reason for post natal care's low regard is found in the limited significance attached by women to the postnatal period; this becomes apparent when the woman talks of 'it' being over, meaning the labour, as if the birth represents the climactic end of her childbearing experience. Thus, viewed with such disdain on both sides, it is hardly surprising that the postnatal period may be an anticlimax and, for the woman, aggravated by painful echoes of the birth, labour and even pregnancy.

After observing such disregard in medical textbooks, a survey of the type and severity of postnatal pain, assessed the effectiveness of therapeutic interventions (Dewan et al. 1993). These researchers recruited 198 women and interviewed them on the first, second and fourth days postnatally, if the woman remained in hospital. The prevalence of postnatal pain appeared on the first day, when 95% of women complained of at least one type of pain. Its severity is indicated by the proportion (72%) who needed analgesic medication. This study illuminated a much-neglected area and began with a large sample. The generalisability of the findings are questionable, though, in view of the inevitable attrition from the study as women went home. Thus, by day four less than 50% of the women were still responding (n=94). These women probably suffered pathological conditions preventing transfer home, making them unrepresentative.

The pain of suffering: postnatal mental health problems

As I have argued in Chapter 2, the depression often witnessed and experienced during pregnancy and new motherhood may appropriately be regarded as a form of emotional pain. The mental health problems faced during the postnatal period, though, extend beyond depression. The least severe form of disturbance goes by various names, including

Pain in Childbearing and its Control, Second Edition. By Rosemary Mander. Published 2011 by Blackwell Publishing Ltd. © 1998, 2011 Rosemary Mander.

'the blues' (Rondón 2003), and features emotional lability. The psychosocial changes for the woman tend to be discounted in favour of attributing a hormonal cause to this and the new mother's other mental difficulties.

On the other hand, and really deserving to be entitled 'suffering' and 'painful' is the most severe form of puerperal mental illness – psychosis. Recent qualitative research by Elizabeth Edwards and Stephen Timmons shows the extent of that suffering among women with puerperal psychosis and severe depression. Superimposed on their mental state, these women felt that they were stigmatised by being unable to access suitable care and through the guilt which they experienced at being 'bad mothers' (2005: 477).

Pelvic pain

When contemplating postnatal pelvic pain, an immediate reaction is 'Hardly surprising ...'. However, birth trauma is not the only cause. In this section I consider first a pain unrelated to trauma, and then move on to three types of pain which are largely traumatic, but which may cause the woman difficulty in differentiating the source. Although urinary tract infection may cause pain postnatally, I have addressed it already (Chapter 6).

Afterpains

As mentioned in relation to Braxton Hicks' contractions (Chapter 6), women feel uterine contractions painful at particular times in their lives. The postnatal period is another of these times, constituting a painful echo of labour. 'Afterpains' may be known as 'after-birth pains' in North America or 'uterine cramps' (Huang et al. 2002). Chronologically, afterpains are the woman's first hint that, although her baby is born, her pain may be unfinished, because afterpains may begin before the placenta is delivered.

The research and clinical attention focusing on afterpains, like pregnancy-related pain (Chapter 6), is scanty. Thus, I have located minimal evidence on the effectiveness of the remedies used and none on the incidence of afterpains. This disregard contrasts with my observation as a midwife: that some women experience their afterpains as a major burden requiring powerful analgesia.

Afterpains tend to be associated with multiparity and with breastfeeding (Marchant 2009). The former is due to the alleged tendency of an over-worked uterus to relax and the latter through the mediation of oxytocin facilitating the let-down reflex. The reality of this association is uncertain, although Christa Kelleher's feminist study of women's post-natal challenges suggests that afterpains are one of the most commonly mentioned forms of breastfeeding-related pain (2006: 2730).

Joyce Vogler (1993) reported the intrauterine pressure during afterpains as 150 mmHg, which is greater than during labour, which peaks at 100 mmHg. The woman's perception of the severity of afterpains, however, has been assessed mainly in two drug trials. Both protocols assessed the woman's pain on entry into the trial. Using a scale of 0–3 to represent none to severe pain respectively, 159 women rated their pain as ranging from 0.09 to 2.53 (Bloomfield et al. 1986). In Norway 64 women completed a 10 cm visual analogue scale (VAS) extending from 'no pain' to 'pain as bad as it can be'; this produced an average score of just below 60 (Skovlund et al. 1991). This is articulated by women as like 'the most challenging moments of their labour' (Kelleher 2006: 2730).

These data provide no indication of the incidence of afterpains, because each study recruited only women experiencing afterpains; they do, however, show how severely women perceive such pain. Because each trial was time-limited neither do they indicate the duration of afterpains, but this has been 'guesstimated' at 2–3 days (Olds et al. 1996). Olds and colleagues' guesstimate is supported by a Scottish survey which included 'uterine cramps' in the data collection (Dewan et al. 1993). Unsurprisingly, these researchers found that afterpains were felt by more women and more severely on the first day, compared with the second and fourth days. Fewer primigravid women experienced these pains and felt them less severely than their multiparous sisters. The maximal incidence and severity was when afterpains were felt as moderate/severe by 56% of first day multiparous women. By day four no primigravid women were experiencing them as moderate/severe, but 5% of multiparous women still felt them so.

Pharmaceutical companies' obvious interest indicates that analgesic medication is widely used to treat afterpains, and administration has been recommended 'one hour before [breast] feeding her infant' (Olds et al. 1996: 1047); such advice raises a host of questions about breastfeeding practice. Vogler (1993) recommends explanations, warmth, rest, relaxation and keeping the bladder empty rather than medication.

It appears, yet again, that this pain is not considered significant, contrasting with my observation of women's experience. Disconcertingly, afterpains coincide with nipple pain, as both are associated with breastfeeding (Niven & Gijsbers 1996a). This coincidence only increases the risk of the woman discontinuing breastfeeding, as increasing proportions of Scottish mothers do within the first 10 days (ISD 2009). For this, if for no other reason, afterpains deserve more, and more serious, attention.

The pain of perineal repair

Although postnatal perineal pain has quite rightly attracted considerable clinical and research attention (see below), the pain of the repair itself has been neglected. Exceptionally, Green and colleagues' large, wide-ranging and authoritative study of labour happened upon women's dissatisfaction with the 'actual suturing' (1988). Only one-third of the women were not caused pain, with 19% reporting severe pain, so that some women remember it as 'the worst thing about the entire birth' (1988: 6.21). Subsequently, Ann Wraight (1993) referred to women being dissatisfied with pain control during their 'stitching'; this study found the large proportion of women who underwent this procedure with inadequate analgesia. These are the one third of the sample who used only nitrous oxide and oxygen or nothing at all. More recently, Julia Sanders and colleagues' authoritative study demonstrates the continuing existence of this problem and that women 'endure high levels of pain' (2002: 1067; 2005). These researchers' longitudinal data collection indicates that women's recollection of pain increased with time, perhaps due to their greater honesty after transfer home.

These women's problems were impressed on me when I was involved in a home birth prior to midwives being permitted to suture the perineum. The general practitioner who we were required to call to suture the laceration declined to infiltrate with local anaesthetic, so nitrous oxide and oxygen was used with limited effect. Thus, my impression is that perineal suturing is painful and that effective analgesia is crucial. It may be, though, that if a laceration is small, local anaesthesia causes more problems than it solves. We should question, however, whether a laceration too small to need local anaesthetic really requires suturing.

The issue of limited or non-suturing of perineal lacerations attracts interest, more because of its effect on subsequent perineal pain than the pain of suturing. Christine Kettle and Susan Tohill conclude that not suturing the skin predisposes to gaping of the wound but the pain of the wound and dyspareunia may be reduced (2008). The evidence relating to non-suturing of first and second degree lacerations is even more limited and is only permissible at the woman's explicit request (Kettle & Tohill 2008).

Tissue adhesives have been introduced in surgery and might eliminate the pain of perineal repair. These substances, applied to the edges of the skin wound, mimic the final stages of coagulation to form a fibrin clot which is both haemostatic and adhesive. Tissue adhesives' value in perineal repair is uncertain, because their main advantage is their cosmetic effect. Additionally, using these adhesives still requires suturing of the deep layers as the adhesive is applied only to the skin wound (Rogerson 2000). Having found no evidence on the relative painfulness of suturing the deep layers, I cannot imagine that non-suturing of just the skin would greatly improve the woman's experience.

Perineal pain

Postnatal perineal pain matters, not only in itself, but also for its effect on the woman's relationships with those she loves. This applies initially to her ability to relax sufficiently to breastfeed and later to her resumption of sexual activity (see 'Dyspareunia', below). The occurrence and severity of perineal pain has been studied in relation to certain interventions, which may resolve birth-related trauma. Additionally, many remedies have been suggested and used to reduce perineal pain, some of which have been researched.

Perineal damage

Following longstanding claims to justify routine episiotomy (Banta & Thacker 1982), a major research project sought its short and long term effects (Sleep 1984). A randomised controlled trial (RCT) distinguished the effects of more liberal and more restrictive use of episiotomy. The sample comprised 1000 women, randomised late in the second stage. No significant differences emerged between the two groups' perineal pain at 10 days or at 3 months, but the women in the restrictive group tended to resume sexual intercourse earlier. While establishing benefits of neither laceration nor episiotomy, this study showed that restricting episiotomy allows more women to birth without perineal damage. A follow-up study, 3 years later, sought the long term effects of the different policies (Sleep & Grant 1987a) and, again, no clear differences manifested themselves.

Suture technique/material

Since midwives assumed responsibility for perineal repair in the 1980s they have been able to decide the most appropriate suture material and method of suturing. Unlike some of the topics which are important to childbearing women the most appropriate suture material/technique has attracted considerable research attention. This research has measured outcomes such as perineal pain, analgesic medication, need for suture removal, need for resuturing, resumption of sexual intercourse and dyspareunia. As mentioned already, not suturing the skin has been shown to convey some benefit in terms of the woman's pain. Kettle and Tohill's authoritative systematic review shows that the evidence supporting the use of synthetic suture material, rather than catgut, is persuasive (2008). Even more pronounced are the advantages of using fast-absorbing polyglactin 910 for perineal suturing.

After reviewing research on the techniques, Adrian Grant (1989b) recommended unambiguously the superiority of subcuticular sutures, which has been endorsed more recently (Kettle & Tohill 2008). The improvements are further enhanced by a continuous suturing technique being used for the suturing of the deeper perineal layers.

It is difficult to avoid the conclusion that the reason for the wealth of research into perineal suture materials relates to the costs involved. The link between suture techniques/materials and perineal pain emerged from a cost effectiveness analysis (Howard et al. 1995b). These health economists analysed the cost effectiveness of perineal repair techniques. The factors affecting costs were categorised according to suture material and technique, and related to outcomes with cost implications. Valid research on non-absorbable and absorbable sutures relied predominantly on pain to evaluate benefits, such as short term and long term pain and dyspareunia. Additionally, analgesic medication use, removal of absorbable material and resuturing had been evaluated. Short term pain and analgesia use differed markedly, with non-absorbable sutures being associated with pain in 32% of women compared with 22% with absorbable sutures, giving an odds ratio of 0.60. Analgesia use was also significantly different. Scrutiny of the research on techniques of skin suturing, found clearly better outcomes in relation to short term pain with continuous suturing, with an odds ratio of 0.68. Additionally, suture material was more likely to need removal, incurring major costs, because of tightness and/or pain, when interrupted suturing was used. Without specifying it, these researchers introduced an argument persuasive to the current UK health care system; this states that greater pain increases health care costs and that such costs are reduced by applying research appropriately.

Local measures

Although bathing has traditionally been recommended as a remedy for both perineal pain and healing, empirical data do not support this. An uncontrolled study (Sleep & Grant 1988a) found that 93% of women questioned on the tenth day agreed that bathing had relieved their perineal pain. These researchers, though, when measuring perineal pain at 10 days and 3 months, found no difference in pain reports between women who were adding salt, Savlon (chlorhexidine gluconate 1.5% wv and cetrimide ph eur 15% wv in an aqueous solution) or neither to their bath. Replicating this study and including a 'shower' group would clarify the value of bathing, but a 'bidet' group would be necessary to control for the psychological benefits of immersion and flowing water.

Local measures comprise the perineal application of a variety of preparations. Ice packs have been used in 84% of maternity units, but their benefit lasts only while frozen (Sleep & Grant 1988b). Gel-filled pads have been marketed as preferable and user-satisfaction has been recorded (Steen 2000; Punasundri 2008). The potentially harmful effects on wound healing associated with temporary ischaemia or ice burns when ice packs are used has not been reported for gel pads.

Pharmacological preparations, such as local anaesthetic gel, have been subjected to research with some possible benefit (Corkill et al. 2001). As found by an authoritative systematic review, these products' benefits are uncertain and their implications for healing require research attention (East et al. 2007).

Physical remedies

The multiplicity of physical interventions recommended for postnatal problems is under-researched and, hence, of uncertain benefit. Postnatal exercises are one example of such an intervention. The effect of pelvic floor exercises on urinary and faecal incontinence was evaluated by Jenny Sleep and Adrian Grant (1987b). The compliance of the sample women verged on enthusiasm, which makes the findings less valid by raising the spectre of the Hawthorne effect. One group was taught the usual pelvic floor exercises in the usual way, whereas the experiment group received individual tuition by a midwife and kept a health diary for a month. Despite methodological problems, it is noteworthy that perineal pain was significantly less in the experiment group at 3 months, although there were no significant differences in any other symptoms. Postnatal exercises have had many claims made for them, but pain control is not one; this research suggests that pain control may be their only benefit.

The air ring or ring cushion has found its way from nursing elderly people to easing postnatal perineal pain. In both situations the aim is to reduce pressure on a limited area by raising it from hard surfaces. Sarah Church and Patricia Lyne (1994) argued that the damage hypothesised as occurring in elderly tissues by the displacement of pressure by air rings is unproven. They suggested that new mothers should not be deprived of this potential source of comfort because our nursing cousins have overreacted to a specious argument.

Various forms of energy, such as infra-red light, have been applied to the perineum to assist healing and reduce pain. Ultrasound and pulsed electromagnetic energy treatment have been shown not to make any difference.

Systemic preparations

The range of oral analgesics available to remedy perineal pain is immense, but their unwanted side-effects, for both woman and baby, demand careful consideration. Suitable only to treat less intense pain, these medications may result in the woman seeking other more effective remedies, such as rectally administered medication, including NSAIDs. Although likely to be effective, suppositories' long term and other effects need attention (Hedayati et al. 2003) and acceptability of this route of administration also deserves consideration.

Complementary therapies

The main focus of complementary remedies in postnatal perineal care is on herbal preparations to assist healing. Substances such as comfrey, lavender and calendula are infused in water and then used for a sitz bath. Because these are 'complementary' interventions and midwives are unlikely to have been taught about their use, comprehensive consultation with recognised herbalists and pharmacists is essential to protect the midwife using them.

Further, regarding knowledge of their effects, herbal preparations should be treated with the same caution that we apply to pharmacological interventions. However, that 'evidence is required that they are both safe and therapeutic' (Sleep 1991: 8) is a counsel of perfection which has been applied less than stringently to their pharmacological equivalents.

Evidence has been sought about lavender oil, a form of aromatherapy, which is widely used for its healing and antiseptic properties but may also be added to bath water to reduce perineal pain (Dale & Cornwell 1994). These researchers' double blind RCT involved 635 women, of whom one group added pure lavender oil to their bath, the second group used synthetic lavender oil and the third used an inert placebo. Six drops were added to the daily bath until the tenth postnatal day. Data were collected using visual analogue scales which the woman completed 30 minutes after her bath and which sought information on mood and perineal pain. On the tenth day the woman and midwife completed questionnaires on perineal healing. The data showed that 90% of mothers reported feeling better after a bath and in 74% the perineum was healed by day ten; these findings, like the women using pure lavender oil having lower pain scores, did not reach statistical significance. That no side-effects were identified suggests the safety of this therapy.

Summary

Since the early 1980s and due largely to one team, midwives' research-based knowledge of perineal damage and associated pain has increased exponentially. Similarly, our knowledge of the causes, treatment and implications of perineal pain has expanded. Longstanding changes in practice have resulted. Our attention, however, has been drawn to the inconsistent and idiosyncratic use of research findings in practice (Harris 1992). Harris interviewed a sample of 76 practitioners, mainly midwives, about the research basis of their perineal care. She found that the questionably relevant ideas on air rings were most frequently quoted. This contrasted with the pertinent and authoritative studies on suture material and technique, such as those mentioned above, which were not reported. Thus, 'inappropriate' research utilisation has been identified and midwives' educational needs are widely recognised, but may not be prioritised (Hundley et al. 2000).

While certain forms of painful perineal damage, such as episiotomy and severe laceration, are easily identifiable and hence researchable, others are less so. This means that certain forms of perineal damage and ensuing pain are under-researched. Examples are bruising and oedema about which women complain and which midwives not infrequently observe; together with the less common haematoma, midwives seek to advise the woman about these forms of trauma. Research is long overdue to increase our knowledge of and improve our care for women with these equally challenging but far from glamorous problems.

Haemorrhoids

Haemorrhoids, usually known as 'piles', are a particular problem in pregnancy and the postnatal period. They are largely due to physiological changes in the pregnant woman's cardiovascular system. In spite of the changes originating with pregnancy, I include haemorrhoids in the 'Pelvic pain' section, rather than with pain in the circulatory system (see 'Thromboembolic pain', this chapter) because, in my experience, women find difficulty distinguishing the pain of haemorrhoids from other perineal pain. Although haemorrhoids are often said to present for the first time during pregnancy, they are thought to be aggravated by the birth. Women are also said to be more aware of this problem postnatally, and for these reasons it is included here rather than with pregnancy pain (Chapter 6, 'Pain of cardiovascular origin').

During childbearing varicose veins may affect a number of sites in the woman's body, such as legs, abdomen and vulva, but when the anal canal is affected haemorrhoids ensue. The incidence of this problem is uncertain, but a large majority of women seeking treatment for haemorrhoids have experienced at least one pregnancy (Quijano & Abalos 2005). Although the association with childbearing is clear, the incidence of haemorrhoids and their development are less certain. The increased venous blood pressure in the dependent parts of the woman's body is likely to be at least partly responsible. Superimposed on this rise in pressure is a 50% increase in the venous distensibility or degree of dilatation at a given pressure, due to placental oestrogens. The development of haemorrhoids has been linked with diet and constipation (Olds et al. 1996), but the empirical evidence supporting these links is unclear. Based on this assertion, women are advised to ensure adequate dietary fibre and a high fluid intake. The pain of haemorrhoids is said to be continuous, being exacerbated by straining, sitting and walking; it is associated with a mucoid discharge and sometimes bleeding, which stains toilet paper and underclothing, as well as anal pruritis (Olds et al. 1996).

Local palliative remedies, such as ice or ointments, are recommended to reduce the size and hence pain of haemorrhoids, but haemorrhoidectomy may be necessary. The literature on haemorrhoids in childbearing tends towards reassurance; as Olds and colleagues state: '[haemorrhoids] usually become asymptomatic after the early postpartal period' (1996). Like many statements relating to haemorrhoids, there is no indication of its research basis. As these authors indicate, and is generally accepted, the expulsive efforts of the second stage are thought to exacerbate haemorrhoids, but again evidence is lacking.

Research on the postnatal period by Christine MacArthur and colleagues (1991) has been roundly criticised for the unrepresentative sample, but it does illuminate a widely neglected area of care. A more recent and authoritative systematic review (Quijano & Abalos 2005) produced similar findings, albeit with the possibility of drug remedies whose safety remains uncertain.

On the basis of the earlier findings, I proposed, with a multidisciplinary team, to seek answers prospectively to the still-outstanding questions about haemorrhoids in childbearing. The funding bodies greeted the research proposal with deafening silence, leading to the conclusion that a problem as fundamental as this holds little attraction for grant-givers. Thus, our lack of authoritative empirical knowledge about this pervasive problem persists and will continue as long as funding bodies direct resources towards acute problems which are perceived as sexy and amenable to high-tech interventions.

Dyspareunia

As emerged in the section on perineal pain, the woman's ability to enjoy coitus is often used to indicate perineal healing. Thus, we should consider first the pathophysiological factors associated with postnatal dyspareunia, which occurs in a majority of new mothers (Kettle et al. 2005).

A widely recognised factor with the potential to make intercourse painful for a woman is the lack of vaginal lubrication, which occurs at various times in her life. This 'dryness' is associated with 'soreness and irritation' during intercourse or afterwards, assuming that it is not severe enough to prevent penetration. Vaginal dryness postnatally, and extending through lactation, is associated with oestrogen deficiency. Thus, the vaginal wall not only becomes drier, but also thinner due to atrophy (Bancroft 1994).

Perineal damage has been implicated in changes in sexual function postnatally. While occasionally thought to be positive, the negativity of these changes is now more widely accepted (Kitzinger 1995). In a survey involving 89 women, suturing of the perineum was identified as the crucial predictor of dyspareunia rather than the intentionality of the damage (Fleming & Schafer 1989). These researchers did, however, find a significantly higher level of long term dyspareunia in women who had an episiotomy. They surmise that the cause is the more extensive tissue damage which an episiotomy incurs, which is due to the incision being made prior to the physiological separation of muscle tissue.

Fear of dyspareunia after vaginal birth may now contribute to the epidemic of 'tocophobia' whose only remedy is caesarean (Mander 2007). Michael Klein and colleagues (2005), however, found that caesarean offers no effective protection from dyspareunia, as women giving birth vaginally with an intact perineum experienced less dyspareunia than women having caesareans.

A study on perineal pain focused on dyspareunia in relation to the suture material (Sleep et al. 1989). Chromic softgut, which was compared with chromic catgut, was 33% more likely to be associated with dyspareunia, even though the timing of resuming sexual intercourse showed no inter-group difference. These findings indicate the significance that women attach to their sexual relationships following the birth and their need to return to 'normal' functioning. This significance reflects the research emphasis on penetrative sex postnatally, resulting in the considerable general concern with female dyspareunia. The lighthearted feminist stance adopted by Sheila Kitzinger (1995) reminds us that sexuality is not limited to one particular act between two people of different genders, but includes a range of activities, attitudes and orientations. The woman's attitudes contribute to how comfortable she is to resume sex; for example, erotic/maternal self-conflict and feelings of territoriality of certain body parts such as her breasts and genitalia may be inhibitory.

Research on postnatal sexuality focuses narrowly on dyspareunia as a problem of the only 'acceptable' sexual behaviour, that is penetration by a male (Ussher 1996: 177). On this basis a feminist plea is made for a more complete or holistic view of women's sexuality giving due regard to the wide ranging sexual needs of the new mother. Jane Ussher's plea is that the topic of postnatal sexuality should be opened up, by being both more inclusive and more openly discussed. This need for openness contrasts with observations in a medical postnatal setting that women who dared mention sex had their questions ignored (Porter & Macintyre 1989). While women may be recommended to seek expert advice about postnatal sexual problems, the recommendation that 'couples can be encouraged to express their affection and love through kissing, holding and talking' (Olds et al. 1996: 1082) seems a sensible preliminary. Perhaps adopting new positions for lovemaking in order to avoid tender spots or including the application of a lubricant as part of the foreplay may be an opportunity for the couple to regain their sexual relationship.

Until relatively recently the woman was recommended to abstain from sexual inter-course until after her 6-week postnatal check. As a student, I was taught that this was to prevent some unspecified 'infection'. It is necessary to contemplate whether this recom-mendation served more to protect staff by preventing questions about painful sex, by delaying the manifestation of such problems beyond 6 weeks.

Thromboembolic pain

The pain of thromboembolism is another example, mentioned in Chapter 6, 'Pain of cardio-vascular origin', of pain *per se* being relatively insignificant. Thromboembolic conditions are, rightly, viewed more seriously than the pain that initially indicates their presence. I use here 'thromboembolism' to denote serious conditions involving thrombosis and/or embolism.

While thromboembolism happens occasionally in pregnancy and sometimes in labour, there is a ball park figure of two-thirds of thromboembolic episodes occurring postnatally, supported by CEMACH data (Drife 2007). These figures also show the significance of thromboembolism. It is the UK's major single cause of maternal death, being equal in absolute numbers to deaths due to the second and third most common causes of mortality, namely hypertension and haemorrhage, respectively (Lewis 2007). As well as mortality, thromboembolism contributes to morbidity in the forms of pulmonary hypertension and abnormal lung function.

Superficial thrombophlebitis

Not warranting inclusion with thromboembolism because it is relatively benign, throm-bophlebitis is still painful. It appears by about day four as swelling over the affected blood vessel, usually one of the superficial saphenous veins. Warmth, reddening and tension feature due to local inflammation and the woman may have a low grade pyrexia and tachycardia. Treatment is by a correctly-applied support stocking without limitation of mobility. The woman should elevate the affected leg when stationary to reduce swelling. Local heat and systemic analgesics may reduce pain, but anticoagulant therapy is unnec-essary. Although superficial thrombophlebitis carries no risk of embolism, the woman vulnerable to this condition is also vulnerable to deep vein thrombosis (DVT), because she is likely to be older, parous and overweight. Clearly, vigilance is essential.

Thromboembolic conditions

DVT and the embolus that it may release constitute the threat to maternal life with which I introduced this topic. The embolus may find its way to the lungs to cause pulmonary embolism or to the cerebral circulation.

Pathophysiology

Certain physiological mechanisms protect the woman from excessive bleeding during childbirth. These mechanisms include increased plasma fibrinogen, decreased fibrino-lytic activity, increased circulating volume and myometrial contractility. Unfortunately, the first two of these mechanisms may be too effective and put the woman in jeopardy of excessive blood coagulation. Immobility or other factors leading to slow circulation in the dependent body parts, such as pelvis or legs, may be sufficient to initiate haemostasis.

Thrombosis begins with the aggregation of platelets in a blood vessel, such as the femoral vein, possibly where there is endothelial damage. The thrombus thus formed may not threaten health as, outwith pregnancy, fibrinolysis would destroy it. A surviving thrombus, however, grows to occlude the lumen and the blood beyond it becomes static and coagulates, forming a 'tail' of clot, anchored only at its origin. Clearly, portions of this tail may detach forming emboli, which lodge in pulmonary or cerebral arterioles causing dreadful pain and other clinical features.

The commonly mentioned complication of DVT is pulmonary embolism. The reason for this exclusivity is unclear in view of the likelihood of cerebral embolism (Drife 2007). Pulmonary embolism's dire effects are due to the occlusion of the pulmonary circulation by the thrombus, producing hypoxia, acute pulmonary hypertension, right ventricular failure and cardiogenic shock. The local effect of pulmonary occlusion is exacerbated by the production of serotonin, prostaglandins and histamine, which further constrict circulation. While massive pulmonary embolism causes the woman to collapse suddenly and die, she may survive the initial episode and be transferred for intensive care. She may, however, die in the intensive care unit from associated conditions, such as acute respiratory distress syndrome or multiple organ failure.

In a seriously ill woman, perhaps with a condition such as placental abruption (Chapter 6), coagulation failure is linked with disseminated intravascular coagulation (DIC). This involves clotting throughout the circulation; clotting factors and platelets are consumed, leading to a 'vicious circle' of clotting and life-threatening bleeding. In DVT, thrombus formation may be associated with local inflammation, causing pain and tenderness in the affected vein. The structures surrounding the affected vein may also be inflamed and painful, including muscles, tendons and other perivascular tissues. The severity of the pain in these other structures is so severe that, even after the inflammation of the affected vein resolves, postphlebitis pain often lingers.

Should pulmonary embolism occur, the pain is comparable with the stereotypical myocardial infarction, being deep, retrosternal and crushing. The crucial difference is that pulmonary embolism pain never radiates. The pain is thought to be due to the sudden distension of the pulmonary artery. The nature of the pain of cerebral thrombosis depends on its site; if cortical the headache increases gradually, whereas if the sagittal sinus is occluded cerebral hypertension and raised intracranial pressure ensue.

Risk factors

Although increasing age and high multiparity have long been incriminated as predisposing to thromboembolism, two risk factors deserve particular attention. Excess weight, or obesity currently termed high body mass index (BMI), has attracted undeserved media attention and has had the effect of drawing attention away from the possibly more significant impact of caesarean (Drife 2007). In the seven triennial reports since 1985, in only two did the number of deaths due to pulmonary embolism following vaginal births exceed the number following caesarean. It appears easier to blame obese women for these deaths than interventive and iatrogenic medical practice.

Diagnosis

Thromboembolic disorders are initially diagnosed on the basis of the clinical picture, but ultrasound, doppler flow studies and contrast radiography confirm the diagnosis (Burns 2000). Pulmonary embolism varies considerably in its effects, depending on the size of the embolism and area of lung affected. Clinical signs indicate the need for radiographic investigations, such as pulmonary angiography. In pregnancy the fetal effects of radiological investigations must be balanced against the potentially dire maternal outcome.

Although diagnosis appears straightforward, the techniques commonly employed are inadequate. The tragic outcomes resulting from diagnostic difficulties emerged in the *Confidential Enquiries* (Drife 2007). The number of women with major or minor substandard care associated with thromboembolic conditions constituted the majority of cases with such shortfalls. The observation that women 'did not have their complaints taken seriously and were not investigated' (Drife 2007: 59) is tragically all too familiar. Women died of pulmonary embolism, having been treated for respiratory infection after complaining to a general practitioner or another of breathlessness or chest pain soon after giving birth.

Diagnostic difficulties are further hampered by communication problems with women whose first language is not English (Drife 2007). An example is the case of a woman categorised as an asylum seeker who 'saw her general practitioner early in pregnancy but did not receive a booking appointment until after five months had elapsed' (Drife 2007: 57). The argument for professional interpreters who are fluent, health-oriented and trustworthy is irrefutable in this situation (Schott & Henley 1996). The woman's partner and children may have roles, but not to translate.

Prophylaxis and treatment

The main approach to thromboembolic disorders is prevention. This comprises routine pharmacological prophylaxis using anticoagulant therapy in women at risk (Burns 2000). Prophylactic nursing interventions, such as passive movement and early mobilisation, are particularly significant in this group of women (HMSO 1996). Ethnic minority users of the maternity services also contribute to thromboembolism statistics in other ways. Problems relating to mobilisation are familiar. The culture-based belief widely held among certain groups of mothers of the need for prolonged and complete postnatal rest may make a mother wary of mobilising after an operative birth.

In women with perineal trauma, air rings have been condemned as predisposing to thromboembolism and have been withdrawn. Church and Lyne (1994) question the evidence on air rings, which I have seen many women welcome as a godsend. They conclude that empirical evidence does not justify denying new mothers this crumb of comfort.

The emergency interventions in the event of pulmonary embolism focus on oxygenation, medical aid, analgesia and resuscitation, followed by long-term anticoagulant therapy (Allotey & Louca 1997).

Summary

Although, as I mentioned in my introduction, thromboembolic pain is relatively insignificant, we ignore it at our peril. This doggerel reminds midwives, like our nursing cousins, of the danger:

A little pain behind the calf
Just seemed to make the nurses laugh.
But then to their intense surprise
I died.
They didn't realise
A CLOT
Was what
I'd got.

                                     Douglas 1968: 413

The pain of motherhood

One way of coping with pain is by ascribing it a meaning or purpose (Chapter 1). It may serve as a warning of pathology or, as in labour, alert the woman to the impending birth. Pain postnatally, though, is surprising in its pointlessness. Perhaps women should be prepared for such pain during their childbirth education. I focus here on certain forms of postnatal pain which relate particularly to the woman's baby care.

Breast pain in the non-breastfeeding woman

Women decide not to breastfeed for many reasons, but the woman who feeds her baby only with formula is still vulnerable to pain due to her breasts becoming full and, perhaps, engorged. A study of postnatal pain identified how many 'bottle-feeding mothers' developed breast pain (Dewan et al. 1993). While the proportions of primigravid and multiparous women who experienced mild breast pain were similar, more multiparous women developed moderate to severe pain.

Oestrogen preparations have been used historically to impede the action of prolactin to inhibit lactation. They not only fail to prevent the milk 'coming in', but also increase the risk of thromboembolic disease. For these reasons, non-pharmacological methods of inhibiting lactation are widely recommended.

Perhaps because by definition there are no commercial interests, the non-pharmacological methods are relatively under-researched. Such ignorance is of particular concern after the woman's transfer home, when her support changes markedly. An exception to the lack of research is a study comparing lactation inhibition using bromocriptine mesylate with three non-pharmacological methods, that is, surgical compression binder, standardised support bra and fluid limitation (Brooten et al. 1983). The 68 women in the sample were 'divided' among these four intervention groups. The outcomes (engorgement, pain and leakage) were significantly less in the bromocriptine group, but the binder was associated with the most rapid decrease in pain in the non-pharmacological intervention groups. These findings may be questioned because of the small sample and non-random allocation. The researchers did, however, show that breast pain for the non-breastfeeding woman is greatest from day 3 to 5. This clearly has implications for our teaching, as this woman will almost certainly have transferred home before this pain begins. Immaculada Pertegaz and colleagues (2002) have shown that an ergot-related drug, cabergoline, is effective in inhibiting lactation in those women in whom any lactation might actually be harmful, such as women with mental health problems.

There remains a dearth of evidence relating to the care of the non-breastfeeding woman. Although oestrogens are no longer administered, current drug interventions also have problems of rebound lactation and leakage. This unsatisfactory knowledge-base is unlikely to improve as long as commercial interests control this research.

The pain of breastfeeding

It is difficult to explain logically why breastfeeding is painful. How can it be that an activity so fundamentally beneficial to the baby, and also the woman, may cause her such pain? It has been argued that pain and other problems associated with breastfeeding result from incorrect care, in the form of ignorance about positioning and misguided hospital regimes, making it another example of iatrogenic pain. Such attitudes have been summarised: 'breastfeeding should not hurt at all' (Inch & Renfrew 1989: 1375). The considerable evidence to the contrary suggests that this statement constitutes a counsel of perfection. One of these authors, though, subsequently recanted: 'A few mothers feel acute pain as the baby begins to suckle' (Henschel & Inch 1996: 80). Negative pressure on the milk ducts is blamed by the latter authors for the woman's pain prior to the 'let down' reflex operating.

The frequency of breastfeeding pain has been catalogued by various authoritative sources, beginning with Mavis Gunther (1945) who reported 64% of breastfeeding mothers experiencing nipple pain. Rob Drewett and colleagues (1987) recorded the prevalence of nipple pain among breastfeeding mothers as peaking at 65% on day two. A larger study identified an incidence as high as 96% in the US (Ziemer et al. 1990). Christa Kelleher's more recent qualitative study suggests that at least 63% of women who breastfeed experience pain and/or discomfort (2006: 2730). Despite these data, breast pain in breastfeeding women is not generally accepted, even less expected.

Nipple pain

The nipple pain which women who are breastfeeding may experience is often referred to as 'sore nipples'. This term is valuable because, while underestimating the pain, it does recognise its traumatic origin. This pain is usually due to poor positioning and insufficient breast tissue being taken into the baby's mouth to form, effectively, a teat (Woolridge 1986; Tait 2000). The friction caused by this inadequate teat slipping in and out as the baby sucks was graphically compared with 'a heel in an ill-fitting new shoe' (Henschel & Inch 1996: 81).

Sore nipples may be prevented by teaching the woman, during pregnancy and early motherhood, how to position her baby to minimise friction. If nipple damage occurs, various remedies have been suggested, including local healing agents and mechanical aids. An RCT of interventions to relieve nipple pain found no differences between applying expressed breast milk, modified lanolin, warm water compresses and education only (Pugh et al. 1996). All of the women (n = 177) were taught individually about techniques of positioning the baby and this alone was as effective as any application in preventing soreness.

Nipple shields have long been recommended to reduce trauma and pain and allow healing. An RCT, however, which investigated the treatment of sore nipples showed no significant difference in the rate of healing between resting, using a nipple shield and continuing feeding with supervision (Nicholson 1985). This study did show, however, that the nipple shield was the least acceptable, carrying the likelihood of declining milk supply (Inch & Renfrew 1989). This disadvantage, however, may be reduced with the introduction of ultra-thin nipple shields. The crucial role of teaching, however, cannot be overstated; creams, sprays and mechanical aids may not be harmful, but they are not the complete answer in preventing or resolving nipple pain.

Breast pain in the breastfeeding woman

Breast engorgement is associated with two physiological phenomena which may aggravate each other and which are further exacerbated by inappropriate care. These phenomena are the increasing blood supply to the breasts, possibly associated with some oedema, and the secretion of milk within the alveoli (Henschel & Inch 1996). Any limitation of the baby's frequency and duration of access to the breast by misguided policies further aggravates the physiological changes. Milk secretion operates on a demand–supply principle, so that production ceases if milk is not removed; hence, the serious consequences of uncorrected engorgement for a woman wishing to breastfeed. The problem is intensified by the baby's difficulty in fixing on to the full, tense breast and inability to empty it. The near-physiological nature of engorgement appears in data showing that 40–45% of breastfeeding women experience it within four days of giving birth (Nikodem 1993).

The pain of engorgement is 'throbbing and aching' and the woman is unable to rest, except when lying flat on her back and very still; this makes sleeping difficult, as the usual turns and movements rouse her painfully. Multiparous and primigravid breastfeeding women are likely to experience engorgement pain of a similar intensity, with the most severe pain being experienced by primigravid women on day four (Dewan et al. 1993). The pain of engorgement has been linked with nipple pain, leading to suspicions that the same misguided regimes engender both painful conditions. Thus, engorgement is a further example of iatrogenic pain.

While palliative measures, such as a firm bra or binder and hot/cold bathing, ease the woman's pain to some extent, the baby's unrestricted access to the breast is most effective in both preventing and treating engorgement. This remedy may be compared with pharmacological interventions whose dangers are clearer than their benefits.

A palliative approach to engorgement is the local application of cabbage leaves. Anecdotal evidence suggests that the woman appreciates this low-tech intervention and risks due to pesticide contamination are slight. We are reminded, though, that this is nothing more than palliative and no substitute for prevention by teaching. The effect of cabbage leaves was studied in relation to women's perceptions of engorgement and breastfeeding duration (Nikodem et al. 1993). The leaves were applied for 20 minutes after three feeds per day when engorgement was greatest. In this RCT (n=120) no significant differences emerged, although the experiment group did continue breastfeeding for longer.

Mastitis

The nature of mastitis is contentious because it comprises an essentially dynamic process. One of the few consistent features, as this condition progresses from blocked ducts, through inflammation to infective mastitis and possibly to breast abcess and septicaemia, is pain and local tenderness. The mechanism suggested by Gunther (1958) and later endorsed (Inch & Fisher 1996) is that pressure on the duct system of the breast is responsible for initiating this process. The pressure might be either internal, such as oedema, or external, possibly from clothing, manual pressure or poor positioning, and may lead to obstruction of the milk ducts. This obstruction causes increasing pressure behind the blockage and milk secreted there is forced into surrounding tissues. The local reaction is an immune response, which is recognised by the woman as painful and tender hardening and reddening, that is, inflammation. Damage, such as a cracked nipple, or hygiene problems in combination with a neonatal or family infection may allow the ascent of pathogens, such as staphylococcus aureus or candida albicans; this changes the clinical picture to infective mastitis, carrying the risk of breast abcess and septicaemia (Jahanfar et al. 2009).

As with the other painful problems of breastfeeding discussed here, teaching the woman to position her baby, to permit the breast to be effectively 'milked' and emptied, is thought to prevent mastitis or at least its progression. This recommendation derives from research which classified the progression of mastitis not by milk culture which is notoriously misleading, but by leucocyte and bacterial counts (Thomsen et al. 1984). On the basis of these investigations the women with symptoms were allocated to either continue to breastfeed or to additionally express the affected breast after feeding. In the 'blocked duct' group additional expression did not improve the good outcomes of those who just continued feeding. Where non-infectious inflammation had become established, expression significantly improved the outcome and lessened the likelihood of infective mastitis developing. In the group in whom infective mastitis had been diagnosed, the women who expressed were more successful in their lactation and none developed breast abscesses; this compared with the 9% of the breastfeeding-only women who developed an abscess.

As well as positioning and local phenomena predisposing to mastitis, other factors have been suggested. By studying the relation between 'handedness' and which breast is affected, Sally Inch and Chloe Fisher (1996) demonstrated the importance of manual dexterity in positioning the baby at the breast. These data reinforced the significance of teaching the woman manual breastfeeding skills. Additionally, a Dutch study showed, unsurprisingly, the increased likelihood of a woman developing mastitis if she had had it before or if she had local problems such as breast pain or damaged nipples (Foxman et al. 1994). More interestingly, this study showed that women denied daytime rest were more vulnerable to mastitis. While the prevalence of tiredness for the new mother is generally recognised, and particularly for the breastfeeding woman, she may need to be taught to identify and access effective support (McQueen & Mander 2003).

Back pain

Although back pain in pregnancy has received appropriate research attention (see Chapter 6) and the same now applies to certain post-intervention pain (see below), there is a long-standing lack of data on postnatal back pain. While preparing for a major study, Garcia and Marchant (1993) found that women considered back pain to be a minor problem, even though it was reported as having been experienced by 20% of new mothers (n=90) 8 weeks after the birth. To explain the significance of this pain, Jo Garcia and Sally Marchant

(1993) remind us of the interaction between physical and emotional aspects of well-being, without mentioning the downward spiral which may develop if either is lacking. These researchers illustrate the significance of problems such as back pain by discussing the interdependence of family members, in physical and emotional terms, at challenging times, such as after the birth. On a purely bodily level it is helpful to contemplate the changes in the woman's lifestyle which may influence back pain shortly after the birth. These include child-lifting/carrying, feeding and the demands of extra laundry. Although these examples are physical, they are also fundamental to the maternal role, making it likely that any difficulty with them affects the woman's self-perception of herself as a mother.

The dearth of evidence relating to back pain postnatally is beginning to be addressed. Roshni Patel and colleagues (2007) investigated the relationship between type of birth and subsequent back pain. While demonstrating that the majority of women still experienced back pain 8 months after the birth, it is unsurprising that these researchers' findings were overwhelmingly reassuring for women experiencing interventive births. This study, however, may have forfeited detail of, for example, difficulty of birth and severity of pain, in the interests of obtaining an authoritatively large data set (n = 14 663).

In considering maternal back pain, we need to remember that back pain is also common among those who provide care (Karahan et al. 2009). While probably still more prevalent among our nursing cousins, increasingly interventive obstetric practice resulting in the mother being less mobile may cause this problem to affect more midwives.

Summary

The pain of motherhood is dominated by pain associated with infant feeding, particularly breastfeeding. Although some regard breastfeeding pain as unnecessary, even iatrogenic, this paradoxical pain is the common experience of a large majority of women who breastfeed (Kelleher 2007). The extent to which women should be warned of the likelihood of experiencing pain during breastfeeding is uncertain. On the one hand this information may constitute negative advertising, which may deter women from even attempting breastfeeding (Watson & Mander 1995), but the largely successful move towards breastfeeding through the Baby Friendly Hospital Initiative (BFHI) (Mander 2008), may mean that the painful penalty all too frequently demanded of the woman may be overlooked.

Postintervention pain

Pain that is experienced postnatally often results from events that began during pregnancy and labour. Afterpains (this chapter) relate to physiological processes, indicating that the uterine expansion of pregnancy is being reversed and that the contractions of labour are continuing and reducing the risk of haemorrhage. Other postnatal pain may be due to spontaneous, variably physiological processes, such as the pain, felt as dysuria, of perineal damage. Interventions used during labour, thought or known to be associated with postnatal pain, are to a greater or lesser extent iatrogenic. In Chapter 12, I consider various types of childbearing pain which may be iatrogenic, but because these intrapartum interventions give rise to postnatal pain, I consider them specifically here.

Postepidural back pain

Although the effects of epidural analgesia on the progress of labour are long-recognised (Williams et al. 1985), the findings of Christine MacArthur and her colleagues on the long term effects of this intervention were disconcerting for obstetric anaesthetists (1991). This retrospective, low-response study showed an increased incidence of new back pain following epidural analgesia in labour; to the extent that 18.9% of women in whom an epidural had been used developed back pain, whereas only 10.5% of women with no epidural did so (Chapter 9, 'Epidural analgesia (and combined)'). This revelation struck at obstetric anaesthetists' very *raison d'être* (Mander 1993) and was hastily greeted with attempts to limit the damage. This damage limitation exercise produced various results, depending on the research method and the sample. One group of studies, such as MacLeod and colleagues (1995), not only endorsed MacArthur and colleagues' findings, but exceeded them. A second reaction is exemplified by Robin Russell and colleagues (1993), whose retrospective study achieved a 63% response rate and findings comparable with those of MacArthur and colleagues. These researchers sought to explain away their unwelcome findings with a number of strategies. First, 'psychological' factors were blamed by linking the back pain with depressed state. Second, the validity of the responses was questioned, stating that 'these women were prone to tick boxes' (p. 1302). Third, the back pain was played down by dismissing it as 'postural and not severe'. Fourth, other explanations for the women's back pain were suggested, such as dislocated/fractured coccyx. Fifth, the woman's poor posture was a cause. Sixth, re-entering the realms of psychology, these researchers blamed the woman's projection of her disappointment with her labour onto the epidural. The final explanation which these researchers offer for their findings was the 'self-fulfilling prophecy' (Russell et al. 1993:1388), due to the media exposure of MacArthur and colleagues' findings. While the latter might possibly apply to Russell and colleagues' data, it is disproved by a subsequent publication (MacLeod et al. 1995), the data collection for which pre-dated the media attention and whose findings exceeded MacArthur and colleagues'.

A third group of studies, originally from North America, have refuted a causal association between epidural and back pain (Ostgaard & Andersson 1992; Howell et al. 2001; Anim-Somuah et al. 2005). The expectation of back pain, though, persists (Wong & To 2007). The intervention which is epidural analgesia and its potential for causing problems clearly raises many fundamental issues, the essence is succinctly summarised by an 'anaesthesiologist':

> The practice of obstetric anaesthesia is unique in medicine in that we use an invasive and potentially hazardous procedure to provide a humanitarian service to healthy women undergoing a physiological process. (Bogod 1995)

Post-general anaesthetic neck/shoulder pain

In a survey of postnatal pain, a small proportion complained of neck and/or shoulder pain (Dewan et al. 1993). Like MacArthur and colleagues (1991), these researchers related their findings to having had a general anaesthetic (GA). They found a significant difference in the proportions of women experiencing this pain following GA compared with others (64% as opposed to 24%). These symptoms are attributed to the positioning and manipulation necessary to make GA safer, together with the ligamentous laxity of pregnancy.

Post-caesarean pain

There is a disconcerting trend towards regarding caesarean as just an alternative method of birth (Mander 2007), which is only encouraged by the diminutive terms applied to it, such as 'c-section'. Despite this, we should recall that caesarean comprises major abdominal surgery and 'is not a risk-free procedure and can cause problems in current and future pregnancies' (Lewis 2007: xii).

Research by Hillan (1992) on caesarean involved 100 women and a multiplicity of data collection methods. She emphasised the woman's difficulty in coping postnatally with 'the physical and psychological impact of major surgery, which may have occurred on top of a long and exhausting labour' (1992a: 160). These difficulties were compounded by the women's perception that 'the midwives were unaware of the difficulties [the women] had … in coping with the "aftermath" of this method of delivery' (p.168). Hillan's groundbreaking findings have been endorsed by Swedish researchers (Karlström et al. 2007). The Swedish women reported their difficulty with infant care, which related to lifting/handling and feeding the baby. Whereas emergency caesarean is usually found to attract more problems, these researchers found no difference between the women who had experienced elective and emergency surgery. The women's perception of their problems being denigrated by staff is supported by the Swedish data, indicating that the women's pain was under-treated (2007: 436). These data lead to the conclusion that the underestimation of caesarean pain may prevail among staff.

The woman's reality of experiencing the 'aftermath' of caesarean contrasts sharply with the medical practitioner's aims (Minzter 1993). In deciding medication, the anaesthetist seeks to ensure analgesia and minimal sedation while ensuring the woman's ability to ambulate. Fast-acting pain control is recommended to permit minimal drug transfer during breastfeeding. In achieving this, intramuscular (IM) opioids are discounted as providing inadequate analgesia, whereas opioids administered by patient/parturient controlled analgesia (PCA) either intravenously (IV) or epidurally are more effective. Although my experience supports this observation regarding short term pain control, I have found that nausea and vomiting are problematic for the woman using PCA. This may be due to the 'routine' administration of antiemetics with IM opioids, but not accompanying PCA administration.

Minzter is complacent about the safety of the effects of opioids on the nursing mother, which contrasts sharply with concerns expressed by Freeborn and colleagues (1980; see the section on 'Breastfeeding' in Chapter 9). The importance of maternal–newborn interaction following caesarean section is correctly emphasised by Minzter, but such interaction is only effective if the woman's pain control is adequate, which should be assessed as objectively as possible. Research has shown the benefits of intrathecal opioids and patient controlled analgesia, although both carry the risks of pruritis (itching) as well as nausea and vomiting. Wound infiltration with local anaesthetic has been evaluated experimentally, but its effectiveness remains uncertain (Pearce & Dodd 2004).

While Minzter showed very clearly the potential for a high standard of care following caesarean, the reality may fall short. This is associated with observations by Wraight (1992) and Linda Rajan (1993) of the limitations inherent in anaesthetic services (Chapter 2, 'Pain intervention research').

Resources are finite and operating theatre activities are, probably appropriately, prioritised. These researchers draw our attention to the problems of labouring women, and the midwives caring for them, in locating anaesthetic personnel to provide specialist interventions. Inevitably, lower priority is given to women who have already given birth but are still using, for example, PCA. It is my experience that the needs of this woman fall a long way behind those of her sisters in theatre and in labour. The ethical dilemma of offering care, without staff to provide it (Wraight 1992; Audit Commission 1997), emerges again. This is endorsed by US findings which expose the 'myth of the pain-free caesarean' (Declercq et al. 2002: 2), which serves to entice women along the road to painful disillusionment.

Summary

These examples of pain following interventions to facilitate the birth vary in their intensity and causality. There is also huge variation in our knowledge of the link between intervention and pain. Such gaps need to be filled, if, for no other reason, to be able to help women to prepare for and cope with the experience. It is necessary to continue asking: 'If women were fully informed would so many still agree so willingly?' (Newson 1984).

Musculoskeletal pain

Back pain is the puerperal musculoskeletal pain that attracts most attention, possibly because it is so common, but also because there are many important issues related to it. Back pain has been discussed elsewhere (Chapter 6 and above). While there is a variety of other pains of musculoskeletal origin, that associated with the symphysis pubis (Chapter 6) now seems to be attracting the research and clinical attention that it deserves. Pain over the symphysis pubis is not unique to the puerperium, but, because this joint may be damaged during childbirth, such pain may begin postnatally or pre-existing pain may be aggravated (Shepherd & Fry 1996). Postnatal symphysis pubis diastasis/dysfunction (SPD) is most likely to be due to traumatic separation during the birth, which may be associated with the second cause, which is the non-infectious inflammation of the symphysis, pubic bones and nearby structures, known as osteitis pubis. The traumatic separation of the symphysis during childbirth and has been attributed to 'precipitous (sic) labour, difficult instrumental delivery, cephalo-pelvic disproportion, previous or existing pelvic abnormality and multiparity' (Shepherd & Fry 1996:200) and the lithotomy position (Cockshoot 1995). In such situations, this cartilaginous joint is overstretched or torn (Lowery 1995) and the pain manifests itself suddenly, within hours after the birth.

Little attention has been given to the recurrence risk. That this needs researching became clear to me when caring for a woman who had experienced symphysial pain following her previous birth. Her anxiety was profound and, despite my best efforts, marred an otherwise satisfactory birth experience. She was eventually convinced when, following the birth, she almost danced painlessly to the shower.

Pain control in the puerperium

The limited attention given to the postnatal period in general and to pain in particular is, not surprisingly, reflected in the scanty research on pain control; although the work of Colleen Stainton and her colleagues represents an important exception to this observation (1999).

Non-pharmacological methods

I have referred to various non-pharmacological methods of pain control in the specific sections, such as those on breast pain and perineal pain. With the exception of work such as that by Ailsa Dale and Sheila Cornwell (1994) on using lavender oil to reduce perineal pain, the non-pharmacological methods have attracted little research attention. Thus, midwives are unable to confidently recommend their use.

Pharmacological methods

The pharmacological methods have attracted marginally more interest than their non-pharmacological counterparts in controlling postnatal pain. In their study of health after childbirth, MacArthur and colleagues (1991) found that general practitioners were keen to treat some painful conditions, such as haemorrhoids, migraine and headaches. It may be assumed that treatment included analgesic drugs. The relative benefits of two widely used oral analgesic agents (mefenamic acid and paracetamol) were the focus of Dewan and colleagues' discussion of pain relief (1993); they concluded that the former is more effective, and that 'side effects and concentrations in breast milk are negligible' (p. 66). In her account of analgesia after caesarean, Minzter (1993) considered only pharmacological methods, with a focus on PCA. Her criteria for recommending certain medications related to the mother's ability to interact with her baby, rather than these drugs' transfer via breast milk.

Minzter drew attention to the mother's need to assume some degree of control after surgery and uses this argument to advocate PCA. Similar logic has been applied more widely by our nursing cousins, who have introduced and evaluated self-administration of medicine (SAM) programmes (Furlong 2008). Although many of these programmes have been introduced in medical wards and areas where each patient is prescribed a multiplicity of drugs, other areas have also been studied. Jones and colleagues (1996) undertook part of their SAM study in a gynaecology ward, whose drug administration and client population may bear comparison with the maternity area. Having established that a majority of the women would be happy to self-administer, a system to test out the feasibility of SAM was operationalised. Most of the medications were analgesics, initially dispensed in bottles containing one day's supply and kept in the bedside locker. These researchers found that, as well as reducing anxiety by increasing their control, patients experienced less delay in medication administration and that time and confusion were reduced during medicine rounds. Contrary to staff anxieties, Jones and colleagues (1996) found that 'mistakes, stealing and misuse' did not feature. The disadvantages of staff administration by drug rounds of postnatal analgesia is spelt out by Alison Mynick (1981), who introduced a SAM programme in the maternity area. Like more recent nurse researchers, Mynick found that the women were satisfied and that staff time was utilised more efficiently. Thus, it appears that such an innovation might provide both woman and midwife with learning opportunities.

Conclusion

The limited interest in the postnatal period is a continuing source of concern. Researchers have suggested that this lack of interest leads to services failing to meet consumers' needs (Glazener et al. 1993). These researchers also drew attention to the increased risk of maternal morbidity and mortality associated with interventive techniques. In more general terms, responsibility for postnatal ill-health has been attributed to society at large (Garcia & Marchant 1993). This claim is based on society fostering such high expectations among women of getting 'back to normal' (1993) that women are prevented from seeking help when they do not 'match up with the images in the popular media' (1993: 3). Thus, maternal ill-health remains under-reported and under-treated. Of particular significance, Jo Garcia and Sally Marchant maintained, was the lack of any systematic feedback to maternity staff. For this reason, a potential stimulus to change practice is unutilised.

I have shown that the pain that a woman experiences postnatally may relate to her care of her child, or to pathophysiological changes during or after the birth, labour or pregnancy. The duration of the pain is even less certain. Even though it is increasing, there remain huge gaps in our knowledge of the duration of painful postnatal problems. Whether these gaps are filled depends on the preparedness of researchers and funding agencies to invest time and money in research which may at first sight appear pedestrian to the point of being boring. As has been observed:

> many of the problems are not major but diminish the quality of life.
>
> Glazener et al. 1993: 136

These researchers did not elucidate whose quality of life is diminished, but the effects are likely to extend beyond the woman herself. It is only through such basic research that the first weeks, months and perhaps years of motherhood may become less painful for all.

Chapter 11

Fetal/neonatal pain

It is relatively recently that the subject of pain experienced by the neonate has been opened up to debate; and it is only now resulting in serious attention being given to the closely related topic of fetal pain. Thus, many complex issues are being brought to light. In this chapter, in the hope of teasing out these issues, I focus first on the pathophysiology and then approach the ethical quagmire in which fetal/neonatal pain is submerged; I end by summarising the issues in the form of the practical applications of this material. Because the mother does, I use the term 'baby' here to indicate the fetus and the neonate; additionally, when considering fetal age, I use postmenstrual rather than postconceptual age.

Traditionally, health care workers have chosen to believe that the baby does not suffer or experience pain, and continued to do so at least until 1986 (Rawlinson 1996). Such beliefs, constituting denial, are attributable to ignorance, insensitivity, personal bias or an inability to cope with the alternatives (Fletcher 1990). Such denial may be compounded by the nature of pain, which is essentially subjective. Thus, the emotional component of pain may not be identified in the fetus/neonate, leading to the concept of nociception, that is, the reception of harmful stimuli, being preferred by some authorities.

Pathophysiological issues

In purely anatomical terms these traditional beliefs do not stand up to scrutiny. An example is the incomplete myelination of the peripheral nervous system, which has been cited to refute the existence of fetal/neonatal pain. Incomplete myelination has also been said to indicate neurological immaturity. While poor myelination may reduce the speed of conduction, one must remember that, in such small beings, the distances involved are not great so the time taken for the passage of impulses is unlikely to be greatly affected (Anand & Hickey 1987). Following animal studies, Maria Fitzgerald (1994) suggested that any early deficiency in myelination is corrected by the third trimester of fetal life or, after preterm birth, its neonatal equivalent.

Another example of a questionable belief is the lack of structural integrity of the neonatal nervous system. Fitzgerald's suggestion that the component parts and their connections are functional by the time of birth is progressed by Marc Van de Velde and colleagues, who consider the pain perception pathways to be completely developed by

Pain in Childbearing and its Control, Second Edition. By Rosemary Mander. Published 2011 by Blackwell Publishing Ltd. © 1998, 2011 Rosemary Mander.

26 weeks' gestation (2006). In contrast, though, the organisation of the responses may be incomplete, giving rise to less easily recognisable manifestations of pain, especially for those more accustomed to adult responses.

Another belief supporting the denial of fetal/neonatal pain is the suggestion that absence of memory of any painful event negates the potential for harm. It has been shown, however, that disturbed feeding and sleeping behaviour may follow inflicted or iatrogenic pain. Fitzgerald and Anand (1993) have extended this argument to suggest that responses to subsequent pain may also be affected. The Rawlinson report (1996) explained this phenomenon in terms of noxious fetal/neonatal stimuli modifying gene expression in the spinal cord to reduce pain thresholds. Such a reduction means that throughout life this person would experience greater pain following minor injury than she or he would otherwise have done. Thus, the potential for pain experience has been established, but the existence of that pain is harder to verify. It is necessary to be wary of attributing intentionality to the fetus when behaviour that is later characteristic of emotional states is observed. Despite this caution, skin stimulation to the fetus clearly produces responses, even if they are not clearly or easily recognisably organised.

The difficulty of assessing fetal/neonatal pain (Van de Velde et al. 2006) may have provided another rationale for denying its existence. While this suggestion is contradicted by some caring intensively for the neonate, who claim to be able to describe accurately neonatal pain expression (Penticuff 1989; Carter 1990; Hamblett 1990), the implementation of formal pain assessment is slow (Harrison et al. 2006).

Apart from the anatomical and physiological data already mentioned, the evidence for fetal/neonatal pain experience depends largely on hormonal and metabolic measures of stress (Van de Velde et al. 2006). An early study to provide fetal evidence was undertaken on babies subjected to 'intrauterine needling' for the sampling or transfusion of blood (n = 30) (Giannakoupoulos et al. 1994). In the control group the needle was introduced at the insertion of the cord into the placenta; when this site was unavailable, intra-abdominal insertion was necessary, providing the experiment group. Babies who underwent intra-abdominal injection showed increased cortisol and beta-endorphin levels, which correlated positively and significantly with the duration of the procedure. These authors interpreted their data as evidence of fetal pain and recommended pain control medication prior to such interventions. It may be that the fetal stress response to this intervention was simply that and the stress response would manifest itself even in the presence of adequate analgesia, making it a less than valid proxy for pain measurement.

Ethical issues

Discussion of fetal and, to a lesser extent, neonatal pain inevitably raises a number of serious ethical issues. These relate initially to the status of the fetus, but may be broadened to the ethics of pain control more generally. While debates about fetal status are based on religious or secular principles, I consider here only secular arguments. The 'personhood' of the fetus has been used to justify her or his privileged position (Gillon 1994). A more convincing argument in defence of the fetus' moral status may, however, be found in Raanan Gillon's 'consequentialist' argument. This view depends on the consideration extended to the fetus having the potential to benefit the person into whom she or he develops (Benn 1984). This argument requires the identification of the fetus with the person she or he will eventually become. Thus, fetal appearance is crucial, so that the more mature fetus is more likely to benefit (Engelhardt 1986). While arguments about the moral status of the fetus tend to focus on the conflict between maternal and fetal rights associated with termination of pregnancy and other aspects of maternal choice, the consequentialist view clearly facilitates the serious consideration of fetal pain.

Fetal muscle relaxants have been administered to facilitate intrauterine intervention, demonstrating the feasibility of fetal medication (Fan et al. 1994) and this has been followed by Nicholas Fisk and colleagues' demonstration of the effectiveness of fetal analgesia (2001). The question that arises in this context is 'Because we can, must we?' In other words, is there any ethical imperative, obligation or compulsion for those who are able to control pain to do so?

Any attempt to answer this question must begin with the twin principles that underpin health care ethics, that is beneficence and non-maleficence. These principles may be summarised in terms of *primum non nocere*, which is translated as 'Above all do no harm'. Within these safeguards the obligation to treat permits limited flexibility. The conditions for overriding the general obligation to treat include pointless treatment and situations where the costs outweigh the benefits (Beauchamp & Childress 2001). Thus, the practitioner is morally allowed not to obey a 'perfect duty' only when there is adequate justification for disobedience. Again, the balance of costs and benefits determines the decision of whether to treat. Unfortunately, the participant to whom the costs and benefits accrue is not always as clear. In clinical neonatal care, these principles were applied by Gary Walco and colleagues; they argued that 'Denial of relief from pain … must be judged an ethically unjustified harm, unless such deprivation serves a substantially greater good' (1994: 542). This 'greater good' should be in terms of 'defined therapeutic benefits' (p. 543) and not the traditional and largely unsubstantiated beliefs with which this section opened.

Clinical applications and debates

Our increasing ability to observe the fetal condition, and particularly potentially life-threatening states, has led inevitably and inexorably to more and more complex intrauterine interventions (MacKenzie & Adzick 2001). Fetal haematological investigations and treatment have made way for fetal surgery such as vesico-amniotic shunt, to prevent pathological sequelae associated with obstructive uropathy. Intrauterine interventions will only be facilitated by maternal–fetal or fetal medication, such as that recounted by Van de Velde and colleagues (2010).

Of an entirely different order is the more routine yet potentially discomforting intervention, whose effects have yet to be systematically investigated, ultrasound (Beech & Robinson 1994). The not infrequent reports of maternal recognition of changes in the pattern of fetal movement during ultrasound exposure remain anecdotal. The mother may attribute such a change in behaviour to unpleasant sensations:

The scan upset the baby.

The baby jumped away every time the ultrasound probe was positioned.

Beech & Robinson 1994: 16

A blind study by Heddwyn David and colleagues concluded that 'ultrasound increases fetal activity' (1975: 63), but no explanation was forthcoming as to the reason. This research has not been pursued, possibly due to the huge potential of ultrasound to facilitate medical intervention.

Our increasing awareness of the likelihood of fetal pain may lead us to reassess some of the interventions which may be undertaken with little regard for the fetal effects. An example is the ubiquitous abdominal palpation which, as those of us who work in centres where fetal breathing observations are used know only too well, are associated with adverse changes in the pattern of fetal breathing.

Questions about neonatal pain have focused mainly on interventions such as circumcision in North America (Brady-Fryer 2004) and heelprick in the UK (Jain et al. 2001). Pharmacological remedies have been subjected to medical research (Aranda et al. 2005), while more low-tech remedies have been studied by nursing personnel (Ward-Larson et al. 2004). Joy Penticuff (1989) extended these questions to include the cumulative effects of months of interventive activity on the vulnerable and ineffectually protesting sick neonate. The behaviourally immature pain responses associated with prolonged neonatal unit care have been clearly demonstrated (Johnston & Stevens 1996).

The observation and assessment of neonatal pain have shown huge strides forward recently (Brahnam 2007), but their use clinically has not kept pace (McGrath & Unruh 1994; Harrison et al. 2006). Perhaps the multiplicity of neonatal pain scoring systems is indicative of the difficulty of devising one that is reliable, valid and acceptable to practitioners (Herr et al. 2006). The validated tools available include the Neonatal Facial Coding System (Lehr et al. 2007), the premature infant pain profile (Jonsdottir & Kristjansdottir 2005) and CRIES, which resembles the more familiar APGAR scoring system (Krechel & Bildner 2007):

C – Crying;
R – Requires increased oxygen administration;
I – Increased vital signs;
E – Expression;
S – Sleeplessness.

The Distress Scale for Ventilated Newborn Infants (DSVNI) was developed from the neonatal infant pain score (NIPS) because of the latter's unsuitability for ventilated infants (Sparshott 1997). The DSVNI may be used during any invasive procedure. A pain score for the ventilated neonate should assume, as the DSVNI does, that the baby has experienced many invasive procedures and may have given up reacting healthily. When using the DSVNI, observations of facial expression and body movement, as well as recordings of heart rate, blood pressure, oxygen saturation and temperature are made before, during and after the intervention. The DSVNI demonstrates to the carer the extent to which the baby has been disquieted by the intervention as well as whether the baby has returned to a steady state subsequently. Such scoring systems were devised for and have been used to advantage in research situations. Despite this and in spite of evidence of their clinical reliability, these techniques are infrequently used in the neonatal unit because they are time-consuming and require experienced coders. The result of this lack of assessment is that neonatal pain is not well-managed (Bakewell-Sachs & Blackburn 2003).

As well as needing to assess the effect of painful invasive stimuli on a baby, it is necessary to consider the extent to which other aspects of the neonatal environment may be disturbing or discomforting. Margaret Sparshott (1997) categorised many features of the neonatal unit environment as 'disturbing', such as light, noise, heat and nakedness. She continued by considering the 'discomforting' features of neonatal life, such as physical examination, hunger and rectal temperature taking. Clearly many of these disturbing and discomforting aspects, as well as the painful interventions, feature in the conventional care of the sick newborn; should we regard the responses, including pain, which they engender as iatrogenic? An example which Sparshott omitted was the methods employed to elicit the Moro or startle reflex, which is part of the 'routine' physical examination. Striking the sides of the plastic cot is a fairly standard and probably more anodyne method, but allowing the baby's head to drop or even smacking the baby's head are not unknown.

In the light of our knowledge of neonatal pain there are a number of possibilities for relatively straightforward changes in practice. The contribution of quality assessment should not be underestimated in such change, and this may be facilitated by parental pressure. Heidi Als and colleagues (1994) advocated developmentally sensitive neonatal care which minimises environmental stress and, although no claims are made to reduce pain, they may facilitate coping (Stevens 1996). Sparshott (1997) listed the therapeutic interventions used to prevent or treat pain by pharmacological methods. She also listed the 'consolation' and 'cherishment' activities which are becoming standard, including variation in day/night lighting, noise reduction and facilitating skin-to-skin contact.

Perhaps because it is so often used, the treatment of pain caused by endotracheal suctioning has been well-researched. Twenty preterm babies having suctioning were involved in a randomised crossover trial to assess the effects of 'facilitated tucking' as a consolation activity following this procedure (Axelin et al. 2006). The main outcome measure employed the NIPS score and vital signs were also recorded and the parent's perception of the procedure was assessed by questionnaire. Facilitated tucking by the parent was associated with the infant calming down more quickly. On the basis of this study this intervention is recommended as an effective and safe low-tech pain management technique. A similarly low-tech pain control strategy is the one known as 'non-nutritive sucking', which may have encountered adverse publicity due to its association with 'dummies' or 'pacifiers' (Bakewell-Sachs & Blackburn 2003).

Clearly the major barrier to alleviating neonatal pain is in carers' attitudes, as simple yet effective non-pharmacological remedies have been identified (Bakewell-Sachs & Blackburn 2003). More interventive forms of pain control include the pharmacological approaches, which may be indicated postoperatively or during invasive diagnostic/therapeutic procedures. Their administration may be hampered by pharmacokinetic (movement within the body) and pharmacodynamic (dose-response) complexity in neonates and preterm infants; these phenomena differ markedly between babies and even more from adults. Opioids' benefits are hindered by their lesser analgesic effects, especially when compared with the relative increase in the risk of respiratory depression. The non-opioid analgesics have little role in neonatal care because of problems such as uncertain efficacy and safety and their binding properties aggravating jaundice (Stevens 1996).

Variability in the application of our knowledge of neonatal pain control was brought home to me after I was asked by a concerned mother whether her newborn daughter would be given 'pain killers' after her forthcoming surgery. On the basis of my reading about changing attitudes to neonatal pain, I reassured her. Discussing this with a neonatal nurse colleague later, though, I learned that my confidence had been misplaced. Apparently, the surgical unit to which the baby had been transferred still clung to the outdated attitudes to neonatal pain with which I began this chapter.

Conclusion

I have established the importance of fetal/neonatal pain and have considered the reasons for the variable impact of this knowledge on practice. The issue of fetal pain is so closely linked to the abortion debate, though, that it has effectively been hijacked by the anti-choice lobby (Tobin 2008). This has resulted in it being a 'no go' area in relation to other areas of concern, such as ultrasound and fetal investigations (Peacock & Furedi 1996). Unfortunately, this link in no way explains the limited application of this knowledge in the care of the neonate. These questions become more urgent when we recall that local anaesthesia is now being recommended to be administered routinely prior to intravenous cannulation in adults.

Chapter 12

Conclusion

Having addressed a wide range of aspects relating to the control of pain in childbearing, I draw together the themes of the argument that I am advancing in this book in these concluding reflections, comments and observations.

Research issues

An issue which has emerged repeatedly through this book relates to research. This issue has manifested itself in a number of ways. First, is the limited availability of research which addresses the woman's agendas. This is a reflection of the priorities of funding agencies and of researchers. The question of how the woman makes informed decisions about childbearing without good evidence remains unanswered. The need for research for the childbearing woman and about that woman is in urgent need of attention. Second, a similar observation relates to the midwife and how she is supposed to provide effective, evidence-based care in the absence of suitable research evidence. At the same time evidence about midwifery practice and interventions deserves attention. Although it has been galling to discuss those situations in which the midwife does not make appropriate use of the evidence which does exist.

Believing the woman

The last point may be related to the midwife facing difficulty in understanding how the existing research is relevant to her practice and, hence, in applying it. The problem may also relate to the midwife's difficulty in simply believing the findings, which may sometimes appear inconsistent with previous practice to the point of being counter intuitive. This incredulity may be linked not only to research findings, but also to what the midwife is told by the woman. Anecdotes abound about the woman describing the severity of her pain, only to find her account being questioned by those caring for her. Perhaps this is one occasion when the midwife might learn from her nursing cousins about believing pain stories:

> Pain is whatever the experiencing person says it is, existing whenever [s]he says it does.
> McCaffery 1979

Pain in Childbearing and its Control, Second Edition. By Rosemary Mander. Published 2011 by Blackwell Publishing Ltd. © 1998, 2011 Rosemary Mander.

Significance

Because it matters so much, I consider it necessary to focus on the significance of pain in childbearing. Having examined its individual or personal meanings already (Chapters 1 and 2), considering pain's meaning in more global terms may answer the question 'Why does pain in childbearing matter?' The answer may lie in the words that we use. As I mentioned in the Introduction, pain tends to be mentioned in terms of needing to be 'managed' at best, or more likely needing to be 'challenged', 'defeated' or 'conquered'. Are we really supposed to believe, however, that these attacks on pain are intended only to relieve it? Is it pure humanitarian altruism that underpins these attempts to resolve pain in childbearing? I suspect not.

My suspicion is supported by changing attitudes to pain memories; as the obliteration of the memory of pain, rather than the pain itself, was for the first half of the twentieth century the rationale for remedying childbearing pain (Haultain & Swift 1916). However, although having spent so long seeking to obliterate any memory of labour pain, our medical colleagues now lead the movement to persuade us that it 'is soon forgotten' (Reynolds 1997b). This volte-face endorses my belief that other agendas are operating.

What are these other agendas?

It may be that extending the boundaries of knowledge through research encourages interest in treating childbearing pain. Alternatively, it has been suggested that increasing certain occupational groups' power base may be a factor (Mander 1993b). A third possibility, though, is still less acceptable. This is the rationale that staff encounter difficulty coping with a woman who is 'awake', 'moaning' or frequently 'moving position' (Hardy 1991: 62). Thus, the quiet, smoothly functioning labour ward may be interpreted as a sign of 'professional competence' (Schott & Henley 1996: 167). This quietness has been elevated to an art form, as recounted by an NCT teacher:

> Some years ago I was taken round a labour ward by the sister in charge. She stopped in the corridor and said 'Listen'. I could hear nothing and said so. 'I know', she said, 'aren't epidurals wonderful things?' (Schott & Henley 1996: 167)

Further influencing these attitudes, our medical colleagues' unbearable impotence graphically manifests itself:

> My discomfort in the labour ward has been due to a feeling of barbarism when standing over someone in obvious pain which could easily be avoided or relieved … 'Shouldn't we be doing something?' (Wilson 1994: 447)

Thus, the rationale behind attempts to control childbearing pain may be less than transparent and may not necessarily relate to the feelings of the woman experiencing the pain. The intervention by which pain is controlled, though, may correlate with other interventions in childbearing in a number of ways. First, the prevention of pain may be presented as the rationale for intervention. Next, those interventions may, perhaps inadvertently, engender or aggravate the woman's pain. Additionally, the cultural environment in which the pain occurs may have been subjected to interventions that reduce the individual's ability to cope with pain. I will now examine more closely these three associations.

Intervention intended to prevent pain

The amelioration of the woman's pain, in terms of its intensity and/or its duration, may provide a rationale for interventions which directly aim to avoid the pain or indirectly aim to shorten the labour. The ultimate example of such an intervention is the Dublin protocol (O'Driscoll 1993). Its initiators claimed humane altruism as the reason for the introduction of this battery of interventions, by reducing the duration of the woman's suffering. This claim contradicts the reports of women having labour augmented, who have told me that amniotomy or oxytocic administration brings an unanticipated and abrupt increase in the intensity of their pain. Thus, although pain is an inevitable aspect of physiological childbearing, the challenge which it represents may, because of medical intervention, be aggravated. In this way pain, which in other contexts is inextricably associated with disease, is perceived, like disease, as representing an obstacle to be overcome. This view contrasts with regarding childbearing pain as an integral component of a physiological process with which the woman is able to work and which she employs constructively (Leap et al. 2010).

Pain as a consequence of intervention

As well as happening spontaneously and usually physiologically in childbearing, pain is further significant because it may arise in the course of treatment, that is, following interventions in childbearing which are intended to be beneficial. These are the forms of pain that could appropriately be described as iatrogenic (Penn 1986: 14; Melzack & Wall 1991 Bestetti & Regalia 2006). The augmentation of labour mentioned above may serve as one example, but other examples are better documented.

One example of iatrogenic pain is our use of vaginal examination (VE) in labour, which has been shown to be both distasteful and painful for the woman (Bergstrom et al. 1992; Clement 1994; Hilden et al. 2003) as well as carrying long term consequences (Menage 1993). Uncertainty about the need for this intervention has been aggravated by the serious doubts which have been cast on the value of the information thus obtained (Walsh 2010; Dupuis et al. 2005). The contribution of this 'invasive intervention of as yet unproved value' (Enkin 1992: 20) needs to be subjected to research if its virtually routine use is to continue.

A further example of iatrogenic pain is found in the literature on perineal suturing. That this intervention is painful for the woman is well-known (Wraight 1993), but whether it should be undertaken routinely is less clear (Chapter 10). The need for suturing is further called into question by the increasing body of evidence indicating the hazardous use of particular suture materials and techniques (Kettle & Johanson 2008). Thus, the pain of suturing as well as associated longer term perineal pain proves to be iatrogenic.

Although the possibility of epidural analgesia causing postnatal back pain is no longer supported by research evidence, the risk of this form of pain has been shown to continue to influence women's decision-making.

Cultural iatrogenesis

Having considered examples of iatrogenic pain specific to childbearing, it is now necessary to look more broadly at Western societal attitudes to pain. As Ivan Illich suggests, there is a movement to persuade individuals that they are incapable of coping with or enduring pain, which, he maintains, is largely medically driven and is summarised thus:

> Medical enterprise saps the will of people to suffer their reality (Illich 1976: 127).

As I have discussed (Chapter 1), culture lends meaning to pain, including childbearing pain, which in turn, Illich maintains, imbues the person with the ability to cope with it (1976). Traditional coping skills, which have been developed over centuries and by generations of women, are 'trammelled' by medical progress. Thus, by depriving the person of the suffering, she is denied the opportunity to enjoy the success of coping (1976: 128) and the sense of achievement which it brings with it (Flint 1997). Women find themselves being encouraged not to cope by being told, 'You don't get a medal for being a martyr' (Langford 1997: 6). It may be that Illich's words are particularly apposite in the context of childbearing pain: 'Now an increasing portion of all pain is man-made.' (1976: 135). Thus, this scenario demonstrates the limited extent to which the control of pain control rests with the childbearing woman.

The transformatory nature of pain

In stark contrast to the prospect of iatrogenesis, the pain of childbirth may be interpreted in a very different way. This contrasting view draws on anthropological concepts to recognise giving birth as a rite of passage (van Gennep 1960). Like other major transitions in the woman's life, the meanings inherent in giving birth are profound and marked by well-defined rituals to ensure the woman's safety. Having successfully negotiated such a rite of passage, though, the woman becomes confident that the maturity such negotiation carries will enable her to effectively mother the new individual to whom she has given birth (Mander 2010). If, however, her experience of giving birth is undermined, then her transformation to motherhood may be similarly jeopardised. For these reasons, the woman's control of her pain control is crucial, not only for her experience of childbirth, but also for her becoming a mother, for her longer term parenting and the effect on future generations of mothers.

References

Aaserud, M., Lewin, S., Innvaer, S., Paulsen, E.J., Dahlgren, A.T., Trommald, M., Duley, L., Zwarenstein, M., Oxman, A.D. (2005) Translating research into policy and practice in developing countries: a case study of magnesium sulphate for pre-eclampsia. *BMC Health Services Research* **5**(68). DOI:10.1186/1472-6963-5-68.

Abouleish, E., Depp, R. (1975) Acupuncture in obstetrics. *Anesthetic Analgesia* **54**, 83–8.

Adewuya, A.O., Ologun, Y.A., Ibigbami, O.S. (2006) Post-traumatic stress disorder after childbirth in Nigerian women: prevalence and risk factors. *BJOG: An International Journal of Obstetrics & Gynaecology* **113**(3), 284–8.

Ahlborg, G., Axelsson, J., Bodin, L. (1996) Shift work nitrous oxide exposure and subfertility among Swedish midwives. *International Journal of Epidemiology* **25**(4), 783–90.

Ahmad, W.I.V. (1993) The Politics of 'Race' and Health. University of Bradford.

Allotey, J.C., Louca, O. (1997) Thromboembolic disorders: treatment and diagnosis. *British Journal of Midwifery* **5**(2), 75–9.

Als, H., Lawhon, G., Duffy, F., McAnulty, G.B., Gibes-Grossman, R., Blickman, J.G. (1994) Individualised development care for the very low birth weight preterm infant. *Journal of the American Medical Association* **272**(11), 853–8.

Anand, K.J., Hickey, P.R. (1987) Pain and its effects in the human neonate and fetus. *New England Journal of Medicine* **317**(21), 1321–9.

Ananth, C.V., Wilcox, A.J. (2001) Placental abruption and perinatal mortality in the United States. *American Journal of Epidemiology* **153**(4), 332–7.

Anderson, T. (2007) Stages of labour: bunkum! *The Practising Midwife* **10**(8), 54.

Anderson, K.N. (ed.) (1994) *Mosby's Medical Nursing and Allied Health Dictionary.* Mosby, St Louis.

Anim-Somuah, M., Smyth, R.M.D., Howell, C.J. (2005) Epidural versus non-epidural or no analgesia in labour. *Cochrane Database of Systematic Reviews*, Issue 4. Art. No.: CD000331. DOI: 10.1002/14651858.CD000331.pub2.

Anionwu, E.N., Atkin, K. (2001) The politics of sickle cell disorders and thalassaemia. In: *The Politics of Sickle Cell and Thalassaemia* (eds E.N. Anionwu & K. Atkin), ch. 1, p. 1–7. Open University Press, Buckingham.

Aranda, J.V., Waldemar, C., Hummel, P., Thomas, R., Lehr, T., Anand, K.J.S. (2005) Analgesia and sedation during mechanical ventilation in neonates. *Clinical Therapeutics* **27**(6), 877–99.

Argyle, M., Colman, A.M. (1995) *Social Psychology.* Longman Group, London.

Arndt, G.M.D.F. (1994) *Nurses' Medication Errors: An Interpretative Study of Experiences.* Frankfurt am Main, Peter Lang.

Arthurs, G. (1994) Hypnosis and acupuncture in pregnancy. *British Journal of Midwifery* **2**(10), 495–8.

Audit Commission (1997) *First Class Delivery: Improving Maternity Services in England and Wales.* HMSO, London.

Auvray, A., Myin, E., Spence, C. (2008) The sensory-discriminative and affective-motivational aspects of pain. *Neuroscience and Behavioural Reviews* **34**(2), 214–23.

Avsar, A.F., Ozmen, S., Soylemez, F. (1996) Vitamin B1 and B6 substitution in pregnancy for leg cramps. *American Journal of Obstetrics & Gynecology* **175**(1), 233–4.

Axelin, A., Salantera, S., Lehtonen, L. (2006) Facilitated tucking by parents' in pain management of preterm infants—a randomized crossover trial. *Early Human Development* **82**(4), 241–7.

Ayres, S., Mihan, R. (1969) Leg cramps (systremma) and restless legs syndrome response to vitamin E (tocopherol). *California Medicine* **111**(2), 87–91.

Ayers, S., Pickering, A.D. (2001) Do women get posttraumatic stress disorder as a result of childbirth? A prospective study of incidence. *Birth* **28**(2), 111–8.

Baeza Pertegaz, I., Alberdi, J., Parellada Rodón, E. (2002) Is cabergoline a better drug to inhibit lactation in patients with psychotic symptoms? *Journal of Psychiatry & Neuroscience* **27**(1), 54.

Baker, A., Ferguson, S.A., Roach, G.D., Dawson, D. (2001) Perceptions of labour pain by mothers and their attending midwives. *Journal of Advanced Nursing* **35**(2), 171–9.

Baker, D., Pryce, G., Giovannoni, G., Thompson, A.J. (2003) The therapeutic potential of cannabis. *Lancet Neurology* **2**(5), 291–8.

Bakewell-Sachs, S., Blackburn, S. (2003) State of the science: achievements and challenges across the spectrum of care for preterm infants. *Journal of Obstetric Gynecologic and Neonatal Nursing* **32**(5), 683–95.

Ball, J.A. (1993) Complications of the puerperium. In: *Myles Textbook for Midwives* (eds V.R. Bennett & L.K. Brown), pp. 477–88. Churchill Livingstone, Edinburgh.

Bancroft, J. (1994) *Human Sexuality and Its Problems*, 2nd edn. Churchill Livingstone, Edinburgh.

Bandura, A. (1977) Self-efficacy: towards a unifying theory. *Psychological Review* **84**, 191–215.

Banks, A., Levy, D. (2007) General anaesthesia for operative obstetrics. *Anaesthesia & Intensive Care Medicine* **8**(8), 317–9.

Banks, E. (1992) Labouring in comfort. *Nursing Times* **88**(31), 40–1.

Banta, D., Thacker, S.B. (1982) Benefits and risks of episiotomy. *Birth* **9**(1), 25–30.

Baram, D.A. (1995) Hypnosis in reproductive health care: a review and case reports. *Birth* **22**(1), 37–42.

Barclay, L.M., Everitt, L., Rogan, F., Schmied, V., Wyllie, A. (1997) Becoming a mother – an analysis of women's experience of early motherhood. *Journal of Advanced Nursing* **25**(4), 719–28.

Barclay, L.M., Lloyd, B. (1996) The misery of motherhood: alternative approaches to maternal distress. *Midwifery* **12**(3), 136–9.

Barragán Loayza, I.M., Gonzales, F. (2006) Biofeedback for pain during labour (Protocol). *Cochrane Database of Systematic Reviews*, Issue 4. Art. No.: CD006168. DOI: 10.1002/14651858. CD006168.

Bastiaenen, C.H.G., de Bie, R.A., Bastiaanssen, J.M., Essed, G.G.M., van den Brandt, P.A. (2005) Review: a historical perspective on pregnancy-related low back and/or pelvic girdle pain. *European Journal of Obstetrics & Gynecology and Reproductive Biology* **120**(1), 3–14.

Bastiaenen, C.H.G., de Bie, R.A., Wolters, P.J.M.C., Vlaeyen, J.W.S., Leffers, P., Stelma, F., Bastiaanssen, J.M., Essed, G.G.M., van den Brandt, P.A. (2006) Effectiveness of a tailor-made intervention for pregnancy-related pelvic girdle and/or low back pain after delivery: short-term results of a randomized clinical trial. *BMC Musculoskeletal Disorders* **7**, 19.

Beauchamp, T.L., Childress, J.F. (2001) *Principles of Biomedical Ethics*, 5th edn. Oxford University Press, Oxford.

Beech, B.L. (1998/9) Book review. *AIMS Journal* **10**(4), 21.

Beech, B.L. (2001/2) What is normal birth? Time to stop confusing what is common with what is normal. *AIMS Journal* 2001–2 Winter **13**(4), 1, 3.

Beech, B.L. (1995a) Conscious during a general anaesthetic caesarean operation. *AIMS Journal* **7**(3), 8–10.

Beech, B.L. (1995b) Water labour water birth. *AIMS Journal* **7**(1), 1–3.

Beech, B.L., Robinson, J. (1994) *Ultrasound–Unsound*. Association for the Improvement in Maternity Services, London.

Beil-Hildebrand, M. (1999) Personal communication.

Benatar, S. (1997) Editorial: Social suffering: relevance for doctors. *British Medical Journal* **315**, 1634–5.

Bendelow, G.A., Williams, S.J. (1995) Transcending the dualisms: towards a sociology of pain. *Sociology of Health and Illness* **17**(2), 139–65.

Bendelow, G.A., Williams, S.J. (1998) Natural for women, abnormal for men: beliefs about pain and gender. In: *The Body in Everyday Life* (eds S. Nettleton & J. Watson), ch. 11, pp. 199–217. Routledge, London.

Benn, S.J. (1984) Abortion infanticide and respect for persons. In: *The Problem of Abortion* (ed. J. Feinberg), pp. 135–44. Wadsworth, Belmont.

Bergström, H., Kieler, U., Waldenström (2009) Effects of natural childbirth preparation versus standard antenatal education on epidural rates, experience of childbirth and parental stress in mothers and fathers: a randomised controlled multicentre trial. *BJOG: An International Journal of Obstetrics & Gynecology* **116**(9), 1167–76.

Bergstrom, L., Roberts, J., Skillman L., Seidel, J. (1992) You'll feel me touching you, sweetie. *Birth* **19**(1), 10–18.

Beringer, R.M., Patteril, M. (2004) Puerperal uterine inversion and shock. *British Journal of Anaesthesia* **92**(3), 439–41.

Bernat, S., Woolridge, J.P., Snell, L. (1992) Biofeedback assisted relaxation to reduce stress in labour. *Journal of Obstetric Gynaecological and Neonatal Nursing* **21**(4), 295–303.

Bestetti, G., Regalia (2006) A physiological pain, pathological pain and iatrogenic pain: the quality of pain and women's experience. In: *Coming into the World: A Dialogue between Medical and Human Sciences* (eds G.B. La Sala, P. Fagandini, V. Iori, F. Monti, & I. Blickstein), ch. 25, pp. 341–56. Berlin de Gruyter GmbH & Co, Berlin.

Bewley, C. (2002) Fact or fallacy? Domestic violence in pregnancy: an overview. *MIDIRS Midwifery Digest* **12**(Suppl. 2), S3–S5.

Björklund, K., Bergström, S., Nordström M-L., Ulmsten, U. (2000) Symphyseal distention in relation to serum relaxin levels and pelvic pain in pregnancy. *Acta Obstetricia et Gynecologica Scandinavica* **79**(4), 269–75.

Blair, J.M., Dobson, G.T., Hill, D.A., McCracken, G.R., Fee, J.P.H. (2004) Patient controlled analgesia for labour: a comparison of remifentanil with pethidine. *Anaesthesia* **60**(1), 22–7.

Blanchard, E.B., Ahles, T.A. (1990) Biofeedback therapy. In: *The Management of Pain*, 2nd edn (eds J.J. Bonica, J.D. Loesser, C.R. Chapman & W.E. Fordyce). Lea & Febiger, Philadelphia.

Bloomfield, S.S., Mitchell, J., Cissel, G., Barden, T.P. (1986) Flurbiprofen aspirin codeine and placebo for postpartum uterine pain. *American Journal of Medicine* **24**(80)(a), 65–70.

Blue Skies (2006) New Spaces and Possibilities: The Adjustment to Parenthood for New Migrant Mothers. Blue Skies Report No 13/06 Wellington, New Zealand.

Blumstein, H.A., Moore, D. (2003) Visual analog pain scores do not define desire for analgesia in patients with acute pain. *Academic Emergency Medicine* **10**(3), 211–4.

Bobak, I.M., Jensen, M.D. (1993) *Maternity and Gynecologic Care: The Nurse and the Family*, 5th edn. Mosby, St Louis.

Bogod, D. (1995) Advances in epidural analgesia for labour: progress versus prudence. *Lancet* **345**, 1129–30.

Bond, M.R. (1984) *Pain: Its Nature, Analysis and Treatment*. Churchill Livingstone, Edinburgh.

Bonica, J.J. (1990) *The Management of Pain*, 2nd edn. Lea & Febiger, Philadelphia.

Bonica, J.J., Loeser, J.D. (2001) History of pain concepts and therapies. In: *Bonica's Management of Pain*, 3rd edn (ed. J.D. Loeser), ch. 1. Lippincott Williams & Wilkins, Philadelphia.

Bonica, J.J. (1990) History of pain concepts and therapies. In: *The Management of Pain*, 2nd edn (eds J.J. Bonica, J.D. Loeser, C.R. Chapman & W.E. Fordyce), ch. 1. Lea & Febiger, Philadelphia.

Bonica, J.J. (1994) Labour pain. In: *Textbook of Pain*, 3rd edn (eds P.D. Wall & R. Melzack), pp. 615–41. Churchill Livingstone, Edinburgh.

Booth, B. (1993a) Therapeutic touch. *Nursing Times* **89**(31), 48–50.

Booth, B. (1993b) Hypnotherapy. *Nursing Times* **89**(40), 42–5.

Boothby, R. (2005) Acute abdominal pain in pregnancy. In: *Handbook of Obstetric and Gynecologic Emergencies*, 3rd edn (ed. G.I. Benrubi), ch. 2, pp. 23–37. Lippincott Williams & Wilkins, New York.

Boswell, M.V., Hameroff, S.R. (1996) Theoretical mechanisms of general anesthesia. In: *Physiologic and Pharmacologic Bases of Anesthesia* (ed. V.J. Collins), ch. 25. Williams & Wilkins, Baltimore.

Botting, D. (1997) Review of literature on the effectiveness of reflexology. *Complementary Therapies in Nursing & Midwifery* **3**(5), 123–130.

Bowlby, J. (1969) *Attachment and Loss*. Vol. 1: *Attachment*. Hogarth, London.

Bowler, I.M.W. (1993) Stereotypes of women of Asian descent in midwifery: some evidence. *Midwifery* **9**(1), 7–16.

Bracken, M., Enkin, M., Campbell, H., Chalmers, I. (1989) Symptoms in pregnancy: nausea and vomiting, heartburn, constipation and leg cramps. In: *Effective Care in Pregnancy and Childbirth* Vol.1: Pregnancy (eds I. Chalmers, M. Enkin & M.J.N.C. Keirse), ch. 32, pp. 502–9. Oxford University Press, Oxford.

Brady-Fryer, B., Wiebe, N., Lander, J.A. (2004) Pain relief for neonatal circumcision. *Cochrane Database of Systematic Reviews*, Issue 3. Art. No.: CD004217. DOI 10.1002/14651858. CD004217.pub2.

Brahnam, S., Chuang, C-F., Sexton, R.S., Shih, F.Y. (2007) Machine assessment of neonatal facial expressions of acute pain. *Decision Support Systems* **43**(4), 1242–54.

Brasic, J.R. (1999) Should people with nocturnal leg cramps drink tonic water and bitter lemon? *Psychological Report* **84**(2), 355–67.

Brodie, E.E., Whyte, A., Niven, C.A. (2007) Analgesia through the looking-glass? A randomized controlled trial investigating the effect of viewing a 'virtual' limb upon phantom limb pain, sensation and movement. *European Journal of Pain* **11**(4), 428–36.

Brodwin, P.E., Kleinman, A. (1987) The social meanings of chronic pain. In: *Handbook of Chronic Pain Management* (eds G.D. Burrows, D. Elton & G.V. Stanley). Elsevier, Amsterdam.

Brooten, D.A., Brown, L.P., Hollingsworth, A.O., Tanis, J.L., Donlen, J. (1983) A comparison of four treatments to prevent and control breast pain and engorgement in nursing mothers. *Nursing Research* **32**(4), 225–9.

Brown, S.T., Douglas, C., Flood, L.A.P. (2001) Women's evaluation of intrapartum nonpharmacological pain relief methods used during labor. *Journal of Perinatal Education* **10**(3), 1–8.

Brucker, M.C. (1988) Managing gastrointestinal problems in pregnancy. *Journal of Nurse-Midwifery* **33**(2), 67–73.

Burns, E.E., Blamey, C., Lloyd, A.J. (2000) Aromatherapy in childbirth: an effective approach to care. *British Journal of Midwifery* **8**(10), 639–43.

Burns, M.M. (2000) Emerging concepts in the diagnosis and management of venous thromboembolism during pregnancy. *Journal of Thrombosis and Thrombolysis* **10**(1), 59–68.

Callister, L.C. (2001) Culturally competent care of women and newborns: knowledge, attitude, and skills. *Journal of Obstetric Gynecologic & Neonatal Nursing* **30**(2), 209–15.

Callister, L.C., Khalaf, I., Semenic, S., Kartchner, R., Vehvilainen-Julkunen, K. (2003) The pain of childbirth: perceptions of culturally diverse women. *Pain Management Nursing* **4**(4), 145–54.

Campbell, F.A., Tramèr, M.R., Carroll, D., Reynolds, D.J.M., Moore, R.A., McQuay, H.J. (2001) Are cannabinoids an effective and safe treatment option in the management of pain? A qualitative systematic review. *British Medical Journal* **323**(7303), 13–8.

Cannon, W.B. (1932) *The Wisdom of the Body*. Appleton, New York.

Carter, B. (1990) A universal experience. *Paediatric Nursing* **2**(7), 8–10.

Carty, E.A., Conine, T.A. (1983) *Childbirth Education for Women with Arthritis*. British Columbia Health Care Research Foundation, University of British Columbia.

Carty, E.A., Conine, T.A., Wood-Johnson, F. (1986) Rheumatoid arthritis pregnancy: helping women to meet their needs. *Midwives Chronicle* **99**(1186), 254–6.

Cassell, E.J. (1998) The nature of suffering and the goals of medicine. *Loss, Grief & Care*, 8756:4610, **8**(1), 129–42.

Caton, D. (1985) The secularization of pain. *Anesthesiology* **62**, 493–501.

Caton, D. (1995) In the present state of our knowledge: early use of opioids. *Obstetrics Anesthesiology* **82**(3), 779–84.

Caton, D., Corry, M.P., Frigoletto, F.D., Hopkins, D.P., Lieberman, E., Mayberry, L., Rooks, J.P., Rosenfield, A., Sakala, C., Simkin, P., Young, D. (2002) The nature and management of labor pain: executive summary. *American Journal of Obstetrics and Gynecology* **186**(5) (Suppl.), S1–S15.

CEMACH (2007) Key findings for 2003–05. In: *Saving Mothers' Lives: Reviewing Maternal Deaths to Make Motherhood Safer 2003–05* (ed. G. Lewis). CEMACH, London.

Cervero, F. (2005) The Gate theory: then and now. In: *The Paths of Pain 1975–2005* (eds H. Merskey, D. Loeser & R. Dubner), ch. 3, pp. 33–48. IASP Press, Seattle.

Chalmers, I. (1993) Effective care in midwifery: research, the professions and the public. *Midwives Chronicle* **106** (1260), 3–12.

Chamberlain, G. (1993) The history of pain relief in labour. In: *Pain and Its Relief in Childbirth* (eds G. Chamberlain, A. Wraight & P. Steer), ch. 1. Churchill Livingstone, Edinburgh.

Chamberlain, G., Wraight, A., Steer, P. (1993) *Pain and Its Relief in Childbirth*. Churchill Livingstone, Edinburgh.

Chang, M-Y., Wang, S-Y., Chen, C-H. (2002) Effects of massage on pain and anxiety during labour: a randomized controlled trial. *Taiwan Journal of Advanced Nursing* **38**(1), 68–73.

Chant, S. (2003) Female Household Headship and the Feminisation of Poverty: Facts, Fictions and Forward Strategies. Gender Institute. Issue 9. Accessed 05/09 http://www.lse.ac.uk/collections/genderInstitute/pdf/femaleHouseholdHeadship.pdf

Chao, A., Chao, A., Wang, T., Chang, Y., Peng, H., Chang, S., Chao, A., Chang, C., Lai, C., Wong, A. (2007) Pain relief by applying transcutaneous electrical nerve stimulation (TENS) on acupuncture points during the first stage of labor: a randomized double-blind placebo-controlled trial. *Pain* **127**(3), 214–20.

Chapman, C.R., Gunn, C.C. (1990) Acupuncture. In: *The Management of Pain*, 2nd edn (eds J.J. Bonica, J.D. Loeser, C.R. Chapman & W.E. Fordyce), pp. 1805–21. Lea & Febiger, Philadelphia.

Cheema, K. (2002) Supporting pregnant teenagers. *MIDIRS* **12**(Suppl. 1), S26–29.

Cherian, V.T., Smith, I. (2001) Prophylactic ondansetron does not improve patient satisfaction in women using PCA after caesarean section. *British Journal of Anaesthesia* **87**(3), 502–4.

Cherny, N.I. (2005) The challenge of palliative medicine. The problem of suffering. In: *Oxford Textbook of Palliative Medicine*, 3rd edn (eds D. Doyle, G. Hanks, N.I. Cherny & K. Calman), ch. 1, pp. 7–14. Oxford University Press, Oxford.

Chertok, I.R.A. (2009) Reexamination of ultra-thin nipple shield use, infant growth and maternal satisfaction. *Journal of Clinical Nursing* **18**(21), 2949–55.

Cheung, N.F. (1996) Background and cosmology of Chinese diet therapy in childbearing. *Midwives* **109**(1301) 190–93.

Cheung, N.F. (2000) The childbearing experiences of Chinese and Scottish women in Scotland. Unpublished PhD thesis, University of Edinburgh.

Chung, U.L., Hung, L.C., Kuo, S.C., Huang, C.L. (2003) Effects of L14 and BL67 acupressure on labor pain and uterine contractions in the first stage of labor. *Journal of Nursing Research* **11**(4), 251–60.

Chuntharapat, S., Petpichetchian, W., Hatthakitc, U. (2008) Yoga during pregnancy: effects on maternal comfort, labor pain and birth outcomes. *Complementary Therapies in Clinical Practice* **14**(2), 105–15.

Church, S., Lyne, P. (1994) Research-based practice: some problems illustrated by the discussion of evidence concerning the use of pressure-relieving devices in nursing and midwifery. *Journal of Advanced Nursing* **19**(3), 513–18.

Clark, D. (1999) Total pain, disciplinary power and the body in the work of Cicely Saunders, 1958–1967. *Social Science & Medicine* **49**(6), 727–36.

Clement, S. (2001) The caesarean experience. *Clinical Obstetric and Gynaecology* **15**(1), 165–78.

Cluett, E.R., Burns, E. (2009) Immersion in water in labour and birth. *Cochrane Database of Systematic Reviews*, Issue 2. Art. No.: CD000111. DOI: 10.1002/14651858.CD000111.pub3.

Cockshoot, A. (1995) Diastasis symphysis pubis – a painful problem. *Changing Childbirth Update* **4**, 10.

Cohen, E. (1995) Towards a history of European physical sensibility: pain in the later Middle Ages. *Science in Context* **8**(1), 47–74.

Conduit, E. (1995) *The Body Under Stress: Developing Skills for Keeping Healthy*. Erlbaum Associates, Hove.

Cooper, G., McClure, J. (2007) Anaesthesia. In: *Saving Mothers' Lives: Reviewing Maternal Deaths to Make Motherhood Safer 2003–05* (ed. G. Lewis), ch. 8. CEMACH, London.

Corkill, A., Lavender, T., Walkinshaw, S.A., Alfirevic, Z. (2001) Reducing postnatal pain from perineal tears by using lignocaine gel: a double-blind randomized trial. *Birth* **28**(1), 22–7.

Cox, J.E., Bevill, L., Forsyth, J., Missal, S., Sherry, M., Woods, E.R. (2005) Youth preferences for prenatal and parenting teen services. *Journal of Pediatric and Adolescent Gynecology* **18**,167–74.

Cox, B.M. (1990) Drug tolerance and physical dependence. In: *Principles of Drug Action: The Basis of Pharmacology*, 3rd edn (eds W.B. Pratt & P. Taylor), pp. 639–90. Churchill Livingstone, Edinburgh.

Craig, K.D., Wyckoff, M.G. (1987) Cultural factors in chronic pain management. In: *Handbook of Chronic Pain Management* (eds G.D. Burrows, D. Elton & G.V. Stanley), p. 99. Elsevier, Amsterdam.

Craigin, E.B. (1916) Conservatism in obstetrics. *New York Medical Journal* **104**, 1–3.

Cronk, M. (2005) Hands off that breech! *AIMS Journal* **17**(1), 1& 3–4.

Crowell, M.K., Hill, P.D., Humenick, S.S. (1994) Relationship between obstetric analgesia and time of effective breast feeding. *Journal of Nurse-Midwifery* **39**(3), 150–6.

Crowhurst, J.A., Plaat, F. (2000) Labor analgesia for the 21st century. *Seminars in Anesthesia, Perioperative Medicine and Pain* **19**(3), 164–70.

Cunningham, N. (1999) Primary requirements for an ethical definition of pain. *Pain Forum* **8**(2), 93.

Cunningham, F.G., Lucas, M.J. (1994) Urinary tract infections complicating pregnancy. *Baillière's Clinical Obstetrics and Gynaecology* **8**(2), 353–73.

Cyna, A.M., McAuliffe, G.L., Andrew, M.I. (2004) Hypnosis for pain relief in labour and childbirth: a systematic review. *British Journal of Anaesthesia* **93**(4), 505–11.

Daar, A.S., Merali, Z. (2002) Infertility and social suffering: the case of ART in developing countries. In: *Medical, Ethical and Social Aspects of Assisted Reproduction* (eds E. Vayena, P.J. Rowe & P.D. Griffin), ch. 1, pp. 55–21. WHO, Geneva, Switzerland.

Dahle, L.O., Berg, G., Hammar, M., Hurtig, M., Larsson, L. (1995) The effect of oral magnesium substitution on pregnancy-induced leg cramps. *American Journal of Obstetrics and Gynecology* **173**(1), 175–80.

Dale, A., Cornwell, S. (1994) The role of lavender oil in relieving perineal discomfort following childbirth: a blind randomised controlled trial. *Journal of Advanced Nursing* **19**(1), 89–96.

David, M., Pachaly, J., Vetter, K. (2006) Perinatal outcome in Berlin (Germany) among immigrants from Turkey. *Archives of Gynecology and Obstetrics* **274**(5), 271–8.

David, H., Weaver, J.B., Pearson, J.F. (1975) Doppler ultrasound and fetal activity. *British Medical Journal* **2**, 62–4.

Davidhizar, R., Giger, J.N. (2004) A review of the literature on care of clients in pain who are culturally diverse. *International Nursing Review* **51**(1), 47–55.

Davitz, L.J., Sameshima, Y., Davitz, J. (1976) Suffering as viewed in six different cultures. *American Journal of Nursing* **76**(8), 1296–7.

De Voe, S.T., De Voe, K., Jr, Rigsby, W.V.C., McDaniels, B.A. (1969) Effect of meperidine on uterine contractility. *American Journal of Obstetrics and Gynecology* **105**, 1004–7.

Declercq, E.R., Sakala, C., Corry, M.P., Applebaum, S., Risher, P. (2002) Listening to mothers. Maternity Center Association New York, accessed 12 September 2010. http://www.childbirth connection.com/pdfs/LtMreport.pdf.

Denham, C.R. (2007) TRUST: the 5 rights of the second victim. *Journal of Patient Safety* **3**(2), 107–9.

Dening, F. (1982) The woman's stoole or the parturition chair. *Midwives Chronicle* **95**(1139), 440–2.

Dennis, C.L., Hodnett, E. (2007) Psychosocial and psychological interventions for treating postpartum depression. *Cochrane Database of Systematic Reviews* (4):CD006116.

Derbyshire, S.W.G. (1999) The IASP definition captures the essence of pain experience. *Pain Forum* **8**(2), 106.

Dewan, G., Glazener, C., Tunstall, M. (1993) Postnatal pain: a neglected area. *British Journal of Midwifery* **1**(2), 63–6.

Dhany, A. (2008) Essential oils and massage in intrapartum care. *The Practising Midwife* **11**(5), 34–9.

Di Renzo, G.C. (2003) Tocophobia: a new indication for cesarean delivery? *Journal of Maternal-Fetal & Neonatal Medicine* **13**(4), 217.

Dickens, C. (1839) *The Life and Adventures of Nicholas Nickleby.* Chapman and Hall, London.

Dick-Read, G. (1933) *Natural Childbirth (Revelation of Childbirth).* Heinemann, London.

Dick-Read, G. (1954) *Childbirth Without Fear: The Principles and Practice of Natural Childbirth,* 3rd edn. William Heinemann Medical Books Ltd, London.

Dihle, A., Bjolseth, G., Helseth, S. (2006) The gap between saying and doing in postoperative pain management. *Journal of Clinical Nursing* **15**(4), 469–79.

DIWB (2009) Symphysis Pubis Diastasis Disability Information in West Berkshire, accessed 8 September 2010. http://www.diwb.org/main/directory.php?element=374.

DoH (1993) Changing Childbirth (Cumberlege Report) Part 1: Report of the Expert Maternity Group. Department of Health HMSO.

DoH (2007) Building a safer NHS for patients: implementing an organisation with a memory, accessed 7 September 2010. http://www.dh.gov.uk/en/Publicationsandstatistics/Publications/PublicationsPolicyAndGuidance/Browsable/DH_4916671.

DONA (2005) History and mission, accessed 9 September 2010. http://www.dona.org/aboutus/mission.php.

Doughty, A. (1987) Landmarks in the development of regional anaesthesia in obstetrics. In: *Foundations of Obstetric Anaesthesia* (ed. B.M. Morgan), pp. 1–18. Farrand Press, London.

Douglas, C.P. (1968) Thromboembolic disease in pregnancy and the puerperium. *Midwife, Health Visitor and Community Nurse* **4**, 413–15.

Downe, S. (2004) *Normal Childbirth: Evidence and Debate*. Churchill Livingstone, Edinburgh.

Downe, S. (2009) The transition and the second stage of labour: physiology and the role of the midwife. In: *Myles Textbook for Midwives*, 15th edn (eds D.M. Fraser & M.A. Cooper), ch. 28, pp. 509–30. Churchill Livingstone, Edinburgh.

Dowswell, T., Bedwell, C., Lavender, T., Neilson, J.P. (2009) Transcutaneous electrical nerve stimulation (TENS) for pain relief in labour. *Cochrane Database of Systematic Reviews*, Issue 2. Art. No.: CD007214. DOI: 10.1002/14651858.CD007214.pub2.

Dowswell, T., Neilson, J.P. (2008) Interventions for heartburn in pregnancy. *Cochrane Database of Systematic Reviews*, Issue 4. Art. No.: CD007065. DOI: 10.1002/14651858.CD007065.pub2.

Drewett, R.F., Kahn, H., Parkhurst, S., Whiteley, S. (1987) Pain during breastfeeding: the first three months postpartum. *Journal of Reproductive and Infant Psychology* **5**(3), 183–6.

Drife, J. (2007) Thrombosis and thromboembolism. In: *Saving Mothers' Lives: Reviewing Maternal Deaths to Make Motherhood Safer 2003–05* (ed. G. Lewis), ch. 2. CEMACH, London.

Duley, L., Matar, H.E., Almerie, M.Q., Hall, D.R. (2008) Alternative magnesium sulphate regimens for women with pre-eclampsia and eclampsia (Protocol). *Cochrane Database of Systematic Reviews*, Issue 4. Art. No.: CD007388. DOI: 10.1002/14651858.CD007388.

Dumas, G.A., Reid, J.G., Wolfe, L.A., Griffin, M.P., McGrath, M.J. (1995) Exercise, posture and back pain during pregnancy. *Clinical Biomechanics* **10**(2), 98–103.

Dupuis, O., Ruimark, S., Corinne, D., Simone, T., André, D., René-Charles, R. (2005) Fetal head position during the second stage of labor: comparison of digital vaginal examination and transabdominal ultrasonographic examination. *European Journal of Obstetrics, Gynecology and Reproductive Biology* **123**(1), 193–7.

Dworkin, R.H., Turk, D.C., Revicki, D.A., Harding, G., Coyne, K.S., Peirce-Sandner, S., Bhagwat, D., Everton, D., Burke, L.B., Cowan, P., Farrar, J.T., Hertz, S., Maxi, M.B.,, Rappaport, B.A., Melzack, R. (2009) Development and initial validation of an expanded and revised version of the short-form McGill Pain Questionnaire (SF-MPQ-2). *Pain* **144**(1–2), 35–42.

East, C.E., Begg, L., Henshall, N.E., Marchant, P., Wallace, K. (2007) Local cooling for relieving pain from perineal trauma sustained during childbirth. *Cochrane Database of Systematic Reviews*, Issue 4. Art. No.: CD006304. DOI: 10.1002/14651858.CD006304.pub2.

Edwards, E., Timmons, S. (2005) A qualitative study of stigma among women suffering postnatal illness. *Journal of Mental Health* **14**(5), 471–81.

Edwards, N.P. (2005) *Birthing Autonomy: Women's Experiences of Planning Home Births*. Routledge, Abingdon.

El Halta, V. (1996) Posterior labor – a pain in the back! Its prevention and cure. *Clarion* **11**(1), 6–7, 12–13.

El-Tawil, S., Musa, T.A., El-Tawil, T., Weber, M. (2004) Quinine for muscle cramps (Protocol). *Cochrane Database of Systematic Reviews*, Issue 2. Art. No.: CD005044. DOI: 10.1002/14651858. CD005044.

Engelhardt, H.T., Jr (1986) *The Foundations of Bioethics*. Oxford University Press, New York.

Eriksson, S.L., Gentele, C., Olofsson, C.H. (2003) PCEA compared to continuous epidural infusion in an ultra-low-dose regimen for labor pain relief: a randomized study. *Acta Anaesthesiologica Scandinavica* **47**(9), 1085–90.

Erskine, A., Morley, S., Pearce, S. (1990) Memory for pain: a review. *Pain* **41**, 255–65.

Escott, D., Slade, P., Spiby, H., Fraser, R.B. (2005) Preliminary evaluation of a coping strategy enhancement method of preparation for labour. *Midwifery* **21**(3), 278–91.

Escott, D., Spiby, H., Slade, P., Fraser, R.B. (2004) The range of coping strategies women use to manage pain and anxiety prior to and during first experience of labour. *Midwifery* **20**(2), 144–56.

Evans, M. (2006) The 'pain relief talk': is it informing, frightening or empowering – time to re-evaluate the focus. *MIDIRS Midwifery Digest* **16**(2), 265–8.

Everitt, H., Kumar, S., Little, P. (2003) A qualitative study of patients' perceptions of acute infective conjunctivitis. *British Journal of General Practice* **53**(486), 36–41.

Evron, S., Sadan, O., Ezri, T. (2003) The incidence of urinary retention during labor with two methods of epidural analgesia: an ultrasound-guided study. *American Journal of Obstetrics and Gynecology* **189**(6), S198.

Fadaizadeh, L., Emami, H., Samii, K. (2009) Comparison of visual analogue scale and in measuring acute postoperative pain. *Archives of Iranian Medicine* **12**(1), 73–5.

Fan, S.Z., Susetio, L., Tsai, M.C. (1994) Neuromuscular blockade of the fetus with pancuronium and pipecuronium for intrauterine procedures. *British Journal of Anaesthesia* **49**(4), 284–6.

Finlayson, M. (2009) Pelvic girdle pain: symphysis pubis dysfunction (SPD). *AIMS Journal* **21**(2), 12–4.

Fisk, N.M., Gitau, R., Teixeira, J.M., Giannakoulopoulos, X., Cameron, A.D., Glover, V.A. (2001) Effect of direct fetal opioid analgesia on fetal hormonal and hemodynamic stress response to intrauterine needling. *Anesthesiology* **95**(4), 828–35.

Fitzgerald, M., Anand, K.J.S. (1993) Developmental neuroanatomy and neurophysiology of pain. In: *Pain in Infants, Children and Adolescents* (eds N.L. Schechter, C.B. Berde & M. Yaster). Williams & Wilkins, Baltimore.

Fleming, N., Schafer, A.W. (1989) Postpartum perineal pain and sexual function in women with and without episiotomies. In: *The Free Woman* (eds E.V. van Hall & W. Everaerd). Parthenon, Carnforth.

Fleming, V.E.M. (1992) Client education: a futuristic outlook. *Journal of Advanced Nursing* **17**(2), 158–63.

Fletcher, V. (1993) Pain and the neonate. In: *Midwifery Practice: A Research-Based Approach* (eds J. Alexander, V. Levy & S. Roch), ch. 8. Macmillan, London.

Fleuren, M., Grol, R., De Haan, M., Wijkel, D. (1994) Care for the imminent miscarriage by midwives and G.P.s. *Family Practice* **11**(3), 275–81.

Fogarty, V. (2008) Intradermal sterile water injections for the relief of low back pain in labour: a systematic review of the literature. *Women and Birth* **21**(4),157–63.

Fordyce, W.E., Roberts, A.H., Sternback, R.A. (1988) The behavioral management of pain: a critique of a critique. *Pain* **33**(3), 385–9.

Forna, F., Gülmezoglu, A.M. (2009) Surgical procedures to evacuate incomplete miscarriage. Issue 1. Art. No.: CD001993. DOI: 10.1002/14651858.CD001993.

Fox, H. (1978) *Pathology of the Placenta*. W.B. Saunders, London.

Foxman, B., Schwartz, K., Looman, S.J. (1994) Breastfeeding practices and lactation mastitis. *Social Science and Medicine* **38**(5), 755–61.

Frank, A.W. (2001) Can we research suffering? *Qualitative Health Research* **11**, 353–62.

Freeborn, S.F., Calvert, R.T., Black, P. (1980) Saliva and blood pethidine concentrations in the mother and newborn baby. *British Journal of Obstetrics and Gynaecology* **87**, 966–9.

Freeman, M.P. (2007) Antenatal depression: navigating the treatment dilemmas. *American Journal of Psychiatry* **164**(8), 1162–5.

Freire, P., Shor, I. (1987) A pedogogy for liberation: dialogues on transforming education Basing stoke, Macmillan.

Friedewald, M. (2007) Facilitating discussion among expectant fathers: is anyone interested? *Journal of Perinatal Education* **16**(2), 16–20, accessed 7 September 2010. http://www.pubmed-central.nih.gov/articlerender.fcgi?artid=1893085

Friedewald, M. (2008) Discussion forums for expectant fathers: the perspectives of male educators. *Journal of Perinatal Education* **17**(3), accessed 7 September 2010. http://www.pubmedcentral.nih.gov/articlerender.fcgi?artid=2517183

Furlong, S. (2008) Do programmes of medicine self-administration enhance patient knowledge, compliance and satisfaction? *Journal of Advanced Nursing* **20**(6), 1254–62.

Gagnon, A.J., Sandall, J. (2007) Individual or group antenatal education for childbirth or parent-hood, or both. *Cochrane Database of Systematic Reviews*, Issue 3. Art. No.: CD002869. DOI: 10.1002/14651858.CD002869.pub2.

Garcia, J., Marchant, S. (1993) Back to normal? Postpartum health and illness 1992. Research and the Midwife Conference Proceedings, 1990, University of Manchester.

Garfield, R.E., Maner, W.L. (2007) Physiology and electrical activity of uterine contractions. *Seminars in Cell & Developmental Biology* **18**, 289–95.

Garland, D. (2000). *Waterbirth – An Attitude to Care*, 2nd edn. Books for Midwives, London.

Garshasbi, A., Zadeh, S.F. (2005) The effect of exercise on the intensity of low back pain in preg-nant women. *International Journal of Gynecology and Obstetrics* **88**(3), 271–5.

Gaston-Johansson, F., Fall-Dickson, J.M., Bakos, A.B., Kennedy, M.J. (1999) Fatigue, pain, and depression in pre-autotransplant breast cancer patients. *Cancer Practice* **7**(5), 240–7.

Giannakoupoulos, X., Sepulveda, W., Kourtis, N.M. (1994) Fetal plasma cortisol and beta-endorphin response to intrauterine needling. *Lancet* **344**(8915), 77–8.

Gillon, R. (1994) *Principles of Health Care Ethics*. John Wiley & Sons, Chichester.

Glazener, C.M.A., MacArthur, C., Garcia, J. (1993) Postnatal care: time for a change. *Contemporary Reviews in Obstetrics and Gynaecology* **5**(3), 130–6.

Glucklich, A. (2001) *Sacred Pain: Hurting the Body for the Sake of the Soul*. Oxford University Press, Oxford.

Grabowska (2001) Alternative therapies for pain relief. In: *Pain in Childbearing: Key Issues in Management* (ed. M. Yerby), ch. 8, p. 97. Baillière Tindall, Edinburgh.

Grant, A. (1989b) The choice of suture materials and techniques for repair of perineal trauma: an overview of the evidence from controlled trials. *British Journal of Obstetrics and Gynaecology* **96**(11), 1281–9.

Green, C. (1993) Hospital staff culture, pathology and the patient. *Psychiatric Bulletin* **17,** 111–2.

Green, J.M., Baston, H.A. (2003) Feeling in control during labor: concepts, correlates, and conse-quences. *Birth* **30**(4), 235–47.

Green, J., Coupland, V.A., Kitzinger, J.V. (1988) *Great Expectations: A Prospective Study of Women's Expectations and Experiences of Childbirth*. Child Care and Development Group, University of Cambridge, Cambridge.

Green, J.M., Kitzinger, J.V., Coupland, V.A. (1990) Stereotypes of childbearing women: a look at some evidence. *Midwifery* **6**(3), 125–32.

Greenhalgh, R., Slade, P., Spiby, H. (2000) Fathers: coping style, antenatal preparation and experiences of labor and the postpartum. *Birth: Issues in Perinatal Care* **27**(3), 177–184.

Gross, M.M., Hecker, H., Keirse, M.J.N.C. (2005) An evaluation of pain and 'fitness' during labor and its acceptability to women. *Birth* **32**(2), 122–8.

Gunther, M. (1945) Sore nipples: causes and prevention. *Lancet* **2**, 590–3.

Gunther, M. (1958) Discussion on the breast in pregnancy and lactation. *Proceedings of the Royal Society of Medicine* **51**, 506–9.

Gutmann, C. (2001) *The Legacy of Dr. Lamaze The Story of the Man Who Changed Childbirth*. St. Martin's Press, Tr Benderson B. New York.

Haldeman, S. (1989) Manipulation and massage for the relief of pain. In: *Textbook of Pain* (eds P.D. Wall & R. Melzack), pp. 942–51. Churchill Livingstone, Edinburgh.

Halldorsdottir, S., Karlsdottir, S.I. (1996) Journeying through labour and delivery: perceptions of women who have given birth. *Midwifery* **12**(2), 48–61.

Hallgren, A., Kihlgren, M., Norberg, A., Forslin, L. (1995) Women's perceptions of childbirth and childbirth education before and after education and birth. *Midwifery* **11**(3), 130–7.

Hamblett, D. (1990) Pain in the neonate. *Paediatric Nursing* **2**(1), 14–15.

Hamilton, A. (2009) Comfort and support in labour. In: *Myles Textbook for Midwives*, 15th edn (eds D.M. Fraser & M.A. Cooper), ch. 27, pp. 483–507. Churchill Livingstone, Edinburgh.

Hanser, S.B., Thompson, L.W. (1994) Effects of music therapy strategy on depressed older adults. *Journal of Gerontology* **49**(6), 265–9.

Hardy, J. (1991) A randomised controlled trial into the use of TENS in labour. Research and the Midwife Conference Proceedings, 1990, University of Manchester.

Harmon, T.M., Hynan, M.T., Tyre, T.E. (1990) Improved obstetric outcomes using hypnotic analgesia and skill mastery combined with childbirth education. *Journal of Consulting and Clinical Psychology* **58**(5), 525–30.

Harris, M. (1992) The impact of research findings on current practice in relieving postpartum perineal pain in a large district general hospital. *Midwifery* **8**(3), 125–31.

Harrison, D., Loughnan, P., Johnston, L. (2006) Pain assessment and procedural pain management practices in neonatal units in Australia. *Journal of Paediatrics and Child Health* **42**, 1–2 6–9.

Harvey, T. (2002) When a healer harms: the impact and implications of Shipman and Allitt. *British Journal of Health Care Management* **8**(8), 310.

Haultain, F.W.N., Swift, B.H. (1916) The morphine-hyoscine method of painless childbirth. *The British Medical Journal* October **2**(2911), 513–5.

HCNTO (2006) National Occupational Standards for Aromatherapy Health Care National Training Organisation. QCA & SQA http://www.aromatherapycouncil.co.uk/index_files/NOS%20review%202006.pdf

Healthcare Commission (2007) Women's experiences of maternity care in the NHS in England: key findings from a survey of NHS trusts carried out in 2007. Commission for Healthcare Audit and Inspection, London. Available from: http://tinyurl.com/HC-NHSSurvey–2007

Hedayati, H., Parsons, J., Crowther, C.A. (2003) Rectal analgesia for pain from perineal trauma following childbirth. *Cochrane Database of Systematic Reviews*, Issue 3. Art. No.: CD003931. DOI: 10.1002/14651858.CD003931.

Helman, C.G. (2007) Pain and culture. In: *Culture, Health and Illness*, 5th edn, ch. 7. Hodder Arnold, London.

Henschel, D., Inch, S. (1996) *Breastfeeding: A Guide for Midwives*. Hale Books for Midwives Press, Manchester, and the Royal College of Midwives, London.

Herr, K., Coyne, P.J., Key, T., Manworren, R., McCaffery, M., Merkel, S., Pelosi-Kelly, J., Wild, L. (2006) Pain assessment in the nonverbal patient: position statement with clinical practice recommendations. *Pain Management Nursing* **7**(2), 44–52.

Hibbard, B.M., Scott, D.B. (1990) The availability of epidural anaesthesia and analgesia in obstetrics. *British Journal of Obstetrics and Gynaecology* **97**, 402–5.

Hicks, J.B. (1871) On the contractions of the uterus throughout pregnancy: their physiological effects and their value in the diagnosis of pregnancy. *Transactions of the Obstetrical Society of London* **13**, 216–31.

Higgins, C. (1995) Microbiological examination of urine in urinary tract infection. *Nursing Times* **91**(11), 33–5.

Hilden, M., Sidenius, K., Langhoff-Roos, J., Wijma, B., Schei, B. (2003) Women's experiences of the gynecologic examination: factors associated with discomfort. *Acta Obstetricia et Gynecologica Scandinavica* **82**(11), 1030–6.

Hilgard, E.R. (1973) A neodissociation theory of pain reduction in hypnosis. *Psychological Review* **80**, 396–411.

Hilgard, E.R., Hilgard, J.R. (1986) *Hypnosis in the Relief of Pain*, 2nd edn. Kaufmann, Los Altos.

Hillan, E. (2000) The aftermath of caesarean delivery. *MIDIRS Midwifery Digest* **10**(1), 70–2.

Hillan, E.M. (1992) Research and audit: women's views of caesarean section. In: *Women's Health Matters* (ed. H. Roberts), pp. 157–75. Routledge, London.

Hodnett, E.D., Gates, S., Hofmeyr, G.J., Sakala, C. (2007) Continuous support for women during childbirth. *Cochrane Database of Systematic Reviews*, Issue 3. Art. No.: CD003766. DOI: 10.1002/14651858.CD003766.pub2.

Holdcroft, A., Maze, M., Doré, C., Tebbs, S., Thompson, S. (2006) A multicenter dose-escalation study of the analgesic and adverse effects of an oral cannabis extract (Cannador) for postoperative pain management. *Anesthesiology* **104**(5), 1040–6.

Hollister, L.E. (1992) Drugs of abuse. In: *Basic and Clinical Pharmacology* (ed. B.G. Katzung), pp. 437–51. Lange, Connecticut.

Hope-Allan, N., Adams, J., Sibbritt, D., Tracy, S. (2004) The use of acupuncture in maternity care: a pilot study evaluating the acupuncture service in an Australian hospital antenatal clinic. *Complementary Therapies in Nursing and Midwifery* **10**(4), 229–32.

Hosking, R.D., Zajicek, J.P. (2008) Therapeutic potential of cannabis in pain medicine. *British Journal of Anaesthesia* **101**(1), 59–68.

House of Commons (1992) Health Committee Second Report. Maternity Services, HMSO, London.

Howard, R.J., Tuck, S.M., Pearson, T.C. (1995a) Pregnancy and sickle cell disease in the UK. *British Journal of Obstetrics and Gynaecology* **102**(12), 947–51.

Howard, S., McKell, D., Mugford, M., Grant, A. (1995b) Cost-effectiveness of different approaches to perineal suturing. *British Journal of Midwifery* **3**(11), 587–90, 603–5.

Huang, Y-C., Tsai, S-K., Huang, C-H., Wang, M-H., Lin, P-L., Chen, L-K., Lin, C-J., Sun, W-Z. (2002) Intravenous tenoxicam reduces uterine cramps after cesarean delivery. *Canadian Journal of Anesthesia* **49**(4), 384–7.

Hughes, T.W., Kosterlitz, H.W., Fothergill, L.A., Morgan, B.A., Morris, H.R. (1975) Identification of two related pentapeptides from the brain with potent opiate agonist activity. *Nature* **258**, 577–5.

Hundley, V., Milne, J., Leighton-Beck, L., Graham, W., Fitzmaurice, A. (2000) Raising research awareness among midwives and nurses: does it work? *Journal of Advanced Nursing* **31**(1), 78–88.

Hunt, S., Symonds, A. (1995) *The Social Meaning of Midwifery*. Macmillan, London.

Hytten, F.E. (1991) The alimentary system. In: *Clinical Physiology in Obstetrics* (eds F.E. Hytten & G. Chamberlain), ch. 5. Blackwell Science, Oxford.

IASP (2009) The International Association for the Study of Pain. Accessed 4 September 2010 http://www.iasp-pain.org/AM/Template.cfm?Section=General_Resource_Links&Template=/CM/HTMLDisplay.cfm&ContentID=3058#Pain

Idvall, E., Brudin, L. (2005) Do health care professionals underestimate severe pain more often than mild pain? Statistical pitfalls using a data simulation model. *Journal of Evaluation in Clinical Practice* **11**(5), 438–43.

Impey, L., Hughes, J. (1995) Abdominal pain in pregnancy: who needs to be admitted? *Journal of Obstetrics and Gynaecology* **15**(6), 263–5.

Inch, S., Fisher, C. (1996) Mastitis: infection or inflammation? *Practitioner* **239**, 472–6.

Inch, S., Renfrew, M.J. (1989) Common breastfeeding problems. In: *Effective Care in Pregnancy and Childbirth* (eds I. Chalmers, M. Enkin & M.J.N.C. Keirse), pp. 1375–89. Oxford University Press, Oxford.

Isaacs, D., Garsia, R., Peat, B. (2003) HIV in pregnancy: interests of the mother and the baby. *Journal of Paediatrics and Child Health* **39**(1), 60–3.

ISD (2009) Child Health. Accessed 02.10 http://www.isdscotland.org/isd/ch-breastfeeding.jsp?pContentID=1914&p_applic=CCC&p_service=Content.show&

Iverson, L. (1979) *The Brain: Scientific American Book*. McGraw Hill Publishing, New York.

Lowe, N.K. (1992) Differences in first and second stage labor pain between nulliparous and multiparous women. *Journal of Psychosomatic Obstetrics & Gynaecology* **13**, 243–53.

Jackson, M. (2003) *Pain: The Fifth Vital Sign*. Crown Publishers, New York.

Jahanfar, S., Ng, C.J., Teng, C.L. (2009) Antibiotics for mastitis in breastfeeding women. *Cochrane Database of Systematic Reviews*, Issue 1. Art. No.: CD005458. DOI: 10.1002/14651858. CD005458.pub2.

Jain, A., Rutter, N., Ratnayaka, M. (2001) Topical amethocaine gel for pain relief of heel prick blood sampling: a randomised double blind controlled trial. *Archives of Disease in Childhood Fetal Neonatal* **84**, F56–F59.

Jain, S., Eedarapalli, P., Jamjute, P., Sawdy, R. (2006) Symphysis pubis dysfunction: a practical approach to management. *The Obstetrician & Gynaecologist* **8**(3), 153–8.

Jamieson, L. (1993) Preparing for parenthood: daily life in pregnancy. In: *Myles Textbook for Midwives* (eds V.R. Bennett & L.K. Brown), pp. 106–122. Churchill Livingstone, Edinburgh.

Jauncey, L. (2008) The Second Stage: What Women Say About Labour Nursing, Midwifery and Allied Health Professions. Research Unit University of Stirling.

Jeffery, P. (1989) *Labour Pains and Labour Power: Women and Childbearing in India*. Zed Books, London.

Jensen, T.S., Gebhart, G.F. (2008) New pain terminology: a work in progress. *Pain* **140**(3), 399–400.

Johnson, P. (1996) Birth under water – to breathe or not to breathe. *British Journal of Obstetrics & Gynaecology* **103**(3), 202–8.

Johnston, C.C., Stevens, B.J. (1996) Experience in an NNICU affects pain response. *Pediatrics* **98**(5), 925–30.

Jones, L., Arthurs, G.J., Sturman, E., Bellis, L. (1996) Self-medication in acute surgical wards. *Journal of Clinical Nursing* **5**(4), 229–32.

Jonsdottir, R.B., Kristjansdottir, G. (2005) The sensitivity of the premature infant pain profile – PIPP to measure pain in hospitalized neonates. *Journal of Evaluation in Clinical Practice* **11**(6), 598–605.

Jordan, B. (1978) *Birth in Four Cultures*. Monographs in Women's Studies. Eden Press, Vermont.

Joseph, S., Bailham, D. (2004) Traumatic childbirth: what we know and what we can do. *Midwives* **7**(6), 258–61.

Jouppila, R., Jouppila, P., Moilanen, K., Pakarinen, A. (1980) The effect of segmental epidural analgesia on maternal prolactin during labour. British Anderson T 2007 Stages of labour: bunkum! *The Practising Midwife* **10**(8), 5.

Jowers Ware, L., Epps, C.D., Herr, K., Packard, A. (2006) Evaluation of the Revised Faces Pain Scale, Verbal Descriptor Scale, Numeric Rating Scale, and Iowa Pain Thermometer in Older Minority Adults. *Pain Management Nursing* **7**(3), 117–25.

Kao, M.J., Hsieh, Y.L., Kuo, F.J., Hong, C.Z. (2006) Electrophysiological assessment of acupuncture points. *American Journal of Physical Medicine & Rehabilitation* **85**(5), 443–8.

Kappesser, J., Williams, A., Prkachin, K. (2006) Testing two accounts of pain underestimation. *Pain* **124**(1), 109–16.

Karahan, A., Kav, S., Abbasoglu, A., Dogan, N. (2009) Low back pain: prevalence and associated risk factors among hospital staff. *Journal of Advanced Nursing* **65**(3), 516–24.

Karlström, A., Engström-Olofsson, R., Norbergh, K-G., Sjöling, M., Hildingsson, I. (2007) Postoperative pain after cesarean birth affects breastfeeding and infant. *Journal of Obstetric Gynecologic and Neonatal Nursing* **36**(5), 430–40.

Kayani, S.I., Walkinshaw, S.A., Preston, C. (2003) Pregnancy outcome in severe placental abruption. *BJOG: An International Journal of Obstetrics and Gynaecology* **110**(7), 679–83.

Keirse, M.J.N.C., Chalmers, I. (1989) Methods for inducing labour. In: *Effective Care in Pregnancy and Childbirth* (eds I. Chalmers, M. Enkin & M.J.N.C. Keirse), ch. 62. Oxford University Press, Oxford.

Keirse, M.J.N.C., Enkin, M., Lumley, J. (1989) Social and professional support during childbirth. In: *Effective Care in Pregnancy and Childbirth* (eds I. Chalmers, M. Enkin & M.J.N.C. Keirse), ch. 49. Oxford University Press, Oxford.

Kelleher, C.M. (2006) The physical challenges of early breastfeeding. *Social Science & Medicine* **63**(10), 2727–38.

Kendall-Tackett, K. (2004) Trauma associated with perinatal events: birth experience, prematurity and childbearing loss. In: *Handbook of Women Stress and Trauma* (ed. K. Kendall-Tackett), ch. 3, pp. 53–74. Taylor & Francis, New York.

Kettle, C., Johanson, R. (2008) Absorbable synthetic versus catgut suture material for perineal repair. *Cochrane Database of Systematic Reviews* 1999, Issue 4. Art. No.: CD000006. DOI: 10.1002/14651858.CD000006.

Kettle, C., Tohill, S. (2008) Perineal Care. *BMJ Clinical Evidence*, accessed February 2010.

Kettle, C., Ismail, K., O'Mahony, F. (2005) Dyspareunia following childbirth. *The Obstetrician & Gynaecologist* **7**(4), 245–9.

Khamashta, M.A. (2006) Systemic lupus erythematosus and pregnancy. *Best Practice & Research Clinical Rheumatology* **20**(4), 685–94.

Khamashta, M.A., Hughes, G.R. (1996). Pregnancy in systemic lupus erythematosus. *Current Opinions in Rheumatology* **8**(5), 424–9.

Kimber, L., McNabb, M., Mc Court, C., Haines, A., Brocklehurst, P. (2008) Massage or music for pain relief in labour: a pilot randomised placebo controlled trial. *European Journal of Pain* **12**(8), 961–9.

King, S. (2000) The classification and assessment of pain. *International Review of Psychiatry* **12**(2), 86–90.

Kinsella, M., Dob, D., Holdcroft, A. (2007) Regional anaesthesia. In: *Crises in Childbirth – Why Mothers Survive. Lessons from the Confidential Enquiries into Maternal Deaths* (eds D. Dob, A. Holdcroft & G. Cooper), ch. 4, pp. 67–86. Radcliffe Publishing, Abingdon.

Kirkham, M. (1989) Midwives and information giving during labour. In: *Midwives, Research and Childbirth* 1 (eds S. Robinson & A.M. Thomson). Chapman & Hall, London.

Kirkman, M. (2001) Thinking of something to say: public and private narratives of infertility. *Health Care for Women International* **22**(6), 523–35.

Kitzinger, J. (1989) Strategies of the early childbirth movement: a case study of the National Childbirth Trust. In: *The Politics of Maternity Care: Services for Childbearing Women in Twentieth-Century Britain* (eds J. Garcia, R. Kilpatrick & M.P.M. Richards). Clarendon Press, Oxford.

Kitzinger, S. (1978) Pain in childbirth. *Journal of Medical Ethics* **4**, 119–21.

Kitzinger, S. (1987a) *Giving Birth: How It Really Feels*. Gollancz, London.

Kitzinger, S. (1987b) *Some Women's Experiences of Epidurals: A Descriptive Study*. National Childbirth Trust, London.

Kitzinger, S. (1992) Reply to a letter. *Birth* **19**(2), 110–111.

Kitzinger, S. (1995) Sexuality in the postpartum period: a review. *MIDIRS Midwifery Digest* **5**(4), 451.

Kitzinger, S. (1996) *The Complete Book of Pregnancy and Childbirth*. Alfred A. Knopf, New York.

Kitzinger, S. (2006) *The Politics of Birth*. Elsevier, Amsterdam.

Klein, M.C., Kaczorowski, J., Firoz, T., Hubinette, M., Jorgensen, S., Gauthier, R. (2005) A comparison of urinary and sexual outcomes in women experiencing vaginal and caesarean births. *Journal of Obstetrics and Gynaecology of Canada* **27**(4), 332–9.

Kleinman, A., Brodwin, P., Good, B., Delvecchio-Good, M. (1992) Pain as human experience: an introduction. In: *Pain as Human Experience: An Anthropological Perspective* (eds M. DelVecchio, P. Brodwin, B. Good & Kleinman), pp. 1–28. Berkeley University of California Press, California.

Knight, P.R., Bacon, D.R. (2002) An unexplained death: Hannah Greener and chloroform. *Anesthesiology* **96**, 1250–3.

Köder, E.E., Köder, K. (1997) An overview of reflexology. *European Journal of General Practice* **3**(2), 52–7.

Koebnick, C., Leitzmann, R., Garcia, A.L., Heins, U.A., Heuer, T., Golf, S., Katz, N., Hoffmann, I., Leitzmann, C. (2005) Long-term effect of a plant-based diet on magnesium status during pregnancy. *European Journal of Clinical Nutrition* **59**(2), 219–25.

Konotey-Ahulu, F.I.D. (1991) *The Sickle Cell Disease Patient*. Macmillan, London.

Koppel, G.T., Kaiser, D. (2001) Fathers at the end of their rope: a brief report of fathers abandoned in the perinatal situation. *Journal of Reproductive and Infant Psychology* **19**(3), 249–51.

Koshy, M. (1995) Sickle cell disease and pregnancy. *Blood Reviews* **9**(3), 157–64.

Krechel, S.W., Bildner, J. (2007) CRIES: a new neonatal postoperative pain measurement score. initial testing of validity and reliability. *Pediatric Anesthesia* **5**(1), 53–61.

Kreiger, D., Kunz, D. (2004) *The Spiritual Dimension of Therapeutic Touch*. Bear & Co, Vermont.

Krieger, D. (1979) *The Therapeutic Touch: How to Use Your Hands to Help or Heal*. Prentice Hall, New Jersey.

Krishnan, V. (2002) Spinal anesthesia for caesarean. *International Journal of Obstetric Anaesthesia* **11**(4), 322.

Kristiansson, P., Svardsudd, K., von Schoultz, B. (1996) Back pain during pregnancy: a prospective study. *Spine* **21**(6), 702–9.

Kübler-Ross, E. (1970) *On Death and Dying*. Tavistock Publications, London.

Kumasaka, P.G. (2005) Pelvic pain. In: *An Introduction to Clinical Emergency Medicine: Guide for Practitioners in the Emergency Department* (eds S.V. Mahadevan & G.M. Garmel), ch. 29, pp. 427–42. Cambridge University Press, New York.

Labrecque, M., Nouwen, A., Bergeron, M., Rancourt, J.F. (1999) A randomized controlled trial of nonpharmacologic approaches for relief of low back pain during labor. *Journal of Family Practice* **48**(4), 259–63.

Langford, J. (1997) The legendary pain of labour. *New Generation* **16**(1), 6–7.

Larsson, A.-K., Dykes, A.-K. (2008) Care during pregnancy and childbirth in Sweden: perspectives of lesbian women. *Midwifery*. DOI:10.1016/j.midw.2007.10.004, accessed July 2009.

Lasch, K.E. (2000) Culture, pain, and culturally sensitive pain care. *Pain Management Nursing* **1**(3), (Suppl. 1), 16–22.

Lauzon, L., Hodnett, E.D. (2001) Labour assessment programs to delay admission to labour wards. *Cochrane Database of Systematic Reviews*, Issue 3. Art. No.: CD000936. DOI: 10.1002/14651858. CD000936.

Lavender, T., Walkinshaw, S.A. (1998) Can midwives reduce postpartum psychological morbidity? *Birth* **25**(4), 215–9.

Lawrence, A., Lewis, L., Hofmeyr, G.J., Dowswell, T., Styles, C. (2009) Maternal positions and mobility during first stage labour. *Cochrane Database of Systematic Reviews*, Issue 2. Art. No.: CD003934. DOI: 10.1002/14651858.CD003934.pub2.

Leap, N. (1996) A midwifery perspective on pain in labour. Unpublished MSc Dissertation South Bank University, London.

Leap, N. (1997) Birthwrite. Being with women in pain – do midwives need to rethink their role? *British Journal of Midwifery* **5**(5), 263.

Leap, N. (1998) A fresh approach to pain in labour. *New Zealand College of Midwives Journal* **19**, 17–18.

Leap, N. (2000a) Pain in labour: towards a midwifery perspective. *MIDIRS Midwifery Digest* **10**(1), 49–53.

Leap, N. (2000b) The less we do, the more we give. In: *The Midwife-mother Relationship* (ed. M. Kirkham), ch. 1, p. 1. Macmillan, London.

Leap, N., Anderson, T. (2004) The role of pain in normal birth and the empowerment of women. In: *Normal Childbirth: Evidence and Debate* (ed. S. Downe), ch. 2, p. 25. Churchill Livingstone, Edinburgh.

Leap, N., Dodwell, M., Newburn, M. (2010) Working with pain in labour: an overview of evidence. *Perspective* **6**, 9–12.

Lebovits, A.H., Zenetos, P., O'Neill, D.K., Cox, D. (2001) Satisfaction with epidural and intravenous patient-controlled analgesia. *Pain Medicine* **2**(4), 280–6.

Lechner, W., Jarosch, E., Solder, E., Waitz-Penz, A., Mitterschiffthaler, G. (1991) Beta-endorphins during childbirth under transcutaneous electric nerve stimulation [Verhalten von Beta-Endorphin wahrend der Geburt unter transkutaner elektrischer Nervenstimulation]. *Zentralblatt fur Gynakologie* **113**(8), 439–42.

Leder, D. (1986) Toward a phenomenology of pain. *Review Existential Psychologist and Psychiatry* **19**(2), 255–66.

Lee, G. (1998) Minor disorder: 'at last someone is taking me seriously...'. *Practising Midwife* **1**(3), 13.

Lee, M.H.M., Itoh, M., Yang, G.F.W., Eason, A. (1990) Physical therapy and rehabilitation medicine. In: *The Management of Pain*, 2nd edn (ed. J.J. Bonica). Lea & Febiger, Philadelphia.

Leeners, B., Richter-Appelt, H., Imthurna, B., Rath, W. (2006) Review article: influence of childhood sexual abuse on pregnancy, delivery, and the early postpartum period in adult women. *Journal of Psychosomatic Research* **61**(2), 139–51.

Lehr, V.T., Zeskind, P.S., Ofenstein, J.P., Cepeda, E., Warrier, I., Aranda, J.V. (2007) Neonatal facial coding system scores and spectral characteristics of infant crying during newborn circumcision. *The Clinical Journal of Pain* **23**(5), 417–24.

Leslie, K.K., Koil, C., Rayburn, W.F. (2005) Chemotherapeutic drugs in pregnancy: cancer complicating pregnancy. *Obstetrics and Gynecology Clinics of North America* **32**(4), 627–640.

Lesnik-Oberstein, M. (1982) Iatrogenic rape of a fourteen-year-old girl: a note. *Child Abuse and Neglect* **6**, 103–4.

Lewin, K. (1935) *Dynamic Theory of Personality*. McGraw Hill, New York.

Lewis, G. (2007) Domestic abuse. In: *Saving Mothers' Lives: Reviewing Maternal Deaths to Make Motherhood Safer 2003–05* (ed. G. Lewis), ch. 13. CEMACH, London.

Lewis, G., Macfarlane, A. (2007) Which mothers died, and why? In: *Saving Mothers' Lives: Reviewing Maternal Deaths to Make Motherhood Safer 2003–05* (ed. G. Lewis), ch. 1. CEMACH, London.

Lewis, C.S. (1940) *The Problem of Pain*. Century Press, London.

Lewis, J. (1990) Mothers and maternity policies in the twentieth century. In: *The Politics of Maternity Care: Services for Childbearing Women in Twentieth-Century Britain* (eds J. Garcia, R. Kilpatrick & M.P.M. Richards), ch. 1. Clarendon Press, Oxford.

Lieberman, E. (1999) No free lunch on labor day: the risks and benefits of epidural analgesia during labor. *Journal of Nurse-Midwifery* **44**(4), 394–8.

Lindsay, E.N. (2006) Asymptomatic bacteriuria: review and discussion of the IDSA guidelines. *International Journal of Antimicrobial Agents* **28S**, (Suppl.), S42–S48.

Lipson, J.G., Rogers, J.G. (2000) Pregnancy, birth, and disability: women's health care experiences. *Health Care for Women International* **21**, 11–26.

Lipton, J.A., Marbach, J.J. (1984) Ethnicity and the pain experience. *Social Science and Medicine* **19**(12), 1279–98.

Littlewood, J., McHugh, N. (1997) *Maternal Distress and Postnatal Depression: The Myth of Madonna.* Macmillan, London.

Llewellyn-Jones, D. (1973) *Fundamentals of Obstetrics and Gynaecology.* Faber & Faber, London.

Lloyd, G., McLauchlan, A. (1994) Nurses' attitudes towards management of pain. *Nursing Times* **90**(43), 40–3.

Locsin, R.G.R.A.C. (1981) The effect of music on the pain of selected post-operative patients. *Journal of Advanced Nursing* **6**(1) 19–25.

Loeser, J.D. (2005) Introduction. In: *The Paths of Pain, 1975–2005* (eds H. Marskey, J.D. Loeser & R. Dubner). IASP Press, Seattle.

Loos, M.J.A., Houterman, S., Scheltinga, M.R.M., Roumen, R.M.H. (2008) Evaluating post-herniorrhaphy groin pain: Visual Analogue or Verbal Rating Scale? *Hernia* **12**, 147–51.

Lothian, J.A. (1988) Relaxation: therapeutic touch. In: *Childbirth Education: Practice, Research and Theory* (eds F.H. Nichols & S.S. Humenick), ch. 10. W.B. Saunders, Philadelphia.

Lowdon, G. (1995) Of no consequence. *NCT New Generation Digest* p. 14.

Lowe, N.K. (2002) The nature of labor pain: the nature and management of labor pain. *American Journal of Obstetrics & Gynecology* **186**(5), (Suppl.), S16–S24.

Lowery, C.L. (1995) Sudden joint and extremity pain in pregnancy. *Obstetrics and Gynecology Clinics of North America* **22**(1), 173–90.

Lukse, M., Vacc, N. (1999) Grief, depression, and coping in women undergoing infertility treatment. *Obstetrics & Gynecology* **93**(2), 245–51.

Lythgoe, J., Metcalfe, A. (2008) Birth of a midwifery acupuncture service. *The Practising Midwife* **11**(5), 25–9.

MacArthur, C., Lewis, M., Knox, E.G. (1991) *Health After Childbirth.* HMSO, London, and University of Birmingham.

Machover, I. (1995) The mobile epidural … is it such good news? *AIMS Journal* **7**(2), 10–11.

Macintyre, P.E., Schug, S.A. (2007) *Acute Pain Management: A Practical Guide*, 3rd edn. Saunders, Edinburgh.

MacKenzie, T.C., Adzick, N.S. (2001) Advances in fetal surgery. *Journal of Intensive Care Medicine* **16**(6), 251–62.

Mackey, R.B. (1995) Discover the healing power of therapeutic touch. *American Journal of Nursing* **95**(4), 27–32.

Macleod, J., Macintyre, C., McClure, J.H. (1995) Backache and epidural analgesia. A retrospective survey of mothers one year after childbirth. *International Journal of Obstetric Anaesthesia* **4**(1), 21–5.

Macones, G.A. (2008) Clinical outcomes in VBAC attempts: what to say to patients? *American Journal of Obstetrics & Gynecology* **199**(1), 1–2.

Magpie Trial Collaborative Group (2002) 'Do women with pre-eclampsia, and their babies, benefit from magnesium sulphate? The Magpie Trial: a randomised placebo-controlled trial'. *Lancet* **359**, 1877–90.

Main, C.J., Spanswick, C.C. (2000) Models of pain. In: *Pain Management: An Interdisciplinary Approach* (eds C.J. Main & C.C. Spanswick), ch. 1, pp. 3–17. Churchill Livingstone, Glasgow.

Maldonado, A., Barger, M. (1995) Comprehensive assessment of common musculoskeletal disorders. *Journal of Nurse-Midwifery* **20**(2), 202–12.

Malfertheiner, S.F., Maximilian, A., Malfertheiner, V., Mönkemüller, K., Röhl, F.W., Malfertheiner, P., Costa, S.D. (2009) Gastroesophageal reflux disease and management in advanced pregnancy: a prospective survey. *Digestion* **79**(2), 115–20.

Mander, R. (in Press) 'Being with woman': the care of the childbearing woman with cancer. In: *Perspectives on Cancer Care* (eds J.N. Fawcett & A. McQueen). Routledge, London.

Mander, R. (1993) Epidural analgesia 1: recent history. *British Journal of Midwifery* **1**(6), 259–64.

Mander, R. (1994) epidural analgesia 2: research basis. *British Journal of Midwifery* **2**(1), 12–16.

Mander, R. (1995) The relevance of the Dutch system of maternity care to the UK. *Journal of Advanced Nursing* **22**, 1023–26.

Mander, R. (1998a) A reappraisal of Simpson's introduction of chloroform. *Midwifery* **14**(3), 181–90.

Mander, R. (1998b) Analgesia and anaesthesia in childbirth: obscurantism and obfuscation. *Journal of Advanced Nursing* **28**(1), 86–93.

Mander, R. (1998c) *Pain in Childbearing and Its Control*. Blackwell Scientific, Oxford.

Mander, R. (2000) The meanings of labour pain or the layers of an onion? A woman oriented view. *Journal of Reproductive & Infant Psychology* **18**(2), 133–42.

Mander, R. (2001) *Supportive Care and Midwifery*. Blackwell Science, Oxford.

Mander, R. (2002) The transitional stage: pain and control. *Practising Midwife* **5**(1), 10–12.

Mander, R. (2004a) Failure to deliver – ethical issues relating to epidural analgesia in uncomplicated labour. In: *Ethics and Midwifery: Issues in Contemporary Practice*, 2nd edn (eds l. Frith & H. Draper). Books for Midwives, Edinburgh.

Mander, R. (2004b) *Men and Maternity*. Routledge, London.

Mander, R, (2006) *Loss and Bereavement in Childbearing*, 2nd edn. Routledge, London.

Mander, R. (2007) *Caesarean: Just Another Way of Birth?* Routledge, London.

Mander, R. (2008) Baby friendly–mother friendly? Policy issues in breastfeeding promotion. *MIDIRS* **18**(1), 104–6 & 108.

Mander, R. (2010) Skills for working with (the woman in) pain. In: *Essential Midwifery Practice: Intrapartum Care* (eds D. Walsh & S. Downe), ch. 8, pp. 125–40. Wiley Blackwell, Chichester.

Mander, R., Murphy-Lawless, J., Edwards, N. (2010) Reflecting on good birthing: an innovative approach to culture change (Part 2). *MIDIRS* **20**(1), 25–9.

Mander, R., Smith, G.D. (2008) A systematic review of medical diagnosis in Ogilvie's syndrome in childbearing. *Midwifery* available online 18 November 2008, http://dx.doi.org/10.1016/j.midw.2008.09.003

Man-Son-Hing, M., Wells, G. (1995) Meta-analysis of efficacy of quinine for treatment of nocturnal leg cramps in elderly people. *British Medical Journal* **310**(6971), 13–17.

Marchant, S. (2009) Physiology and care in the puerperium. In: *Myles Textbook for Midwives*, 15th edn (eds D.M. Fraser & M.A. Cooper), ch. 34, p. 651. Churchill Livingstone, Edinburgh.

Marck, P.B. (1994) Unexpected pregnancy. In: *Uncertain Motherhood: Negotiating the Risks of the Childbearing Years* (eds P.A. Field & P.B. Marck), pp. 82–138. Sage, London.

Mardorossian, C.M. (2003) Laboring women, coaching men: masculinity and childbirth education in the contemporary United States. *Hypatia* **18**(3), 113–34.

Marrero, J.M., Goggin, P.M., de Caestecker, J.S., Pearce, J.M., Maxwell, J.D. (1992) Determinants of pregnancy heartburn. *British Journal of Obstetrics and Gynaecology* **99**, 731–4.

Marris, P. (1986) *Loss and Change*. Routledge Kegan Paul, London.

Mårtensson, L., McSwiggin, M., Mercer, J.S. (2008) US midwives' knowledge and use of sterile water injections for labor pain. *Journal of Midwifery & Women's Health* **53**(2), 115–22.

Mårtensson, L., Wallin, G. (2006) Use of acupuncture and sterile water injection for labor pain: a survey in Sweden. *Birth* **33**(4), 289–96.

Martí-Carvajal, A.J., Peña-Martí, G.E., Comunián-Carrasco, G., Martí-Peña, A.J. (2009) Interventions for treating painful sickle cell crisis during pregnancy. *Cochrane Database of Systematic Reviews*, Issue 1. Art. No.: CD006786. DOI: 10.1002/14651858.CD006786.pub2.

Martin, E. (1989) *The Woman in the Body*. Open University Press, Milton Keynes.

Matthews, M.K. (1989) The relationship between maternal labour analgesia and delay in the initiation of breast feeding in healthy neonates in the early neonatal period. *Midwifery* **5**(1), 3–10.

Maude, R.M., Foureur, M.J. (2007) It's beyond water: stories of women's experience of using water for labour and birth. *Women and Birth* **20**(1), 17–24.

McAllister, G., Farquhar, M. (1992) Health beliefs: a cultural division? *Journal of Advanced Nursing* **17**, 1447–54.

McCaffery, M. (1979) *Nursing Management of the Patient with Pain*. Lippincott, Philadelphia.

McConahay, T., Bryson, M., Bulloch, B. (2005) Clinically significant changes in acute pain in a pediatric ED using the Color Analog Scale. *American Journal of Emergency Medicine* **25**(7), 739–42.

McCourt, C., Pearce, A. (2000) Does continuity of carer matter to women from minority ethnic groups? *Midwifery* **16**(2), 145–54.

McCrea, B.H. (1996) An Investigation of Rule-Governed Behaviours in the Control of Pain Management During the First Stage of Labour. Unpublished D. Phil. thesis, University of Ulster.

McGrath, P.J., Unruh, A.M. (1994) Measurement and assessment of paediatric pain. In: *Textbook of Pain*, 3rd edn (eds P.D. Wall & R. Melzack), ch. 16. Churchill Livingstone, Edinburgh.

McIntosh, J. (1989) Models of childbirth and social class: a study of eighty working class primigravidae. In: *Midwives, Research and Childbirth 1* (S. Robinson & A.M. Thomson), ch. 10. Chapman & Hall, London.

McKenzie, A.M., Parris, W.C.V. (1997) *Historical Perspectives in Parris WCV Cancer Pain Management*. Butterworth-Heinemann, Boston.

McLintock, A.H. (1876) *Treatise on the Theory and Practice of Midwifery 2*. New Sydenham Society, London.

McManus, A.J., Hunter, L.P., Renn, H. (2006) Lesbian experiences and needs during childbirth: guidance for health care providers. *Journal of Obstetric Gynecologic and Neonatal Nursing* **35**(1), 13–23.

McManus, T.J., Calder, A. (1978) Upright posture and the efficiency of labour. *Lancet* **1**(14), 72–4.

McQueen, A., Mander, R. (2003) Tiredness and fatigue in the postnatal period. *Journal of Advanced Nursing* **42**(5), 463–9.

Melzack, R. (1975a) The McGill pain questionnaire: major properties and scoring methods. *Pain* **1**, 277–99.

Melzack, R. (1975b) How acupuncture can block pain. In: *Pain: Clinical and Experimental Perspectives* (ed. M. Weisenberg), pp. 251–7. Mosby, St Louis.

Melzack, R. (1983) Concepts of pain measurement. In: *Pain Measurement and Assessment*, pp. 1–5. Raven Press, New York.

Melzack, R. (1987) The short-form McGill pain questionnaire. *Pain* **30**, 191–7.

Melzack, R. (1993) Pain: past present and future. *Canadian Journal of Experimental Psychology* **47**(4), 615–29.

Melzack, R., Katz, J. (2006) Pain in the 21st century: the neuromatrix and beyond. In: *Psychological Knowledge in Court* (eds G. Young, K. Nicholson & A.W. Kane), ch. 7. Springer, US.

Melzack, R., Wall, P.D. (1965) Pain mechanisms: a new theory. *Science* **150**, 971–9.

Melzack, R., Wall, P.D. (1991) *The Challenge of Pain*, 2nd edn. Penguin, London.

Melzack, R., Wall P. (1965) Pain mechanisms: a new theory. *Science* **150**, 971–79.

Melzack, R., Taenzer, P., Feldman, P., Kinch, R.A. (1981) Labour is still painful after prepared childbirth training. *Canadian Medical Association Journal* **125**, 357–63.

Melzack, R., Kinch, P., Dobkin, M., Lebrun, P., Taenzer (1984) Severity of labour pain: influence of physical as well as psychological variables. *Canadian Medical Association Journal*, **130**.

Melzack, R., Taenzer, P., Feldman, P., Kinch, R.A. (1981) Labour is still painful after prepared childbirth training. *Canadian Medical Association Journal* **125**(5), 357–63.

Menage, J. (1993) Post-traumatic stress disorder in women who have undergone obstetric and/or gynaecological procedures. *Journal of Reproductive and Infant Psychology* **11**(4), 221–8.

Mendez-Bauer, C., Arroyo, J., Garcia-Ramos, C., et al. (1975) Effects of standing position on spontaneous uterine contractility and other aspects of labour. *Journal of Perinatal Medicine* **3**, 89–100.

Merskey, H. (2005) Psychiatry and pain: causes effects and complications. In: *The Paths of Pain 1975–2005* (eds H. Merskey, J.D. Loeser & R. Dubner), ch. 29, pp.421–32. IASP Press, Seattle.

Meyer, D.J.N., Ringkamp, M., Campbell, J.N., Raja, S.J. (2006) Mechanisms of cutaneous nociception. In: *Textbook of Pain*, 5th edn (eds S.B. Mcmahon & M. Kolentzberg). Elsevier, London.

Miller, R.L., Pallant, J.F., Negri, L.M. (2006) Anxiety and stress in the postpartum: is there more to postnatal distress than depression? *BMC Psychiatry* **6**, 12.

Mills, G.H., Singh, D., Longman, M., O'Sullivan, J., Caunt, J.A. (1996) Nitrous oxide exposure on the labour ward. *International Journal of Obstetric Anaesthesia* **5**(3), 160–164.

Minzter, B. (1993) Analgesia after caesarean delivery. In: *Postoperative Pain Management* (eds F.M. Ferrante & T.R. Vadeboncouer), pp. 519–30. Churchill Livingstone, Edinburgh.

Mobily, P.R., Herr, K.A., Nicholson, A.C. (1994) Validation of cutaneous stimulation interventions for pain management. *International Journal of Nursing Studies* **31**(6), 533–41.

Moffett, J.A.K., Carr, J., Howarth, E. (2004) High fear-avoiders of physical activity benefit from an exercise program for patients with back pain. *Spine* **29**(11), 1167–73.

Moir, D.D. (1973) *Pain Relief in Labour: A Handbook for Midwives*. Churchill Livingstone, Edinburgh.

Mondelli, M., Rossi, S., Monti, E., Aprile, I., Caliandro, P., Pazzaglia, C., Romano, C., Padua, L. (2007) Prospective study of positive factors for improvement of carpal tunnel syndrome in pregnant women. *Muscle & Nerve* **36**(6), 778–83. http://www3.interscience.wiley.com/cgi-bin/fulltext/114297516/PDFSTART.

Mondofacto (2009) *Online Medical Dictionary*, accessed August 2009. http://www.mondofacto.com/facts/dictionary?diastasis.

Montgomery, K.S. (2003) Improving nutrition in pregnant adolescents: recommendations for clinical practitioners. *Journal of Perinatal Education* **12**(2), 22–30.

Monto, M.A. (1996) Lamaze and Bradley childbirth classes: contrasting perspectives toward the medical model of birth. *Birth: Issues in Perinatal Care* **23**(4), 193–201.

Morgan, B.M. (1984) The consumer's attitude to obstetric care. *British Journal of Obstetrics and Gynaecology* **91**, 624–8.

Morgan, B.M. (1987) Mortality and anaesthesia. In: *Foundations of Obstetric Anaesthesia* (ed. B.M. Morgan). Farrand Press, London.

Morris, D.B. (1991) *The Culture of Pain*. Berkeley University of California Press, California.

Morris, D.B. (1996) About suffering: voice, genre, and moral community. *Daedelus* **125**(1), 25–45.

Morrison, C.E., Dutton, D., Howie, H., Gilmour, H. (1987) Pethidine compared with meptazinol in labour. *Anaesthesia* **42**(1), 7–14.

Morse, J.M. (2001) Toward a Praxis theory of suffering. *Advances in Nursing Science* **24**(1), 47–59

Moscucci, O. (2003) Holistic obstetrics: the origins of 'natural childbirth' in Britain. *Postgraduate Medicine Journal* **79**(929), 168–73.

Motha, G., McGrath, J. (1994) The effects of reflexology on labour outcome. In: *Association of Reflexologists. Reflexology Research Reports* (2nd edn). Association of Reflexologists, London.

Moulder, E. (2008) Healthcare associated infection–intervention-related infection. *Hospital Pharmacist* **15**, 13–15.

Mountcastle, V.B. (1980) *Medical Physiology*, 14th edn. Mosby, St Louis.

Moyzakitis, W. (2004) Exploring women's descriptions of distress and/or trauma of childbirth from a feminist perspective. *RCM Evidence Based Midwifery* **2**(1), 8–14.

Mueller, R.F., Young, I.D. (1995) *Emery's Elements of Medical Genetics*, 9th edn. Churchill Livingstone, Edinburgh.

Mulder, E.J.H., Visser, G.H.A. (1987) Braxton Hicks' contractions and motor behaviour in the near-term human fetus. *American Journal of Obstetrics and Gynaecology* **156**(3), 543–9.

Münstedt, K., Brenken, A., Kalder, M. (2009) Clinical indications and perceived effectiveness of complementary and alternative medicine in departments of obstetrics in Germany: a questionnaire study. *European Journal of Obstetrics & Gynecology & Reproductive Biology* **146**(1), 5–54.

Mynick, A. (1981) Instituting a postpartum self medication program. *Maternal and Child Health Nursing Journal* **6**, 422–4.

Myung, H.H., Hee, Y.O., Young, S.P. (2005) Effects of aromatherapy on labor pain and perception of childbirth experience. *Korean Journal of Women Health Nursing* **11**(2), 135–41.

Nair, U. (2005) Acute abdomen and abdominal pain in pregnancy. *Current Obstetrics & Gynaecology* **15**(6), 359–67.

Nash, M., Benham, G. (2001) The truth and the hype of hypnosis. *Scientific American* **285**(1), 47–53.

Nathan, L., Huddleston, J.F. (1995) Acute abdominal pain in pregnancy. *Obstetrics and Gynecology Clinics of North America* **22**(1), 55–67.

Needham, R., Strehle, E.M. (2008) Evaluation of dressings used with local anaesthetic cream and for peripheral venous cannulation. *Paediatric Nursing* **20**(8), 34–6.

Neilson, J. (2007) Pre-eclampsia and eclampsia. In: *Saving Mothers' Lives: Reviewing Maternal Deaths to Make Motherhood Safer 2003–05* (ed. G. Lewis) ch. 3, p. 76. CEMACH, London.

NES (2006) Midwives and medicines Edinburgh NHS Education for Scotland, accessed July 2009. http://www.nes.scot.nhs.uk/documents/publications/classa/MidwivesandMedicines COMPLETE.pdf.

Newson, K. (1984) Care during labour. *British Journal of Obstetrics and Gynaecology* **91** (July), 609–10.

Newton, C. (1992) Hazards of N$_2$O exposure. *Nursing Times* **88**(39), 54.

NICE (2008) Clinical guideline: antenatal care: routine care for the healthy pregnant woman. National Collaborating Centre for Women's and Children's Health, accessed July 2009. http://www.nice.org.uk/nicemedia/pdf/CG62FullGuidelineCorrectedJune2008July2009.pdf.

Nicholson, W. (1985) Cracked nipples in breastfeeding mothers. *Nursing Mothers of Australia Newsletter* **27**, 7–10.

Nikodem, V.C., Danziger, D., Gebka, N., Gulmezoglu, A.M., Hofmeyr, G.J. (1993) Do cabbage leaves prevent breast engorgement? A randomised, controlled study. *Birth* **20**(2), 61–4.

Nissen, E., Widstrom, A.M., Lilja, G., et al. (1997) Effects of routinely given pethidine during labour on infants' developing breastfeeding behaviour. *Acta Paediatrica* **86**(2), 201–8.

Niven, C.A., Murphy Black, T. (2000) Memory for labor pain: a review of the literature. *Birth* **27**(4), 244–53.

Niven, C. (1992) *Psychological Care for Families: Before, During and After Birth*. Butterworth Heinemann, Oxford.

Niven, C., Gijsbers, K. (1984) A study of labour pain using the McGill Pain Questionnaire. *Social Science and Medicine* **19**(12), 1347–51.

Niven, C., Gijsbers, K. (1996a) Perinatal pain. In: *Conception, Pregnancy and Birth* (eds C.A. Niven & A. Walker), pp. 131–47. Butterworth Heinemann, Oxford.

Niven, C., Gijsbers, K. (1996b) Coping with labour pain. *Journal of Pain and Symptom Management* **11**(2), 116–25.

NMC (2004) Midwives rules and standards. London Nursing & Midwifery Council, accessed July 2009. http://www.nmc-uk.org/aDisplayDocument.aspx?documentID=169.

NMC (2005) Circular 25/2005 Midwives Supply Orders. London Nursing and Midwifery Council, accessed July 2009. http://www.nmc-uk.org/aDisplayDocument.aspx?DocumentID=775.

NMC (2008a) Standards for medicines management. Nursing & Midwifery Council, accessed July 2009. http://www.nmc-uk.org/aDisplayDocument.aspx?DocumentID=6228.

NMC (2008b) Code of Professional Conduct. London Nursing & Midwifery Council, accessed July 2009. http://www.nmc-uk.org/aArticle.aspx?ArticleID=3057.

Nolan, M.L. (1997) Antenatal education – where next? *Journal of Advanced Nursing* **25**(6), 1198–204.

Norén, L., Östgaard, S., Johansson, G., Östgaard, H.C. (2002) Lumbar back and posterior pelvic pain during pregnancy: a 3-year follow-up. *European Spine Journal* **11**(3), 267–71.

O'Driscoll, K. (1993) *Active Management of Labour: The Dublin Experience*, 3rd edn. Mosby, London.

O'Sullivan, G. (2004) Analgesia and anaesthesia in labour. *Current Obstetrics & Gynaecology* **15**(1), 9–17.

Oakley, A. (1993) The follow-up survey. In: *Pain and Its Relief in Childbirth: The Results of a National Survey Conducted by the National Birthday Trust* (eds G. Chamberlain, A. Wraight & P. Steer), ch. 10. Churchill Livingstone, Edinburgh.

Oakley, A. (1980) *Women Confined: Towards a Sociology of Childbearing*. Martin Robinson, Oxford.

Oakley, A., Richards, M.P.M. (1990) Some women's experiences of caesarean delivery. In: *The Politics of Maternity Care: Services for Childbearing Women in Twentieth Century Britain* (eds J. Garcia, R. Kilpatrick & M.P.M. Richards). Clarendon Press, Oxford.

Oduncu, F.S., Kimmig, R., Hepp, H., Emmerich, B. (2003) Cancer in pregnancy: maternal-fetal Conflict. *Journal of Cancer Research and Clinical Oncology* **129**(3), 133–146.

Olds, S.B., London, M.L., Ladewig, P.W. (1996) *Maternal–Newborn Nursing – A Family Centred Approach*, 5th edn. Addison-Wesley, California.

Olofsson, C.H., Ekblom, A., Ekman-Ordeberg, G., Hjelm, A., Irestedt, L. (1996) Lack of analgesic effect of systematically administered morphine or pethidine on labour pain. *British Journal of Obstetrics and Gynaecology* **103** (10), 968–72.

Olsen, K.G. (1991) *The Encyclopaedia of Alternative Health Care*. Piatkus, London.

O'Neill, A. (1994) Danger and safety in medicine. *Social Science and Medicine* **38**(4), 497–507.

Ong, C.K., Forbes, D. (2005) Embracing Cicely Saunders's concept of total pain. *British Medical Journal* **2**, 1451–3123.

Orbach, I., Mikulincer, M., Sirota, P., Gilboa-Schechtman, E. (2003) Mental pain: a multidimensional operationalization and definition. *Suicide & Life-threatening Behavior* **33**(3), 219–30.

Osmond, H., Mullaly, R., Bisbee, C. (1984) Mood Pain: a comparative study of clinical pain and depression. *Journal of Orthomolecular Psychiatry* **14**(1), 5–12.

Ogrodniczuk, J.S., Piper, W.E., Joyce, A.S., Weideman, R., McCallum, M., Azim, H.F., Rosie, J.S. (2003) Differentiating symptoms of complicated grief and depression among psychiatric outpatients. *Canadian Journal of Psychiatry* **48**(2), 87–93.

Østensen, M., Villiger, P.M. (2002) Review immunology of pregnancy – pregnancy as a remission inducing agent in rheumatoid arthritis. *Transplant Immunology* **9**, 2–4, 155–160.

Ostgaard, H.C., Andersson, G.B.J. (1992) Postpartum low-back pain. *Spine* **17**(1), 53–5.

Oteng-Ntim, E., Chase, A.R., Howard, J., Khazaezadeh, N., Anionwu, E.N. (2008) Sickle cell disease in pregnancy. *Obstetrics, Gynaecology & Reproductive Medicine* **18**(10), 272–8.

Oxorn, H. (1986) *Human Labor and Birth*, 5th edn. Prentice Hall, Englewood Cliffs.

Papagni, K., Buckner, E. (2006) Doula support and attitudes of intrapartum nurses: a qualitative study from the patient's perspective. *Journal of Perinatal Education* **15**(1), 11–18.

Parisi, L., Pierelli, F., Amabile, G., Valente, G., Calandriello, E., Fattapposta, F., Rossi, P., Serrao, M. (2003) Muscular cramps: proposals for a new classification. *Acta Neurologica Scandinavica* **107**(3), 176–86.

Parsons, L., MacFarlane, A., Golding, J. (1993) Pregnancy, birth and maternity care. In: *'Race' and Health in Contemporary Britain* (ed. W.I.V. Ahmad), ch. 4. Open University Press, Buckingham.

Pastore, P.A., Loomis, D.M., Sauret, J. (2006) Appendicitis in pregnancy. *Journal of the American Board of Family Medicine* **19**, 621–6.

Patel, R.R., Peters, T.J., Murphy, D.J. (2007) Is operative delivery associated with postnatal back pain at eight weeks and eight months? A cohort study. *Acta Obstetricia et Gynecologica Scandinavica* **86**(11), 1322 –7.

Pauka, S., Treagust, D.F., Waldrip, B. (2005) Village elders' and secondary school students' explanations of natural phenomena in Papua New Guinea. *International Journal of Science and Mathematics Education* **3**(2), 213–38.

Peacock, E., Furedi, A. (1996) Women. *The Guardian*, 22 July, p. 5.

Pearce, E.M., Dodd, J.M. (2004) Rectal analgesia for pain relief after caesarean section (Protocol). *Cochrane Database of Systematic Reviews*, Issue 2. Art. No.: CD004738. DOI: 10.1002/14651858. CD004738.

Pearl, M.L., Roberts, J.M., Laros, R.K. (1993) Vaginal delivery from the persistent occipito posterior position: influence on maternal and neonatal morbidity. *Journal of Reproductive Medicine* **38**(12), 955–61.

Pelvic Partnership (2009) Welcome. Accessed August 2009. www.pelvicpartnership.org.uk.

Penn, R.G. (1986) Iatrogenic disease: an historical survey of adverse reactions before thalidomide. In: *Iatrogenic Diseases*, 3rd edn (eds P.F. d'Arcy & J.P. Griffin). Oxford University Press, Oxford.,

Penticuff, J.H. (1989) Infant suffering and nurse advocacy in neonatal intensive care. *Nursing Clinics of North America* **24**(4), 987–96.

Perkins, E.R. (1980) *Education for Childbirth and Parenthood*. Croom Helm, London.

Pertegaz, I.B., Alberdi, J., Rodón, E.P. (2002) Is cabergoline a better drug to inhibit lactation in patients with psychotic symptoms? *Journal of Psychiatry & Neuroscience* **27**(1), 54.

Philipp, E.E. (1964) Minor disorders of pregnancy. *British Medical Journal* **1**(5385), 749–52.

Phoenix, A. (1990) Black women and the maternity services. In: *The Politics of Maternity Care: Services for Childbearing Women in Twentieth-Century Britain* (eds J. Garcia, R. Kilpatrick & M. Richards), pp. 274–99. Clarendon Press, Oxford.

Phumdoung, S., Good, M. (2003) Music reduces sensation and distress of labor pain. *Pain Management Nursing* **4**(2), 54–61.

Porter, J., Jick, J. (1980) Addiction rare in patients treated with narcotics. *New England Journal of Medicine* **302**, 123.

Porter, M., Macintyre, S. (1989) Psychosocial effectiveness of antenatal and postnatal care. In: *Midwives, Research and Childbirth 1* (eds S. Robinson & A.M. Thomson), pp. 72–94. Chapman & Hall, London.

Premberg, A., Lundgren, I. (2006) Fathers' experiences of childbirth education. *Journal of Perinatal Education* 15(2), 21–8.

Price, J., White, W. (2004) The use of acupuncture and attitudes to regulation among doctors in the UK–a survey. *Acupuncture in Medicine* 22(2), 72–4.

Pugh, L.C., Buchko, B.L., Bishop, B.A., Cochran, J.F., Smith, L.R., Lerew, D.J. (1996) A comparison of topical agents to relieve nipple pain and enhance breastfeeding. *Birth* 23(2), 88–93.

Punasundri, T. (2008) Perineal cold gel pad versus oral analgesic to relief episiotomy wound pain. Sigma Theta Tau International Conference, San Francisco.

Pur, R.D., Bijarnia, S., Verma, I.C. (2007) Genetics of sickle cell disease. In: *Hemoglobinopathies* (ed. A. Sachdeva), ch. 42, pp. 269–73. Jaypee, New Delhi.

Pursey, M. (1994) Mobile epidural – the only analgesia without anaesthesia. *Paediatric Post* 3.

Quijano, C.E., Abalos, E. (2005) Conservative management of symptomatic and/or complicated haemorrhoids in pregnancy and the puerperium. *Cochrane Database of Systematic Reviews*, Issue 3. Art. No.: CD004077. DOI: 10.1002/14651858.CD004077.

Quintner, J.L., Cohen, M.L., Buchanan, D., Katz, J.D., Williamson, O.D. (2008) Pain medicine and its models: helping or hindering? *Pain Medicine* 9(7), 824–34.

Radnovich, R. (2005) Massage and soft tissue manipulation. In: *Principles of Manual Sports Medicine* (ed. S. Karangeanes), ch. 9, pp. 56–64. Williams & Wilkins, Philadelphia.

Rajan, L. (1993) Perceptions of pain and pain relief in labour: the gulf between experience and observation. *Midwifery* 9(3), 136–45.

Rajan, L. (1994) The impact of obstetric procedures and analgesia/anaesthesia during labour and delivery on breast feeding. *Midwifery* 10(2), 87–103.

Ralph, C. (1991) Transcutaneous nerve stimulation. Registrar's letter. United Kingdom Central Council for Nursing, Midwifery and Health Visiting, London.

Ranta, P., Jouppila, P., Jouppila, R. (1996) The intensity of labour pain in grand multiparas. *Acta Obstetricia et Gynecologica Scandinavica* 75, 250–4.

Ranta, P., Jouppila, P., Jouppila, R. (1996) The intensity of labor pain in grand multiparas. *Acta Obstetricia et Gynecologica Scandinavica* 75(3), 250–4.

Rawlinson, P. (1996) Human Sentience Before Birth: A Report by the Commission of Inquiry Into Fetal Sentience. Report produced by the CARE Trust, London.

Raz, R., Chazan, B., Dan, M. (2004) Review article: cranberry juice and urinary tract infection. *Clinical Infectious Diseases* 38, 1413–19.

Read, M.D. (1977) A new hypothesis of itching in pregnancy. *Practitioner* 218, 845–8.

Regnard, C.F.B., Badger, C. (1987) Metabolism of narcotics. *British Medical Journal* 288, 460.

Reynolds, F. (ed) (1990) *Epidural and Spinal Blockade in Obstetrics*. Baillière Tindall, London.

Reynolds, F. 1997 Opioids in labour – no analgesic effect. *Lancet* 349(9044), 4–5.

Richardson, A., Mmata, C. (2007) NHS Maternity Statistics, England: 2005–06. The Information Centre, accessed February 2010, http://www.ic.nhs.uk/webfiles/publications/maternity0506/NHSMaternityStatsEngland200506_fullpublication%20V3.pdf.

Ridley, R.T. (2007) Diagnosis and intervention for occiput posterior malposition. *Journal of Obstetric Gynecologic and Neonatal Nursing* 36(2), 135–43.

Roberts, S.J. (2006) Oppressed group behaviour and nursing. In: *A History of Nursing Ideas* (eds L.C. Andrist, K.A Wolf & P.K. Nicholas), ch. 2, pp. 23–31. Jones & Bartlett, Sudbury, MA, accessed July 2009, http://books.google.co.uk/books?id=pJnYFMQLa_MC&printsec=frontcover.

Robertson, A. (2002) *Empowering Women: Teaching Active Birth*. Birth International, Camperdown, Australia.

Robinson, J. (2007) Post traumatic stress disorder. *AIMS Journal* **19**(1), 5–7.

Robinson, J. (1995) Use of heroin in labour – AIMS' concern. *AIMS Journal* **7**(2), 9–10.

Rodriguez, A., Bohlin, G., Lindmark, G. (2001) Symptoms across pregnancy in relation to psycho-social and biomedical factors. *Acta Obstetricia et Gynecologica Scandinavica* **80**(3), 213–23.

Roffe, C., Sills, S., Crome, P., Jones, P. (2002) Randomised, cross-over, placebo controlled trial of magnesium citrate in the treatment of chronic persistent leg cramps. *Medical Science Monitor* **8**(5), 326–30.

Rogers, D.A., Dingus, D., Standfield, J., Dipiro, J.R., May, J.R., Bowden, T.A. (1990) A prospective study of patient controlled analgesia impact on overall

Rooks JP 2007 Nitrous oxide for pain in labor – why not in the United States? *Birth* **34**(1), 3–5.

Rogers, M. (1980) Nursing: a science of unitary man. In: *Conceptual Models for Nursing Practice*, 2nd edn (eds J. Riehl & C. Roy). Appleton-Century Crofts, Norwalk, Connecticut.

Rogerson, L., Mason, G.C., Roberts, A.C. (2000) Preliminary experience with twenty perineal repairs using Indermil tissue adhesive. *European Journal of Obstetrics & Gynecology and Reproductive Biology* **88**(2), 139–42.

Sanders, J., Campbell, R., Peters, T.J. (2002) Effectiveness of pain relief during perineal suturing. *BJOG: An International Journal of Obstetrics and Gynaecology* **109**(9), 1066–8.

Rollman, G.B. (1983) Measurement of experimental pain in chronic pain patients: methodological and individual factors. In: *Pain Measurement and Assessment* (ed. R. Melzack), pp. 251–8. Raven Press, New York.

Rondón, M.B. (2003) Maternity blues: cross-cultural variations and emotional changes. *Primary Care Update for Obstetrics and Gynecology* **10**(4), 167–71

Rosen, M. (2002) Nitrous oxide for relief of labor pain: a systematic review. *American Journal of Obstetrics and Gynecology* **186**(5), (Suppl.), S110–S26.

Rosenbaum, J.F., Biederman, J., Pollock, R.A., Hirshfeld, D.R. (1994) The etiology of social phobia. *Journal of Clinical Psychiatry* **55**(Suppl.), 10–16.

Rowe, R.E., Garcia, J. (2003) Social class, ethnicity and attendance for antenatal care in the United Kingdom: a systematic review. *Journal of Public Health Medicine* **25**(2), 113–19.

Ruiz-Irastorza, G., Lima, F., Alves, J., Simpson, M.J., Hughes, G.R.V., Buchanan, N.M.M. (1996) Increased rate of lupus flare during pregnancy and the puerperium. *British Journal of Rheumatology* **35**, 133–8.

Russell, J.G.B. (1969) Moulding of the pelvic outlet. *Journal of Obstetrics and Gynaecology of the British Commonwealth* **76**, 817–20.

Russell, R., Dundas, R., Reynolds, F. (1996) Long-term backache after childbirth: prospective search for causative factors. *British Medical Journal* **312**, 1384–8.

Russell, R., Groves, P., Taub, N., O'Dowd, J., Reynolds, F. (1993) Assessing long term backache after childbirth. *British Medical Journal* **306**(6888), 1299–303.

Ryding, E.L., Persson, A., Onell, C., Kvist, L. (2003) An evaluation of midwives' counseling of pregnant women in fear of childbirth. *Acta Obstetricia et Gynecologica Scandinavica* **82**(1), 10–7.

Sammons, L.N. (1984) The use of music by women during childbirth. *Journal of Nurse-Midwifery* **29**(4), 266–70.

Sanders, J., Peters, T.J., Campbell, R. (2005) Techniques to reduce perineal pain during spontaneous vaginal delivery and perineal suturing: a UK survey of midwifery practice. *Midwifery* **21**(2), 154–60.

Savage, J.S. (2006) The Lived experience of knowing in childbirth. *The Journal of Perinatal Education* **15**(3), 10–24.

Scarry, E. (1985) *The Body in Pain: The Making and Unmaking of the World*. Oxford University Press, Oxford.

Schieve, L.A., Handler, A., Hershow, R., Persky, V., Davis, F. (1994) Urinary tract infection during pregnancy: its association with maternal morbidity and perinatal outcome. *American Journal of Public Health* **84**(3), 405–10.

Schmidt, L., Christensen, U., Holstein, B.E. (2005) The social epidemiology of coping with infertility. *Human Reproduction* **20**(4), 1044–52.

Schmied, V., Everitt, L. (1996) Postnatal care: poor cousin or priority area? In: *Midwifery; trends and practice in Australia* (eds L.M. Barclay, & L. Jones), pp. 107–27. Churchill Livingstone, Melbourne.

Schott, J., Henley, A. (1996) *Culture, Religion and Childbearing in a Multiracial Society: A Handbook for Health Professionals*. Butterworth Heinemann, London.

Schug, S.A., Watson, D.S.B. (2002) Pain in the acute care setting. In: *Pain: A Textbook for Therapists* (eds J. Strong, A. Unruh, A. Wright & G.D. Baxter) ch. 19, pp. 379–95. Churchill Livingstone, Edinburgh.

Schultz, R., Read, A.W., Straton, J.A., Stanley, F.J., Morich, P. (1991) Genitourinary tract infections in pregnancy and low birth weight: case control study in Australian Aboriginal women. *British Medical Journal* **303**(6814), 1369–73.

Schuman, A.N., Marteau, T.M. (1993) Obstetricians' and midwives' contrasting perceptions of pregnancy. *Journal of Reproductive and Infant Psychology* **11**(2), 115–18.

Scott, M., Wee, M. (2007) General anaesthesia and acid aspiration. In: *Crises in Childbirth – Why Mothers Survive* (eds D. Dob, A. Holdcroft & G. Cooper) ch. 3, pp. 47–66. Radcliffe Publishing, Abingdon.

Scottish Home and Health Department (1996) Obstetric Anaesthesia and Analgesia in Scotland. National Medical Consultative Committee. Scottish Home and Health Department, Edinburgh.

Sechzer, P.H. (1971) Studies in pain with an analgesic demand system. *Anaesthesia and Analgesia* **50**, 1–10.

Semenic, S.E., Callister, L.C., Feldman, P. (2004) Giving birth: the voices of orthodox Jewish women living in Canada. *Journal of Obstetric, Gynecologic, & Neonatal Nursing* **33**(1) 80–7.

Senden, I.P.M., van der Wettering, M.D., Eskes, A., Bierkens, P.B., Laube, D.W., Pitkin, M.D. (1988) Labour pain: a comparison of parturients in a Dutch and an American teaching hospital. *Obstetrics & Gynecology* **71**(4) 451–3.

Sheikh, A.A., Jordan, C.S. (1983) Clinical uses of mental imagery. In: *Imagery: Current Theory, Research and Application* (ed. A.A. Sheikh), ch. 13. John Wiley & Sons, New York.

Sheiner, E., Sheiner, E.K., Shoham-Vardi, I. (1998) The relationship between parity and labor pain. *International Journal Gynaecology Obstetrics* **63**, 287–8.

Sheiner, E.K., Hershkovitz, R., Mazor, M., Katz, M., Shoham-Vardi, I. (2000) Overestimation and underestimation of labor pain. *European Journal of Obstetrics & Gynecology and Reproductive Biology* **91**(1), 37–40.

Shepherd, J., Fry, D. (1996) Symphysis pubis pain. *Midwives* **109**(1302), 199–201.

Shurtz, J.D., Mayhew, R.B., Clayton, T.G. (1986) Depression recognition and control. *Dental Clinics of North America* **30**(Suppl. 4), S55–65.

SIDA (2001) Briefing paper on the 'feminisation of poverty'. Prepared for BRIDGE by Swedish International Development Cooperation Agency (Sida), accessed May 2009, http://www.bridge.ids.ac.uk/reports/femofpov.pdf.

SIGN (2002) Postnatal Depression and Puerperal Psychosis. SIGN Publication No. 60, accessed July 2009, http://www.sign.ac.uk/guidelines/fulltext/60/index.html.

Silverman, J., Decker, M., Reed, E., Raj, A. (2006) Intimate partner violence victimization prior to and during pregnancy among women residing in 26 U.S. states: associations with maternal and neonatal health. *American Journal of Obstetrics and Gynecology* **195**(1), 140–48.

Simkin, P., Bolding, A. (2004) Update on nonpharmacologic approaches to relieve labor pain and prevent suffering. *Journal of Midwifery & Women's Health* **49**(6), 489–504.

Simkin, P.P., O'Hara, M.A. (2002) Nonpharmacologic relief of pain during labor: systematic reviews of five methods. *American Journal of Obstetrics & Gynecology* **186**, S131–59.

Simkin, P. (1989) Non-pharmacological methods of pain relief during labour. In: *Effective Care in Pregnancy and Childbirth* (eds I. Chalmers, M. Enkin & M.J.N.C. Keirse), ch. 56. Oxford University Press, Oxford.

Simmons, S.W., Cyna, A.M., Dennis, A.T., Hughes, D. (2007) Combined spinal-epidural versus epidural analgesia in labour. *Cochrane Database of Systematic Reviews*, Issue 3. Art. No.: CD003401. DOI: 10.1002/14651858.CD003401.pub2.

Singer, M., Snipes, C. (1992) Generations of suffering: experiences of a treatment program for substance abuse during pregnancy. *Journal of Health Care for the Poor and Underserved* **3**(1), 222–34.

Singer, S. (1985) *Human Genetics: An Introduction to the Principles of Heredity*, 2nd edn. Freeman, New York.

Skibsted, L., Lange, A.P. (1992) The need for pain relief in uncomplicated deliveries in an alternative birth center compared to an obstetric delivery ward. *Pain* **48**(2), 183–186.

Skilnand, E., Fossen, D., Heiberg, E. (2002) Acupuncture in the management of pain in labor. *Acta Obstetricia et Gynecologica Scandinavica* **81**(10), 943–8.

Skovlund, E., Fyllingen, G., Landre, H., Nesheim, B.-I. (1991) Comparison of postpartum pain treatments using a sequential trial design: II Naproxen versus paracetamol. *European Journal of Clinical Pharmacology* **40**(6), 539–42.

Sleep, J. (1984) The West Berkshire episiotomy trial. In: *Research and the Midwife Conference Proceedings* (eds A. Thomson & S. Robinson), 1983, University of Manchester.

Sleep, J. (1991) Postnatal perineal care. In: *Postnatal Care: A Research-Based Approach* (eds J. Alexander, V. Levy & S. Roch), pp. 1–17. Macmillan, London.

Sleep, J., Grant, A. (1987a) West Berkshire perineal management trial: three years follow-up. *British Medical Journal* **295**(6601), 749–51.

Sleep, J., Grant, A. (1987b) Pelvic floor exercises in postnatal care. *Midwifery* **3**(4), 158–64.

Sleep, J., Grant, A. (1988a) Routine addition of salt or Savlon bath concentrate during bathing in the immediate postpartum period – a randomised controlled trial. *Nursing Times* **84**(21), 55–7.

Sleep, J., Grant, A. (1988b) The relief of perineal pain following childbirth: a survey of midwifery practice. *Midwifery* **4**(3), 118–22.

Sleep, J., Grant, A., Ashurst, H., Spencer, J.A.D. (1989) Dyspareunia associated with the use of glycerol-impregnated catgut to repair perineal trauma. *British Journal of Obstetrics and Gynaecology* **96**(6), 741–3.

Smaill, F.M., Vazquez, J.C. (2007) Antibiotics for asymptomatic bacteriuria in pregnancy. *Cochrane Database of Systematic Reviews*, Issue 2. Art. No.: CD000490. DOI: 10.1002/14651858. CD000490.pub2.

Small, R., Lumley, J., Donohue, L., Potter, A., Waldenström, U. (2000) Randomised controlled trial of midwife led debriefing to reduce maternal depression after operative childbirth. *British Medical Journal* **321**, 1043–7.

Smith, C., Crowther, C., Beilby, J., Dandeaux, J. (2000) The impact of nausea and vomiting on women: a burden of early pregnancy. *Australian & New Zealand Journal of Obstetrics & Gynaecology* **40**(4), 397–401.

Smith, N., Nolan, M.L. (2009) Antenatal education principles and practice. In: *Myles Textbook for Midwives*, 15th edn (eds D.M. Cooper & M.A. Cooper), ch. 15, pp. 227–41. Churchill Livingstone, Edinburgh.

Snell, C.C., Fothergill-Bourbonais, F., Durocher-Henriks, S. (1997) Patient controlled analgesia and intramuscular injections: a comparison of patient pain experiences and postoperative outcomes. *Journal of Advanced Nursing* **25**(4), 681–90.

Sorenson, D.S. (2003) Healing traumatizing provider interactions among women through short-term group therapy. *Archives of Psychiatric Nursing* **17**(6), 259–69.

Sosa, R., Kennell, J., Klaus, M., Robertson, S., Urrutia, J. (1980) The effect of a supportive companion on perinatal problems, length of labor, and mother-infant interaction. *New England Journal of Medicine* **303**(11), 597–600.

Sparshott, M. (1997) *Pain, Distress and the Newborn Baby*. Blackwell Science, Oxford.

SPCERH (2003) The Scottish Audit of the Management of Early Pregnancy Loss. SPCERH 19, Aberdeen.

Stables, D., Novak, B. (1999) *Physiology in Childbearing: With Anatomy and Related Biosciences*. Baillière Tindall, Edinburgh.

Stacey, M. (2007) General anaesthesia and failure to ventilate. In: *Crises in Childbirth – Why Mothers Survive* (eds D. Dob, A. Holdcroft & G. Cooper), ch. 2, pp. 19–46. Radcliffe Publishing, Abingdon.

Stainton, C., Edwards, M., Jones, B., Switonski, C. (1999) The nature of maternal postnatal pain. *Journal of Perinatal Education* **8**(2), 1–10.

Steele, A.M., Beadle, M. (2003) A survey of postnatal debriefing. *Journal of Advanced Nursing* **43**, 2130–6.

Steen, M. (2000) Femé pad: out of the ice age and into the new millennium. *British Journal of Midwifery* **8**(5), 312–5.

Steer, P. (1993) The methods of pain relief used. In: *Pain and Its Relief in Childbirth* (eds G. Chamberlain, A. Wraight & P. Steer), ch. 6. Churchill Livingstone, Edinburgh.

Steinberg, E.S., Fishman, E.B., Santos, A.C. (1996) Local anesthetics. In: *A Practical Approach to Pain Management* (eds M. Lefkowitz & A.H. Lebovits), pp. 32–40. Little Brown & Co., Boston.

Sternbach, R.A., Tursky, B. (1965) Ethnic differences among housewives in psychophysical and skin potential responses to electric shock. *Psychophysiology* **1**, 241–6.

Stevens, B. (1996) Pain management in newborns: how far have we progressed in research and practice? *Birth* **23**(4), 229–35.

Stewart, M. (2005) 'I'm just going to wash you down': sanitizing the vaginal examination. *Journal of Advanced Nursing* **51**(6), 587–94.

Stone, J., Lee-Treweek, G. (2005) Regulation and control. In: *Complementary and Alternative Medicine: Structures and Safeguards* (eds G. Lee-Treweek, T. Heller, H. MacQueen, J. Stone & S. Spurr), ch. 3, pp. 53–74. Routledge & Open University, Abingdon.

Strandmark, M. (2004) Ill health is powerlessness: a phenomenological study about worthlessness, limitations and suffering. *Scandinavian Journal of Caring Science* **18**(2), 135–44.

Stremler, R., Hodnett, E., Petryshen, P., Stevens, B., Weston, J., Willan, A.R. (2006) Randomized controlled trial of hands and- knees positioning for occipitoposterior position in labor. *Obstetrical & Gynecological Survey* **61**(5), 294–6

Strong, J., Sturgess, J., Unruh, A.M., Vicenzino, B. (2002) Pain assessment and measurement. In: *Pain: A Textbook for Therapists* (eds J. Strong, A.M. Unruh, A. Wright & G.D. Baxter), ch. 7, pp. 126–47. Churchill Livingstone, Edinburgh.

Sutton, J., Scott, P. (1994) *Understanding and Teaching Optimal Foetal Positioning*. Birth Concepts, Tauranga.

Svensson, J., Barclay, L., Cooke, M. (2007) Antenatal education as perceived by health professionals. *The Journal of Perinatal Education* **16**(1), 9–15.

Szasz (1957) *Pain and Pleasure: A Study of Bodily Feelings*. Tavistock, London.

Tait, P. (2000) Nipple pain in breastfeeding women: causes, treatment, and prevention strategies. *Journal of Midwifery & Women's Health* **45**(3), 212–5.

Tasharrofi, A. (1993) Midwifery care in the Netherlands. *Midwives Chronicle* **106**(1267), 286–8.

ten Klooster, P.M., Vlaar, A.P.J., Taal, E., Gheith, R.E., Rasker, J.J., El-Garf, A.K., van de Laar, M.A.F.J. (2006) The validity and reliability of the Graphic Rating Scale and Verbal Rating Scale for measuring pain across cultures: a study in Egyptian and Dutch women with rheumatoid arthritis. *The Clinical Journal of Pain* **22**(9), 827–30.

Thomsen, A.C., Espersen, T., Maigaard, S. (1984) Course and treatment of milk stasis. *American Journal of Obstetrics and Gynecology* **149**, 492–5.

Thomson, A.M., Hillier, V.F. (1994) A re-evaluation of the effect of pethidine on the length of labour. *Journal of Advanced Nursing* **19**(3), 448–56.

Thorne, S. (2009) Natural Healthcare Council Regulation, accessed December 2009, http://www.acupuncture.org.uk/index.php/about-us/statutory-regulation.html.

Thorpe-Raghdo, B. (2005) Muslim women's perception of parentcraft classes: a summary. *MIDIRS Midwifery Digest* **15**(4), 485–91.

Tiran, D. (1996) The use of complementary therapies in midwifery practice: a focus on reflexology. *Complementary Therapies in Nursing & Midwifery* **2**(2), 32–7.

Tiran, D. (2003) Implementing complementary therapies into midwifery practice. *Complementary Therapies in Nursing & Midwifery* **9**, 10–3.

Tiran, D., Mack, S. (2000) *Complementary Therapies for Pregnancy and Childbirth*, 2nd edn. Balliere Tindall, London.

Tobin, H.J. (2008) Confronting misinformation on abortion: informed consent, deference and fetal pain laws. *Columbia Journal of Gender and Law* **17**(1), 111–52.

Tortora G. J., Derrickson B. (2006) *Principles of Anatomy and Physiology*, 11th edn. John Wiley & Sons, US.

Torvaldsen, S., Roberts, C.L., Bell, J.C., Raynes-Greenow, C.H. (2004) Discontinuation of epidural analgesia late in labour for reducing the adverse delivery outcomes associated with epidural analgesia. *Cochrane Database of Systematic Reviews*, Issue 4. Art. No.: CD004457. DOI: 10.1002/14651858.CD004457.pub2.

Tournaire, M., Theau-Yonneau, A. (2007) Review complementary and alternative approaches to pain relief during labor. *Evidence Based Complementary Alternative Medicine* **4**(4), 409–17.

Trevor, A.J., Miller, R.D. (1992) General anaesthetics. In: *Basic and Clinical Pharmacology* (B.G. Katzung). Lange, Connecticut.

Trout, K. (2004) The neuromatrix theory of pain: implications for selected nonpharmacologic methods of pain relief for labor. *Journal of Midwifery & Women's Health* **49**(6), 482–88.

Tsekeris, C. (2008) Sociological issues in culture and critical theorizing. *Humanity & Social Sciences Journal* **3**(1), 18–25.

Tucker, G. (1996) *National Childbirth Trust Book of Pregnancy, Birth and Parenthood*. Oxford University Press, Oxford.

Twycross, R.G. (1994) Opioids. In: *Textbook of Pain*, 3rd edn (eds P.D. Wall & R. Melzack), pp. 943–62. Churchill Livingstone, Edinburgh.

Unruh, A.M., Harman, K. (2002) Alternative and complementary therapies. In: *Pain: A Textbook for Therapists* (eds J. Strong, A. Unruh, A. Wright & G.D. Baxter), ch. 12, pp. 227–44. Churchill Livingstone, Edinburgh.

Ussher, J.M. (1996) Female sexuality and reproduction. In: *Reproductive Potential and Fertility Control* (eds C.A. Niven & A. Walker). Butterworth Heinemann, London.

Vague, S. (2003) Midwives' experiences of working with women in labour: interpreting the meaning of pain. Unpublished MHSc thesis, Auckland University of Technology, http://repositoryaut.lconz.ac.nz/bitstream/10292/72/2/VagueS.pdf.

Van de Velde, M., Jani, J., De Buck, F., Deprest, J. (2006) Fetal pain perception and pain management. *Seminars in Fetal and Neonatal Medicine* **11**(4), 232–6.

Van de Velde, M., Lewi, L., Debuck, F., Vandermeersch, E. (2007) Combined spinal epidural analgesia in labour: does prophylactic intravenous colloid infusion reduce the incidence of hypotension? *Regional Anesthesia and Pain Medicine* **32**(5), 14.

Van de Velde, M., De Buck, F., Van Mieghem, T., Gucciardo, L., De Koninck, P., Deprest, J. (2010) Fetal anaesthesia: is this necessary for fetoscopic therapy? *Fetal and Maternal Medicine Review* **21**(1), 24–35.

Van der Spank, J.T., Cambier, D.C., De Paepe, H.M.C., Danneels, L.A.G., Witvrouw, E.E., Beerens, I. (2000) Pain relief in labour by transcutaneous electrical nerve stimulation (TENS). *Archives of Gynecology & Obstetrics* **264**(3), 131–6.

van Duinena, M., Rickelt, J., Grieza, E. (2008) Validation of the electronic Visual Analogue Scale of anxiety. *Progress in Neuro-Psychopharmacology and Biological Psychiatry* **32**(4), 1045–7.

van Ryn, M., Fu, S.S. (2003) Paved with good intentions: do public health and human service providers contribute to racial/ethnic disparities in health? *American Journal of Public Health* **93**(2), 248–55.

van Teijlingen, E. (1994) A social or medical model of childbirth? Comparing the arguments in Grampian (Scotland) and The Netherlands. Unpublished PhD thesis, University of Aberdeen.

Vangen, S., Stoltenberg, C., Schei, B. (1996) Ethnicity and use of obstetric analgesia. *Ethnicity and Health* **1**(2), 161–7.

Varney Burst, H. (1983) The influence of consumers in the birthing movement. *Topics in Clinical Nursing* **5**, 42–54.

Vazquez, J.C., Villar, J. (2003) Treatments for symptomatic urinary tract infections during pregnancy. *Cochrane Database of Systematic Reviews*, Issue 4. Art. No.: CD002256. DOI: 10.1002/14651858.CD002256.

Vickers, A., Zollman, C. (1999) ABC of complementary medicine: hypnosis and relaxation therapies. *British Medical Journal* **319**(7221), 1346–40.

Vogler, J.H. (1993) The second and third stages of labour. In: *Maternity and Gynecologic Care: The Nurse and the Family*, 5th edn (eds I.M. Boback & M.D. Jensen), ch. 18. Mosby, St Louis.

Walco, G.A., Cassidy, R.C., Schechter, N.L. (1994) Pain, hurt and harm. *New England Journal of Medicine* **331**(8), 541–4.

Waldenström, U. (1988) Midwives' attitudes to pain relief during labour and delivery. *Midwifery* **4**(2), 48–57.

Waldenström, U., Schytt, E. (2009) A longitudinal study of women's memory of labour pain – from 2 months to 5 years after the birth. *British Journal of Obstetrics and Gynaecology* **116**, 577–83.

Walker, A.C., Tan, L., George, S. (1995) Impact of culture on pain management: an Australian nursing perspective. *Holistic Nursing Practice* **9**(2), 48–57.

Wall, P. (1999) *Pain: The Science of Suffering*. Weidenfeld & Nicolson, London.

Wall, P.D., Jones, M. (1991) *Defeating Pain: The War Against a Silent Epidemic*. Plenum, London.

Wall, P.D., Sweet, W.H. (1967) Temporary abolition of pain. *Science* **155**, 108–9.

Walldén, J., Thörn, S-E., Wattwil, M. (2004) Delay of gastric emptying induced by remifentanil is not influenced by posture. *Anesthetic Analgesia* **99**, 429–34.

Walsh, D. (2010) Labour rhythms. In: *Essential Midwifery Practice: Intrapartum Care* (eds D. Walsh & S. Downe), ch. 5, pp. 63–80. Wiley Blackwell, Chichester.

Ward-Larson, C., Horn, R.A., Gosnell, F. (2004) The efficacy of facilitated tucking for relieving procedural pain of endotracheal suctioning in very low birthweight infants. *The American Journal of Maternal/Child Nursing* **29**(3), 151–6.

Ware, L.J., Epps, C.D., Herr, K., Packard, A. (2006) Evaluation of the Revised Faces Pain Scale, Verbal Descriptor Scale, Numeric Rating Scale, and Iowa pain thermometer in older minority adults. *Pain Management Nursing* **7**(3), 117–25.

Warwick, W., Neal, J. (2007) Beyond spinal headache: prophylaxis and treatment of low-pressure headache syndromes. *Regional Anesthesia and Pain Medicine* **32**(5), 455–61.

Waters, B., Raisler, J. (2003) Ice massage for the reduction of labor pain. *Journal of Midwifery & Women's Health* **48**(5), 317–21.

Waters, J., Thomas, V. (1995) Pain from sickle cell crisis. *Nursing Times* **91**(16), 29–31.

Watson, N., Mander, R. (1995) Advertising infant formula in the maternity area. *MIDIRS Midwifery Digest* **5**(3), 338–41.

Way, W.L., Way, E.L. (1992) Opioid analgesics and antagonists. In: *Basic and Clinical Pharmacology* 5th edn (ed. B.G. Katzung). Prentice Hall, Norwalk.

Welford, H. (1996) Postnatal depression: focusing on a neglected issue. *Midwives* **109**(1301), 165–7.

Wen, Y.R., Hou, W.Y., Chen, Y.A., Hsieh, C.Y., Sun, W.Z. (1996) Intrathecal morphine for neuropathic pain in a pregnant cancer patient. *Journal of the Formosan Medical Association* **95**(3), 252–4.

Whitcome, K.K., Shapiro, L.J., Lieberman, D.E. (2007) Fetal load and the evolution of lumbar lordosis in bipedal hominins. *Nature* **450**, 13 December, 1075–8.

Wiesenfeld-Hallin, Z. (2005) Sex differences in pain perception. *Gender Medicine* **2**(3), 137–45.

Wilkie, D.J., Savedra, M.C., Holzemer, W.L., Tesler, M.D., Paul, S.M. (1990) Use of the McGill Pain Questionnaire to measure pain: a meta-analysis. *Nursing Research* **39**(1), 36–41.

Wilkinson, I. (2005) *Suffering: A Sociological Introduction*. Polity Press, Cambridge.

Williams, M., Booth, D. (1985) *Antenatal Education: Guidelines for Teachers*, 3rd edn. Churchill Livingstone, Edinburgh.

Williams, S., Hepburn, M., McIlwaine, G. (1985) Consumer view of epidural anaesthesia. *Midwifery* **1**(1), 32–6.

Willson, H. (2000) Factors affecting the administration of analgesia to patients following repair of a fractured hip. *Journal of Advanced Nursing* **31**(5), 1145–54.

Wilshin, J., Wilson, P. (1991) A question of delivery. *Nursing Times* **87**(43), 52–4.

Wilton, T., Kaufmann, T. (2001) Lesbian mother's experiences of maternity care in the UK. *Midwifery* **17**(3), 203–211.

Wolf, Z.R., Hicks, R.W., Altmiller, G., Bicknell, P. (2009) Nursing student medication errors involving tubing and catheters: a descriptive study. *Nurse Education Today* **29**(6), 681–8.

Wolff, B.B., Langley, S. (1977) Cultural factors and the response to pain. In: *Culture Disease and Healing: Studies in Medical Anthropology* (ed. D. Landy), Section 34, p. 313. Collier Macmillan, London.

Woods, M. (1989) Pain control and hypnosis. *Nursing Times* **85**(7), 38–40.

Woolf C.J., Thompson (1994) Stimulation-induced analgesia: transcutaneous electrical nerve stimulation (TENS) and vibration. In: *Textbook of Pain*, 3rd edn (eds P.D. Wall & R. Melzack). Churchill Livingstone, Edinburgh.

Woolf, V. (1925) On being Ill. In: *Collected Essays*, Vol. IV (V. Woolf). The Hogarth Press, London.

Woolf, V. (1867) On being Ill. *Collected Essays*, Vol. IV (ed. V. Woolf), pp. 193–203. Harcourt, New York.

Woolridge, M.W. (1986) The 'anatomy' of infant sucking. *Midwifery* **2**(40), 164–71.

Wraight, A. (1992) Pain in labour: the 1990 confidential enquiry into the relief of pain in labour. Research and the Midwife Conference Proceedings, 1990, University of Manchester.

Wraight, A. (1993) Coping with Pain. In: *Pain and Its Relief in Childbirth* (eds G. Chamberlain, A. Wraight & P. Steer), ch. 8. Churchill Livingstone, Edinburgh.

Wright, A., Benson, H.A.E., O'Callaghan, J. (2002) Pharmacology of pain management. In: *Pain: A Textbook for Therapists* (eds J. Strong, A. Unruh, A. Wright & G.D. Baxter), ch. 16, pp. 307–24. Churchill Livingstone, Edinburgh.

Wu, W.H., Meijer, O.G., Uegaki, K., Mens, J.M.A., van Dieën, J.H., Wuisman, P.I.J.M., Östgaard, H.C. (2004) Pregnancy-related pelvic girdle pain (PPP), I: Terminology, clinical presentation, and prevalence. *European Spine Journal* **13**(7), 575–89.

Yancey, M.K., Jun, Z., Schweitzer, D.L., Schwarz, J., Klebanoff, M.A. (2001) Epidural analgesia and fetal head malposition at vaginal delivery. *Obstetrics and Gynecology* **97**(4), 608–12.

Yee, G. (2003) *Poor Banished Children of Eve: Woman as Evil in the Hebrew Bible*. Fortress, Minneapolis, Minnesota.

Young, G., Jewell, D. (1997) Antihistamines versus aspirin for itching in late pregnancy. *Cochrane Database of Systematic Reviews*, Issue 1. Art. No.: CD000027. DOI: 10.1002/14651858. CD000027.

Young, G.L., Jewell, D. (2004) Interventions for leg cramps in pregnancy (Cochrane Review). *The Cochrane Library*, Issue 2. John Wiley & Sons, Chichester.

Zborowski, M. (1952) Cultural components in responses to pain. *Journal of Social Issues* **8**, 16–30.

Zhang, J., Klebanoff, M.A., DerSimonian, R. (1999 Epidural analgesia in association with duration of labor and mode of delivery: a quantitative review. *American Journal of Obstetrics and Gynecology* **180**(4), 970.

Ziemer, M.M., Paone, J.P., Schupay, J., Cole, E. (1990) Methods to prevent and manage nipple pain in breastfeeding women. *Western Journal of Nursing Research* **12**(6), 732–44.

Zimmerman, M. (2005) the history of pain concepts and treatment before IASP. In: *The Paths of Pain 1975–2005* (eds H. Merskey, J.D. Loeser & R. Dubner), ch. 1. IASP Press, Seattle.

Index

Pain in Childbearing and its Control, Second Edition. By Rosemary Mander. Published 2011 by Blackwell
Publishing Ltd. © 1998, 2011 Rosemary Mander.